21 Life Lessons
from
Livin' La Vida Low-Carb

21 Life Lessons

from
Livin' La Vida Low-Carb

How The Healthy Low-Carb Lifestyle
Changed Everything I Thought I Knew

Jimmy Moore

Important Medical Disclaimer
for *21 Life Lessons From Livin' La Vida Low-Carb*

This book provides content related to topics about weight loss, nutrition and health. As such, use of this book implies your acceptance of the terms described herein.

You understand that a private citizen without any professional training in the medical, health, or nutritional field authored this content. You understand that this book is provided to you without a health examination and without prior discussion of your health condition. You understand that in no way will this book provided medical advice and that no medical advice is contained within this book or the content provided.

You understand that this book is not intended as a substitute for consultation with a licensed healthcare practitioner, such as your physician. Before you begin any weight loss program, or change your lifestyle in any way, you will consult your physician or other licensed healthcare practitioner to ensure that you are in good health and that the examples contained in this book will not harm you.

If you experience any unusual symptoms after following any information from this book, you will immediately consult with your healthcare practitioner.

You understand that the information and content of this book should not be used to diagnose a health problem or disease, or to determine any health-related treatment program, including weight loss, diet, or exercise.

You understand that there are risks associated with engaging in any activity described in this book. Any action you take implies that you assume all risks, known and unknown, inherent to lifestyle changes, including nutrition, exercise and any other physical activities and/or injuries which may result from the actions you take.

You hereby release Jimmy Moore and the publisher from any liability related to this book to the fullest extent permitted by law. This includes any damages, costs, or losses of any nature arising from the use of this book and the information provided by this book, including direct, consequential, special, punitive, or incidental damages, even if Jimmy Moore have been advised of the possibility of such damages.

Your use of this book confirms your agreement to the above terms and conditions. If you do not agree, you will not utilize this book and will request your full refund within the timeframe specified in your contract of sale.

Acknowledgments

When I wrote my first book in 2005 just months after losing a total of 180 pounds in the prior year, it was a monumental moment in the story of my life. I had always dreamt of writing a book, but never in my wildest dreams did I ever think it would be on the subject of weight loss. But while *Livin' La Vida Low-Carb: My Journey from Flabby Fat to Sensationally Skinny in One Year* was the fulfillment of that dream, it has been my continued journey to better health that has given me the opportunity to come into contact with some of the world's best and brightest people in the field of nutrition and health. The ongoing education I have received from these researchers, doctors, dietitians, nurses, medical professionals, and lay people alike has been illuminating to say the least and I'm so excited to share just a smidgen of what I've learned from them over these past five years.

I couldn't possibly name every single person who has made such an impact on me to inspire another book about healthy low-carb living, but I'm going to list those who have contributed the most: God Almighty who has given me the breath to breathe and a passion for living life to the fullest; my lovely and faithful wife Christine who has stood by me no matter what and willingly joined me on this great adventure; my brother Kevin whose death in October 2008 at the tender age of 41 has only ignited a fire within me to be even more vigilant about sharing the truth; the sensational work of Gary Taubes in his 2007 blockbuster book release *Good Calories, Bad Calories* which will go down in history as one of the greatest books on health and nutrition to ever be written; my podcast producer Kevin Kennedy-Spaien for investing literally hours upon hours making my interviews with the experts sound amazing; and my faithful moderators at my forum LindaSue, Jay, Justin, Amy, Burt, Mary, Christin, Ron, and Patti for sharing in a loving and sympathetic manner to all those who are looking for help with their low-carb lifestyle.

Additionally, a special thank you to all of the outstanding contributions from the low-carb researchers, medical professionals, and authors who are out there putting their careers on the line to expose the untruths that have been made about low-carb living with solid evidence supporting this healthy way of eating, including Dr. Richard Feinman, Dr. Mary C. Vernon, Dr. Eric Westman, Dr. Jeff Volek, Dr. Stephen Phinney, Dr. Donald Layman, Dr. Cassandra Forsythe, Dr. Mary Enig, Dr. Jay Wortman, Jacqueline Eberstein, Dr. Will Yancy, Dr. Malcolm Kendrick, Dr. James E. Carlson, Drs. Mike and Mary Dan Eades, Dr. Jonny Bowden, Dr. Robert K. Su, Dr. James LaValle, Dr. Barry Groves, Dr. William Davis, Dr. Guenther Boden, Veronica Atkins, Dr. Annika Dahlqvist, Dr. Daniel Chong, T.S. Wiley, Dr. Scott Olson, Dr. Barry Sears, Dr. Diana Schwarzbein, Dr. John Salerno, Dr. Loren Cordain, Dr. Duane Graveline, Dr. Doug McGuff, Dr. Dwight Lundell, Dr. Deborah Snyder, Dr. Al Sears, Dr. Larry McCleary, Dr. Annsi Manninen, Dr. John Briffa, Dr. Keith Berkowitz, Dr. Cassandra Forsythe-Pribanic, Dr. David Ludwig, Dr. Jeffry Gerber, Dr. Ron Rosedale, Dr. Nicolas Perricone, Dr. Michael Dansinger, Dr. Richard Bernstein, Dr. Barbara Berkeley, and we can never forget the late great Dr. Robert C. Atkins.

In the few years since I wrote my first book, low-carb blogs and influential health web sites have been popping up everywhere along with many veterans of the online world and I'm proud to be working alongside such high-quality people as Laura Dolson, Fred Hahn, Tom Naughton, Mark Sisson, Dana Carpender (who so graciously penned the fabulous foreword to this book!), Amy Dungan, Regina Wilshire, Judy Barnes Baker, Kent Altena, Karen Rysavy, Carol Bardelli, Rachel Tomkinson, Dave Dixon, Brian Cormier, Richard Nikoley, Kalyn Denny, Monica Reinagel, Adam Campbell, Methuselah, Art DeVany, Nicki Anderson, Jennette Fulda, Dr. Heidi Dulay, Colette Heimowitz, Diane Kress, Sean Croxton, Kat James, Karly Pitman, Nora Gedgaudas, Nina Planck, Julia Ross, Sally Fallon, Valerie Berkowitz, Andrew DiMino, Connie Bennett, Eric Morrison, Christin Sherburne, Rosanna Forzonti, David Mendosa, JJ Virgin, Elaine Payne, Mark McManus, Cameo Watkins, Jason May, David Gillespie, Dr. Joe Leonardi, Richard Morris, Joel Salatin, Josef Brandenburg, Deon Van Der Merwe, Per Wikholm, Gretchen Becker, and so many more!

Thanks are also owed to Karen Floyd and The Palladian Group team of Stan and Carmen especially for their outstanding job on designing the beautiful cover for this book which I am so proud of. Their input and consultation was an invaluable asset to putting the finishing touches on a book I am thrilled to be able to share with the world. Fellow low-carb enthusiast, blogger and author Dana Carpender did an amazing job with the foreword for this book that I can't wait for you to read. Thank you for your support and friendship over the past few years, Dana! A woman who devoted a considerable amount of time editing this book was Nancy Lopez-Marsh. She did a yeoman's job of making my writing style as effective as possible. Kudos are also in order to Lawrence Hunter for his legal assistance and guidance with the manuscript.

I'd be remiss if I didn't express my sincerest gratitude to my publisher Book-Surge.com who has been nothing but wonderful to me through this process. When I needed a company to step up to the plate to give this book a chance to be read by those who need the message I have to share the most, Book-Surge was there. Although most of the traditional publishing world is caught up in creating "sure-thing" books by the most famous authors, BookSurge understands there is a market for books by lesser-known authors who have something worth sharing. THANK YOU for your support of the Livin' La Vida Low-Carb mission, April and the gang!

Finally, I want to acknowledge and share my appreciation for YOU! That's right, YOU! If you picked up a copy of this book that you are holding in your hands right now, then there's a pretty high probability that you have been a regular reader at my LivinLaVidaLowCarb.com/blog for a while, a listener at my Top 20 iTunes health podcast TheLivinLowCarbShow.com/ShowNotes, a faithful member at my LivinLowCarbDiscussion.com forum, a viewer of the videos my wife Christine and I make at YouTube.com/LivinLowCarbMan, or any of the millions of others who have been exposed to the work I've been doing on behalf of livin' la vida low-carb over these past five years. For that, I want to simply say THANK YOU! Without your steadfast support and dedication to continually educating yourself about healthy low-carb living, there would be no reason for me to invest hundreds of hours monthly to this cause. If for no other reason than to open the eyes and change the lives of even a few, then all of the work I've put into the "Livin' La Vida Low-Carb" concept since 2005 has been totally worth it. Keep learning everything you can about low-carb living, encouraging others to apply the lessons in their own lives, and inspiring people with your own example of making livin' la vida low-carb a reality. YOU CAN DO IT!!!

Contents

Foreword by Dana Carpender

At first glance, Jimmy Moore and I are pretty different. I'm a five-foot-two-inch woman; he's a man who tops me by over a foot. He's a Southern gentleman — a goofy Southern gentleman, but a Southern gentleman nonetheless. I'm an unregenerate Yankee with a big mouth and an attitude. I'm, er, middle aged, he's a decade younger. I'm a better dancer; he's a far better karaoke singer. (No joke. Jimmy's great at karaoke.)

But beneath surface appearances, Jimmy and I are practically breathing the same air. Both of us have struggled with our weight all of our lives, though his problem was more severe than mine. Both of us tried to fix our problem with the highly-touted, authority-sanctioned low-fat/high-carb nutritional approach. Both of us had doubts about low carb and whether it would work for us. Both of us tried low-carbing anyway, out of frustration and not a little panic at the worsening of our problems. And both of us discovered low-carbing not only helped our weight problems, but that it improved our health, energy, mood, constant hunger, our *lives* so much that it was like the light coming on after living in the dark, like living in color after a lifetime of black-and-white.

For both of us, our switch to low carb nutrition was an overwhelming, compelling, life-altering experience. And both of us found ourselves wanting, *needing*, to tell other people about it. It's like being the little boy in "The Emperor's New Clothes": You feel like you're the only one seeing the obvious, and you want to yell "Hey, he's naked!" Or, in this case, you want to run up to strangers in the grocery store who are pushing around carts of low-fat food and holler, "NO! DON'T DO IT, BUDDY! IT'S A LIE, IT'S ALL A LIE!"

Which can be a somewhat obnoxious urge, frankly. Not everyone wants to hear your weight loss story, or the whole song-and-dance about how whole grains are not the royal road to health. This stuff can make you unpopular if you take it too far.

On the other hand, when you lose a bunch of weight, people come out of the woodwork wanting to know how you did it. They're hoping you'll say, "I watched television and ate Pringles," of course. But still, they want to know what your secret is. These are the people it's okay to tell.

And once you run through the interested people in your circle of acquaintance, you can find a whole lot more of them by writing on the Internet. Back in 1999, when I got started, there were no blogs; the format of the day was the ezine. So I started an ezine — and had over a thousand subscribers in a couple of months, and over ten thousand in a year. It mushroomed from there, and in a few years I had a publishing contract.

Jimmy, starting in 2004, first started a blog, then a podcast and a YouTube broadcast, and has reached hundreds of thousands, perhaps millions, of people. And I have to hand it to him: He does it every day. Every day! Do you have any idea how tough that is? Heck, I had a weekly column with United Media for a while, and coming up with one column a week was work.

Both Jimmy and I also sat down and wrote a book about our low carb experience out of sheer evangelical joy; both of us risked our own money by self-publishing. Both of us took on the ridiculously unlikely task of promoting such a book without a publishing house behind us. Just so you know, ninety three percent of all "legitimately" published books never sell more than ten thousand copies. The odds stacked against those of us who self-publish are at least an order of magnitude worse, though Amazon.com, bless their hearts, has made it a lot easier.

Did either of us do it for the money? Are you out of your mind? First of all, if I cynically wanted to write a nutrition or weight loss book just for the money, I'd push low-fat, tons of whole grains, maybe even a quasi-vegetarian diet. Do you have any idea how many more such books have been published — and sold — than low carb books? Do you know how much more respect those authors get? Just look at the public image of Dean Ornish compared to Bob Atkins. (And why is it that people feel free to accuse Dr. Atkins of being a hustler who was only in it for the money, but never say that stuff about Dean

Ornish, who has made a ton of money, too, and is just as in-your-face with his marketing and self-promotion?)

No, again, both Jimmy and I sat down and started writing about our low carb experience because we had to tell someone, and our friends were weary of hearing about it.

It turns out that this urge we both had, to go out there and tell everyone who would listen about our life-changing low carb experience, was a very good thing, not just for us, but for a whole lot of people. Why? The information was out there; it's not like it wasn't. There was *Dr. Atkin's New Diet Revolution* and *Protein Power* burning up the best-seller lists, *The Zone* letting athletes know that carb-loading wasn't all it was cracked up to be, *Sugarbusters* making a splash with the ladies' groups. What did the two of us have to offer?

Support. Frequent, sincere, been-there-done-that messages that no, you're not crazy to think that eggs are healthier than oatmeal, that a steak is more slimming than pasta with fat-free sauce. A reminder to those who slip of just how good it can feel to have stable blood sugar and abundant energy, not to mention to never feel hungry. A constant, critical eye to the billion-and-one articles insisting we're nuts, that we're killing ourselves, that our cholesterol will skyrocket and our arteries clog and our kidneys give up if we don't straighten up and fly right — fly right, that is, according to the Food Pyramid. A venue for the less-publicized but frequent studies demonstrating the remarkable health benefits of carb restriction and liberalized fat consumption.

(I've been doing this fourteen years. Fourteen years! When people tell me low carb is going to ruin my health, I make big eyes at them and ask plaintively, "When?")

Turns out this stuff is vital. I took an informal and certainly statistically meaningless but very interesting poll of my readers a couple of years back, asking them how long they'd been low-carbing, how successful they'd been, and what, in their estimation, were the main reasons for their success or lack thereof. Turns out there were two main themes running through the stories from the folks who had stuck with it: Whether they'd started low-carbing for their health or simply to lose weight, they found the health benefits so great that they cared more about maintaining those benefits than about reaching some arbitrary, fashionably skinny size. And they had support. Lots of support.

Some, like Jimmy and me, were fortunate enough to have a supportive spouse. Some had a friend doing it with them. One woman wrote that she and her mother started low-carbing together, while several said that their whole family got on board for the change.

Others were not so lucky. There were stories of spouses who didn't care how beneficial the program was, they wanted their chips and cookies and they wanted them now. Worse, there were spouses who found the low-carber's success threatening, and even ridiculed their attempts. There were plenty of women who felt that it was incumbent on them as a wife and mother to keep all of their kids' favorite junk food in the house, torpedoing their own success, not to mention making it more likely that those kids would eventually fight the same obesity and health problems. There were folks who felt they had to apologize at every turn for being on "that crazy fad diet."

But many people who lacked support at home, and many who had a supportive home environment but faced the constant bad-mouthing of their nutritional program by the rest of the world, found that the greatest help was online support. The folks who were successful long-term, by and large were the ones who regularly read low carb blogs, who participated in message boards, who deliberately sought out reinforcing information. This stuff turned out to be crucial to the success of many, many low carb dieters.

As I learned from an article by Dr. Mike Eades, another blogger you should be reading, studies have now been done imaging the brain while people are subjected to messages trying to sell them on something, versus when they learn the price — the actual price when it's a shopping decision, or the consequences, if it's the decision of what to put in their mouths. Those sales messages, *whatever they are for*, stimulate dopamine in the brain — they literally give us a mini-high, and make us crave whatever is being sold. Messages regarding the price stimulate aversion. Our neurochemical buttons are being pushed.

How many commercial messages do you see and hear every day telling you to eat carby junk? How many more do you get from family and friends: "Oh, it's so good!" "I don't know how you can pass this up!" "It's a holiday/your birthday/the weekend, live a little!" How many images are you exposed to telling you that food is love, that food is how families bond, and that the food that does this best is "comfort food" — you know, mashed potatoes. Macaroni and cheese. Home-baked cookies.

How many more aversive messages are you exposed to from people who tell you you're nuts, that fat is bad, that eggs cause heart disease, that giving up a whole food group obviously means you're on a fad diet. (I always ask these people if that argument means vegetarianism is a fad diet? For that matter, if cutting carbs is faddy, why isn't cutting fat faddy? That's a food group, too, and one for which we have an actual nutritional requirement.)

Seeking out support is pushing your own buttons. By reading this book, and Jimmy's blog, and my blog and books, and all the other great low carb info you can find, you can stimulate dopamine by the thought of a great steak and a salad, or a sugar-free cheesecake, or a snack of macadamia nuts. By reading about the successes of others, you "sell" yourself on low carb success. By reading critiques of the anti-low carb articles, you arm yourself against the negative button pushing. By reading about the great success of low carb diets in controlling not just weight but numerous health issues, you help un-push the "but all that fat is bad for you" button.

So read this book. It will push all the right buttons!

One other thing that marks the successful: They are not even a tiny bit apologetic about eating this way. They are proud. They don't feel like they need to excuse their dietary oddness, they felt like they know a huge, wonderful secret — and they, like Jimmy and me, want to tell other people about it. It's contagious.

Catch the bug! Jimmy will give you a hundred reasons, heck, a couple- hundred, why eating this way is a *brilliant* decision. He'll give you great comebacks for the nay-sayers. He'll show you research the media hasn't been covering, demonstrating the value of carbohydrate restriction.

And heaven knows, he'll give you a clear example of how not to act embarrassed about being low carb.

Jimmy's changing lives. Heck, Jimmy's probably *saving* lives. I'm proud to call him my friend.

Dana Carpender
HoldTheToast.com
August, 2009

Introduction

It's hard to believe that a little more than five years ago I was carrying around over 400 pounds on my body, taking three prescription medications for declining health problems, wearing size 62-inch waist pants, feeling like an elephant in 5XL shirts, and living a decidedly unhealthy lifestyle without even realizing it. But you could say all of that changed dramatically after a major transformation happened in my life when I started livin' la vida low-carb in 2004.

And yet with big changes like the ones I've experienced since losing 180 pounds and getting my life back, it's hard not to look back on the many lessons learned along the way with gratitude, respect, and humility. That's what this book will attempt to impart on you as you travel with me on what my low-carb path has been like since I first started on it in January 2004. While my debut book released in 2005 called *Livin' La Vida Low-Carb: My Journey From Flabby Fat to Sensationally Skinny in One Year* detailed my triple-digit low-carb weight loss success story and all the raw emotion of that tremendous experience that happened in my life, this new book will be the perfect follow-up to show you the evolutionary process that has taken place in both my knowledge and understanding of how this way of eating really works.

On January 1, 2009, I marked my 5-year anniversary of being on the low-carb lifestyle. Note that I describe this way of eating as a "lifestyle" and not a diet and that is by design. If you are ever going to do something about your obesity, then you must face the facts now — the solution is something you can and MUST do for the rest of your life. Period. End of story. No excuses.

I only wish somebody had told me that as I was eating myself up to 410 pounds! Better late than never I suppose.

Little did I know back in 2004 when I began this amazing journey to better health with the Atkins diet after reading *Dr. Atkins' New Diet Revolution* just how much my life would change physically in terms of my weight and health as well as many other areas of my life, including my new career as a full-time low-carb blogger, podcaster, YouTuber, and so much more! It's all been somewhat of a dream world for me to be able to share my success story with literally millions of people worldwide in the past few years alone, most of whom I'll probably never have the opportunity to meet in person.

But the literally hundreds of e-mails pouring into my inbox each week confirm that the work I am doing IS making a positive and lasting impact on the lives of real people who need their own inspiration, motivation and encouragement to take this low-carb journey for themselves. This weight loss and radical change in my health and life was and still is my greatest accomplishment ever. And that includes marrying my lovely wife Christine, graduating from college, writing my first book, and getting my Master's degree. All of those were amazing feats in the course of my lifetime, but none of them could ever surpass the exhilarating experience of what I was able to do in 2004.

Five years seems like such a long time ago, but at the same time it doesn't. Time has flown by since losing 180 pounds in one year and yet there are plenty of opportunities that come up where the old Jimmy Moore comes face to face with the new one. Although I'm finding it more and more difficult to remember what it was like being obese, there are times when a vision of those days will flash in my head giving me the sobering reminder that I am so much better off now than I was before. That is what drives me to keep on livin' la vida low-carb no matter what for the rest of my life.

And here's why: no more struggling to breathe, no more worries about chest pains, no more dreading walking around Wal-Mart with my wife because I'll be out of breath, no more taking three prescription drugs to control high blood pressure, high cholesterol, and wheezing, no more hating going to the movies or sitting in an airplane seat, no more Big & Tall stores, no more ripping the seat of my pants getting into my car, no more relentless sweating even in the dead of winter, no more wishing I could do more with my life, no more regrets, sorrows, feeling like a failure as a man. These days I am doing everything I could ever dream of and more. God is blessing me for the decisions that have led me to where I am now and I am thankful for His continued guidance in my life through my low-carb journey.

I also have the low-carb lifestyle to thank for giving me my life back! While the rhetoric about low-carb dieting prevents so many people from taking advantage of this scientifically-based nutritional approach that is far superior to low-fat diets not just for weight loss but also for health improvements, the fact of the matter is many people who have struggled time and time again on low-fat diets are finding the most success when they turn to low-carb.

You may not hear about it in the media, but millions upon millions of people are cutting out most of the carbohydrates in their diets and replacing them with fat and moderate amounts of protein to satiate their hunger, control the release of insulin (which just so happens to be the #1 reason fat accumulates in the body), and burn stored body fat (not just weight on the scale, but actual body fat that you can measure in inches pouring off your body). This is not a fad diet program — it's a plan based on facts found throughout the medical literature. I highlight this often within the pages of this book.

The past few years have not always been easy for me and I never expected it to be a free ride after decades of battling the obesity monster. When I lost my weight in 2004, everyone was telling me how good I looked and that the work I invested in changing my life was suddenly over. HA! My response back to them at the time was, "The work has only just begun." Little did I know how prophetic that statement truly was as I've experienced all the ups and downs you would expect after going through such a significant weight loss. You'll read about some of those highs and lows in this book because I believe we can all stand to learn from the lessons we've been given in life.

And despite the naysayers from both inside and outside the low-carb community who have stood up against the work I have been doing to help others, I have still kept over 85% of that original weight loss off for over five years. Although my weight may be slightly higher now than it was when I originally lost that 180 pounds, my clothes fit me perfectly and I'm as healthy as an ox. I attribute this to the muscle weight I've gained through regular resistance training and conditioning. My activity level is even higher now than it was when I was a rambunctious teenager! And I can't imagine ever going back to plopping on the couch eating whole boxes of Little Debbie snack cakes while watching *The Biggest Loser*! That's not who I am anymore — thank the good Lord!

I know what you're thinking, though. Sure, Jimmy lost all that weight and kept it off for several years now — but what is his health like, hmmmmm? I enjoy answering this question much more than talking about my weight loss success because this gets into the nitty gritty of why I am so super-excited about sharing with people the positive message of low-carb living in this book. You see, weight loss is merely a side effect of beginning a low-carb way of eating — improving your HEALTH is what it's really all about.

And even the traditional tests like total cholesterol and LDL don't give you the whole picture of what's happening to you. That's why studies like the ones encouraging people to take more and more statin drugs drive me crazy. The fact is my May 2008 cholesterol numbers are stellar when you look at them through the lens of the most modern tests like the NMR LipoProfile from Lipo-Science (NMRLipoprofile.com):

LDL Particle Number: 1453
Small LDL Particle Number: 30

In case those numbers are foreign to you, let me translate what they mean. The small, dense, and dangerous LDL particles are the ones you don't want in your blood because they lead to plaque buildup, inflammation in the arteries, blockages, and eventually atherosclerosis which leads to heart attack, stroke and even death. Of my total LDL particles, a mere two percent are this kind that you don't want. Doctors hope to keep that number below 600, but mine was 30. Yes, my LDL cholesterol number is 250, but 98 percent of that LDL is the large, fluffy, and protective kind that keeps you out of danger of getting heart disease. Add to this that a CT heart scan done in August 2009 showed that I had a calcium score of zero and I'd say this high-fat, low-carb plan I've been following has kept my heart quite healthy!

Plus, the fact that my HDL "good" cholesterol is an outstanding 65 (should be above 40) and my triglycerides are 85 (should be under 150) proves my diet is not making me more unhealthy as low-fat advocates I affectionately refer to as low-fatties like to say — on the contrary, I've really never been more healthy in my entire life! And these changes are a direct result of eating a high amount of fat, even saturated fat, moderate amounts of protein, and very few carbohydrates while supplementing my diet with certain vitamins and minerals as well as getting the right exercise for me. This is a recipe for weight loss and health success like you've never experienced before!

Would I have ever been able to experience these kinds of what I consider miraculous changes in my life had I listened to all those negative comments about low-carb prior to my New Year's resolution to lose weight and get healthy in 2004? Absolutely not! This is why I encourage people these days to try livin' la vida low-carb. Believe it or not, I have my critics to this very day despite my five-year track record of personal weight loss and health success!

If you are reading this and thinking you'd like to go ahead and get started on your own low-carb lifestyle, then let me encourage you to do the following:

1. Read a solid low-carb book like *Dr. Atkins New Diet Revolution*, *Protein Power* by Drs. Mike & Mary Dan Eades, or for a side-by-side comparison of the most popular low-carb diets get Dr. Jonny Bowden's newly-updated 2010 release *Living Low-Carb*.

2. Have your doctor conduct a NMR LipoProfile (NMRLipoprofile.com) blood test to measure your LDL particle size, HDL cholesterol, and triglycerides at baseline so you can see how much improvement low-carb will make on your health.

3. Commit to following your chosen low-carb plan exactly as prescribed for at least three months while continually educating yourself more and more about the low-carb lifestyle (read Gary Taubes' *Good Calories, Bad Calories* for an excellent history of the science behind low-carb).

4. Get active support not just from your friends and family, but by getting involved with others who have been successful eating this way online through low-carb forums like mine (LivinLowCarbDiscussion.com).

5. Most importantly, NEVER, NEVER, EVER GIVE UP! You'll likely face struggles, temptations, cravings, and even some pain early on when you do this. But let me tell you, the payoff in the end is totally worth it if you can just stick it out until you reach your goal. By the time you get there, you'll want to keep on low-carbing for the rest of your life.

As I reflect on the past five years of low-carb living, I can't help but be grateful to all those who encouraged me, gave me strength, and lifted me up when I felt like calling it quits. As a means of paying it forward, I stand ready to help anyone who has any questions or concerns that they want to share with me anytime. I'm always just an e-mail away at livinlowcarbman@charter.net and anyone who has ever contacted me will tell you I'm thrilled to write you back as quickly as I possibly can. It is my pleasure and honor to serve you and be there for you as you strive to become a long-term low-carb success, too. After all, I've been in your shoes and would have loved having a Jimmy Moore to contact when I needed him.

Within the pages of this book you are holding right now, I have armed you with a plethora of information that is a direct result of the literally thousands of hours I have spent researching and studying through a wide variety of medical data and publications sifting through it all and making it palatable for just about anyone to understand. You'll also read about what it has been like being the caretaker of a nutrition and health blog that started out as a simple hobby and quickly turned into something much bigger than I ever expected it to be. That meteoric rise in my blog's popularity brought on a mixed bag of news which you will see didn't always pan out to be great. Regardless, there are certain indelible lessons learned from every experience and the following pages are filled with 21 of them that I'm ready to share with you now. So hold on tight because this is gonna be one big eye-opening adventure for you to see why I'm still livin' la vida low-carb today! Class is now in session.

LESSON #1
Low-carb is much more than a diet, it's a healthy lifestyle change

"Low-carb eating isn't really a diet — it's a return to the type of eating plan we evolved to perform best on — whole foods from the four basic food groups: Food you could hunt, fish, gather or pluck. It's real food for real health."

— Dr. Jonny Bowden, *PhD, CNS* (JonnyBowden.com)
author of *Living Low-Carb* and *The 150 Healthiest Foods on Earth*

The first thing most people think of when you mention you are on a low-carb diet is how well it works for weight loss. There's certainly nothing wrong with a way of eating that helps you shed stored body fat naturally and effectively like livin' la vida low-carb does. It's one of the major attractions to the low-carb plan for the millions who have tried it.

But far too often I believe a heavy emphasis is placed almost exclusively on the weight loss aspect of low-carb living while the tremendous health benefits that come from reducing carbohydrate intake and increasing dietary fat intake are virtually ignored entirely. This is doing a great disservice to all of the amazing low-carb researchers and practitioners who would be proud to stand up for carbohydrate restriction first and foremost as a way to improve health which just happens to have a nice little side effect of weight loss.

Even still, over the past few years I've heard from quite a few people who want to know if a low-carb diet can help them lose a few pounds in time for some special upcoming occasion like a wedding, a high school reunion, or some other special life event. In fact, here's an example of the kind of question that I'll see from time to time:

Hey Jimmy,

I followed the Atkins diet for awhile, and after a month or so I got back into my old habits. What do you think about the South Beach diet? Is that a good diet to lose some weight for summer?

I'm always amused at some of the subtle messages people e-mail to me and they don't even know it. In this example, I had to ask some obvious questions: Why did you only do the Atkins lifestyle for just "awhile" and not stick with it? If you want to see any success on a weight loss plan, then you have to be persistent with it until you reach your goals—and then keep doing it for the rest of your life.

Atkins or South Beach or any of the nutritional choices out there all require a commitment to lifestyle change if they are going to be effective over the long-term.

Going on a "diet" usually makes you feel rotten and that's why most of us low-carbers don't consider Atkins or our chosen low-carb plan to be anything but the healthy lifestyle change that we all know it to be for us. If the mentality is that you need to "get off" your diet once the weight is gone, then absolutely nothing is going to work for you. Until you realize that the eating habits you have right now are dangerous to your health if you are stuck as an overweight or obese person and you aren't doing something about it, then you will never make the transition to the healthy eating habits you will need to enjoy a long and healthy life.

If you started with and became successful by livin' la vida low-carb, then it is the one and only eating plan you should do even after losing your weight. Or, if you choose to do a low-fat diet and find success with it, then that should be your one and only diet for the rest of your life. The point is to find the proven nutritional plan that works for you, follow that plan exactly as prescribed by the author, and then stick with it for the rest of your life.

Losing weight is fun, but what will motivate you once you reach your goal? How are you going to keep on with the "diet" long after the need for doing one is gone? The answer: sustained weight loss and vastly improved health. You must strategize for the inevitable time when you realize that the way you are eating during the weight loss phase is the way you should be eating for the rest of your life and learn to be happy with it. That's why you should pick your plan wisely from an educated perspective and then GO FOR IT!

Of course, this doesn't mean you're not going to "slip-up" from time to time, but you have to be ready to respond the right way when it happens as I discussed in my first book. But livin' la vida low-carb is such a luxurious and pleasurable way of eating that it's easy to get back on it even when you have a slight stumble along the way. That's why so many people have chosen the healthy low-carb lifestyle. We want to stop being an obesity statistic and we want to instead enjoy good foods to bring ourselves to the healthy weight we need to be. We will also be healthier than we have ever been in our entire lives. That's what happened for me starting in 2004 and can happen for anyone reading this right now.

Over the past five years, I've heard just about every excuse you can possibly think of from those well-meaning people in our lives who share why they think it is probably a good idea NOT to eat low-carb. But quite frankly most of the criticism lacks any solid scientific data to support it. See if some of these sound familiar:

Low-carb is just not sustainable over the long-term.

Cutting out an entire food group will make you unhealthy.

You'll get so bored eating meat, eggs, and cheese every day.

You will binge on sugar and carbs as a rebellious act.

When you add carbs back to your diet, you'll gain the weight back.

You know, looking at some of those excuses for NOT going on a low-carb diet, they certainly seem logical and even somewhat reasonable based on the basic knowledge most people have about a weight loss program these days. After all, it's good to have balance in your diet with a variety of foods that keep things interesting enough that you'll want to eat that way for the rest of your life, right? Well, I'm here to testify today that livin' la vida low-carb is all of that and more for me.

And yet what do we hear in the media about low-carb over and over and over again. It's a fad diet that is unhealthy and dangerous. They have been desperately trying to find something (ANYTHING!) different to replace the low-carb lifestyle as the dominant diet, but it hasn't happened. Sometimes I think the media and the current health experts keep repeating the myths about the low-carb lifestyle's demise hoping that people start believing it at some point. But so many people are realizing that livin' la vida low-carb is a great way to lose weight and get your health back in order — for good!

If so many other diets aren't working for people, then why not try low-carb? The only thing you have to lose is a whole lot of weight and most of the health problems that plague you. I got rid of 180 pounds and came off of three prescription medications for high cholesterol, high blood pressure, and breathing problems thanks to livin' la vida low-carb!

There are still tens of millions of people who are eating a low-carb diet in our society today and they are all living proof that it works for weight loss and health improvements.

And yet I've heard it in television news stories about low-carb diets like Atkins where the reporter or interview guest will say something like, "Sure, that low-carb diet is good for weight loss, but it can't be a very healthy way to lose weight with all that fat and protein." I'll be addressing more of these kinds of myths about low-carb in later chapters, because the truth is, the only unhealthy weight loss is weight loss that compromises your health and there is much proof that low-carb is a healthier way to lose weight than low-fat.

There is continued negative focus in the media on the fat and protein content of foods you may have on a low-carb plan, and not enough attention given to studies which prove fat and protein are beneficial.

Might I remind you that scientists have found in their dogged research (as you will see in later chapters of this book) that following a low-carb lifestyle just about guarantees permanent weight loss success if you stick with it for life and that low-carb provides people needing to lose weight and keep it off the metabolic advantage over other diet plans such as vegan, vegetarian, low-fat, low-calorie and portion-controlled diets. If people seriously make livin' la vida low-carb their lifestyle change, then weight loss and maintenance is sure to follow.

If and when you make the decision to make low-carb much more than a diet and more of a permanent and healthy lifestyle change, then you will begin to reap the long-term rewards that this way of eating will afford you. Coming up in the next lesson, you'll find out why the typical blood work at the doctor's office may not be enough. You may not be aware of the tests you should have run to see if you are at risk for cardiovascular problems. And if you're already livin' la vida low-carb, these tests will demonstrate to you just how healthy your low-carb diet is for you!

LESSON #2
Most cholesterol tests by your doctor
are virtually meaningless

"Think you know what your cholesterol is? Think again. The shameful testing inaccuracy introduced by the standard American diet virtually guarantees that you underestimate heart disease risk. The low-fat dietary catastrophe of the last 30 years needs to be reversed."

— **Dr. William Davis, M.D.,** cardiologist and author of the book
Track Your Plaque (TrackYourPlaque.com),
health blogger at HeartScanBlog.blogspot.com

Of all the untruths we have been told about our health over the years, there is one that sticks out as the most egregious of them all because it has failed to be proven by any reputable science or even through human experience. And yet millions upon millions of Americans are currently taking a prescription medication for this condition because that's what their doctor told them they needed to do to prevent the risk of heart disease. I'm referring to the cholesterol hypothesis.

We've all heard it throughout our lifetime that you better keep your total cholesterol below 200 and your LDL below 100 if you want to keep from having clogged arteries which could lead to a heart attack, stroke, or worse. These warnings have come from well-meaning physicians, dietitians, and other medical professionals who are simply repeating what they have been taught in medical school, personal training, and from other sources.

One of the other sources of information that most people don't know about is pharmaceutical companies, which have a vested interest in you and your diagnosed atherosclerosis. One prescription from your doctor and they swoop in to rescue you with their miracle pills. That's exactly what Pfizer has done marketing Lipitor, Astra-Zeneca with Crestor, Merck/Schering-Plough with Zetia, and the latest statin-boosting drug from Abbott Laboratories released in September 2009 called Trilipix which boasts on the front page of its web site that it must be "used along with a low-fat, low-cholesterol diet." These prescription medications are meant to treat "high cholesterol," but there is a gigantic elephant sitting in the room.

WHAT IS THE PROOF THAT HIGH CHOLESTEROL LEADS TO HEART DISEASE?

Surely you jest, Jimmy! Everyone KNOWS that you put yourself at risk when you allow that dastardly LDL "bad" cholesterol to rise above 100 and total cholesterol above 200. Anyone who refuses to take a statin drug when their cholesterol reaches these benchmarks is simply putting themselves at severe risk for some rather serious health consequences down the road. Why not just take your medicine like the rest of us are doing and put yourself out of harm's way?

You'd be surprised how many people believe this to be true. But the fact of the matter is there is plenty of reason not to take statin drugs. Read any of the books by Dr. Duane Graveline (SpaceDoc.net) about the negative neurological and other side effects he experienced taking a statin medication for his high cholesterol.

Although cholesterol numbers have come way down from where they once were, what is the cost to our health that these reductions have produced? In a podcast interview I conducted with Dr. Jim LaValle from the Cincinnati, OH-based LaValle Metabolic Institute (LMIHealth.com) in January 2009, he said that if you put 250 people in a room and put them all on a statin drug and just one of them reduced their risk of heart disease as a result of this therapy, the pharmaceutical companies believe that is a good enough reason to put the pill on the market for the masses. But what about those other 249 people? What is the detrimental impact of a statin drug on their health?!

A shocking six-year observational study of 3,516 Italian patients who took a statin drug to treat their high cholesterol published in the June 2009 issue of *Pharmacological Research* wanted to find out what impact the drug made on preventing a cardiovascular event while lowering cholesterol. Predictably, the statins indeed lowered cholesterol levels in the study participants who took them faithfully as required. But those same patients who took the popular cholesterol-lowering medications day after day also wound up being hospitalized sooner for heart-related complications than the poor adherents and non-adherents to the statin therapy. Despite having lower cholesterol, these people who did what they thought was the right thing by taking the statin everyday still ended up going to the hospital with a heart attack or heart-related health problem. What's the point of artificially lowering cholesterol levels in your body if the statin drug you're taking is not even going to protect your heart from damage?

Pharmaceutical companies have to stay in business, and battling high cholesterol is big business. If word got out that livin la vida low-carb did more to protect against heart disease than statin drugs, they would soon go out of business. The powers that be will not likely allow that to happen.

While we're on the subject, let's talk about why we have given pharmaceutical companies such power In the United States. My understanding is doctors are limited with their time and ability to continue their education into the latest research that comes out about health. But why have we allowed pharmaceutical companies to have so much say in our health? No one else is allowed this freedom to access health care providers to provide them with education on the latest scientific developments in health!

So that's the system we have for now. Doctors rely partly on highly-paid drug company representatives to give them unbiased reporting on what they need to prescribe their patients for high blood pressure, obesity and high cholesterol, but the reports given are anything but unbiased. There is a conflict of interest when the drug testing trials are funded by a pharmaceutical company and it happens much more frequently than people even realize.

When I decided to go on the Atkins diet in 2004, I was sick and tired (literally!) of settling for the conventional wisdom for what constituted a "healthy" diet and instead chose a way of eating that would help me go on to shed 180 pounds. At the time when I still weighed over 400 pounds, I was taking Crestor after a very painful stint on Lipitor to control my "high cholesterol" which was around 250 at the time. They had me so scared of not taking this statin that I felt like it was my only option despite the continued agonizing pain these drugs have been shown to cause in more users than they care to admit.

A few months after my 180-pound low-carb weight loss, I went back to my family doctor for my annual physical checkup. To put it quite bluntly, my doctor was simply amazed and pleased by the complete turnaround in my health for the better although he was shocked when I told him I did it on a low-carb diet. As I previously stated, I was on medications for breathing, high blood pressure and high cholesterol and for the latter I was told that I needed to take a statin drug to get my total cholesterol down.

Although I used to take those statin drugs to get my cholesterol to go lower as my doctor instructed the unbelievably painful joint and muscle pain that I experienced on these dangerous drugs was too much to bear. In fact, these side effects of statin drugs were the subject of an intensive University of California-San Diego "Statin Effects Study" (StatinEffects.com/Info) to help educate doctors about what they are doing to their patients with these risky medications. It's amazing to me that statin drugs are still allowed on the market with so many unanswered questions about the real harm they are doing to people.

Nevertheless, medical professionals have heralded statins as the miracle panacea they've been longing for to lower cholesterol numbers. But what is it doing to the health of the people taking these pills? Sure, their cholesterol has gone down, but now what problems do they have to deal with because of the statin drugs they are taking? Yikes! Which is worse?

I finally decided to stop taking these statins once and for all in August 2004 because I was tired of hurting and became thoroughly convinced that cholesterol drugs are more about money than about improving people's health in an effort to prevent a heart attack or stroke. Plus, with my enormous weight loss on low-carb, I knew my HDL "good" cholesterol would be way up from the lower 20s it used to linger at before and my triglycerides and total cholesterol would be way down the next time I had my blood work done.

You can imagine my anxious anticipation after having my cholesterol checked in late October 2005 when I got the amazing results:

TOTAL CHOLESTEROL: 201
HDL: 71
LDL: 119
TRIGLYCERIDES: 57

To say I was thrilled with these numbers is an understatement. But I didn't realize just how good they were until I read a study by a highly-respected low-carb diet researcher from the University of Connecticut named Dr. Jeff Volek about how the triglyceride/HDL ratio is a much better indicator of heart health than LDL and total cholesterol. Using this newfound equation, my triglyceride/HDL ratio was a mere 0.83! Sure my LDL and total cholesterol were higher than what my doctor would have preferred, but I was much healthier than I was before my low-carb lifestyle.

Yet, at my checkup with my doctor in 2006, I got some cholesterol numbers that had my doctor pulling out the dreaded "s" word yet again:

TOTAL CHOLESTEROL: 254
HDL: 72
LDL: 170
TRIGLYCERIDES: 44

As you can see, my total cholesterol and LDL had both increased while my HDL grew by one point and my triglycerides continued to plummet 13 more points. I was excited about my triglyceride/HDL ratio, though, which actually improved to a microscopic 0.61!

Nevertheless, my doctor was very alarmed about my cholesterol numbers. He didn't care that my HDL was outstanding (his nurse even said to me that my HDL was too high if you can believe that!) nor was he even proud that my triglycerides had continued on their downward path. All he could see was that my LDL was up which had caused my total cholesterol to be up as well. Guess what the first words out his mouth were to treat it again? You guessed it: Statin!

Since I'd already tried Lipitor and Crestor, he wanted to put me on Vytorin! But I refused. I didn't want the pain of statin drug treatment ever again and was unconvinced that a statin drug was necessary.

I talked to my chiropractor at the time, a vocal opponent of statin drugs, about my cholesterol numbers and he said as long as my total cholesterol/HDL ratio is less than 5:1 I should be fine. Using that scale, my ratio was about 3.5:1 so I was okay according to him. When you've got studies showing that the existence of LDL cholesterol is actually good as you get older, it makes you scratch your head wondering if all this commotion about cholesterol in the United States these days is just one big opportunity by the pharmaceutical companies using our medical doctors as their pawns.

In reviewing my latest blood work numbers at the time, my doctor said he was very "concerned" about my LDL being so high. He said ideally the LDL number should be under 100 mg/dL. I braced myself because I knew that was coming, but I retorted back to him with my excellent HDL and triglyceride numbers.

But what about my triglyceride/HDL cholesterol ratio, doc? Doesn't that count for anything in a discussion of cholesterol health and my risk for cardiovascular disease?

Without hesitation, he responded that while those numbers were indeed good and my weight loss had been quite impressive, those are simply "IRRELEVANT" (his exact word) when you are talking about LDL as a separate measuring stick for the risk of heart disease. He acknowledged that most medical professionals give more weight to the LDL than they do HDL or triglycerides these days and that they want to see that LDL number go as low as possible regardless of what the other numbers are.

This seemed rather shortsighted to me. Why even measure HDL or triglycerides if they aren't regarded as important as LDL? Rather than encouraging me with the incredible improvements that I had seen in my HDL going up to 72 from the lower 20s it used to be before I started livin' la vida low-carb and the steady and swift drop in my triglycerides from the 300s down to 42, my doctor dismissed these numbers and ignored the total cholesterol/HDL ratio which at 3.5 was well within what was considered the safe range.

I told my doctor point blank, "I'm NOT going back on a statin drug again, so come up with something else that's natural for me to get my LDL down if it's that important." To my surprise, he did! Well, sort of.

In a pamphlet from the Orlando, FL-based Florida Lipid Institute called "Drug-Free Cholesterol Lowering Plan," Dr. Paul Ziajka developed a program in 2003 to help people like me get our cholesterol down without using prescription drugs. My doctor said he didn't think I'd see much result from this, but I could try it for four months to see if it would help me get my LDL down. However, he was not very confident in the plan.

This pamphlet basically recommended a low-fat "lifestyle change" and said to avoid eating eggs, cheese, butter, and red meat while eating more tofu, baked chicken, low-fat cheese, 1% milk and margarine. Additionally, the plan called for a three-component plan for getting cholesterol down — plant sterols, soy, and soluble fiber. I chuckled at the conclusion made by Dr. Ziajka at the end of his pamphlet.

"Following our plan AND a low cholesterol, low-fat lifestyle can cut your cholesterol level in half! Just remember, these are changes you are going to make the rest of your life."

If I had seriously tried to do this plan my doctor gave me at the time, then I would have had to abandon most of the low-carb lifestyle changes I had made over the previous two years. That was NOT going to happen!

Before I left his office, I asked my doctor about the various kinds of LDL particle sizes and that perhaps my LDL was of the good variety. He said the only way to know that for sure is to have a specialized test done to measure it. There are a few tests that can measure this, including one called the VAP test (TheVAPTest.com) by Atherotech and another one that I really like known as the NMR Lipoprofile test (NMRLipoProfile.com) by Liposcience. These are much better tests to use than the standard Berkeley Heart Test that most doctors' offices utilize with their patients. The detailed breakdown of your cholesterol with either the VAP or NMR Lipoprofile test is very thorough and will give you a better idea about your risks rather than a generic HDL, LDL and total cholesterol test. Dr. James E. Carlson who wrote a fantastic book about low-carb living entitled *Genocide: How Your Doctor's Dietary Ignorance Will Kill You* says knowing your total cholesterol is like knowing the cumulative score of a baseball game. But if it's 25, then you don't know if a team won 13-12 or if it was a blowout score like 24-1. Interesting analogy.

Getting the LDL particle size pattern from these tests is very important or else your doctor is basically flying blind. When I was faced with the prospect of possibly taking a statin drug again in 2006, I solicited the advice of a woman I greatly admire and respect for her work using a low-carbohydrate health plan with her patients on a daily basis — Dr. Mary C. Vernon from Lawrence, Kansas. She shared with me her comments about my cholesterol numbers to help illuminate issues that I was not aware of at the time. Her many years as an experienced low-carb diet practitioner spoke volumes.

"These labs in which the LDL is calculated are not accurate if your triglycerides are below 100," she explained to me at the time. *"The equation used to calculate these numbers makes assumptions which are not accurate when triglycerides are low."*

My triglycerides were 42, a drop of 14 points (25%) from six months prior. The traditional method of cholesterol testing apparently does not factor in someone who is on a low-carb lifestyle. It's possible this is because the tests were originally developed for a person on a low-fat diet.

"Your total cholesterol and LDL can be elevated because intermediate density lipoproteins are being measured as LDLs," Dr. Vernon added. "You must also remember that your high HDL adds to your total."

I hadn't thought about there being an intermediate subset showing up as LDLs. These specialized tests would certainly clarify that issue once and for all. Additionally, Dr. Vernon's comment about my high HDL number adding to my total cholesterol is a valid one indeed. If my HDL were back down in the lower 20s like it was before I started livin' la vida low-carb, then my total cholesterol would have "only" been around 200, considered to be closer to "normal" cholesterol.

Another thought-provoking idea that I didn't know about was that the liver can secrete LDL into the blood when your VLDLs, another specialized subset of your lipid panel, are "very low," Dr. Vernon stated.

"Although it floats at the same density as LDL, it does not imply the same outcome," she noted.

That, along with the intermediate density lipoprotein could have been artificially elevating my LDL numbers. Again, this underlines the importance of having the proper particle size tests done to shed light on the makeup of my LDL pattern. Dr. Vernon pointed to the work of Dr. Jim Otvos from LipoScience (LipoScience.com) who said his research has found that if a patient's triglycerides are 100 or below, then they automatically have the large fluffy LDL, the non-dangerous type. With my triglycerides where they were at the time, I felt confident based on Dr. Otvos' assessment that my LDL was healthy.

Finally, in June 2008, I was able to have the NMR Lipoprofile test conducted on my LDL cholesterol to see what my particle size actually was. Rather than run the risk of upsetting my doctor I instead decided to go see a doctor who specializes in low-carbohydrate nutrition with his patients just a few hours up the road from me in Durham, North Carolina. His name is Dr. Eric Westman from the Duke Lifestyle Medicine Clinic who not only treats patients with a low-carb eating plan, but also conducts some of the most cutting-edge research on carbohydrate restriction in the entire world!

Dr. Westman ran my blood work to get my lipid profile numbers for me and no doubt they would be a bit stunning to someone who looks at cholesterol in a traditional way:

Total Cholesterol - 326
Total LDL - 246
Total HDL - 65
Triglycerides - 77

Yes, my total cholesterol came in at 326 and hopefully now you know why I don't need to take a statin drug like Lipitor or Crestor to lower it. But check out my triglyceride/HDL ratio. It's virtually 1-1 and that's fantastic! Note that my HDL is above 50 and my triglycerides are below 100 — a tell-tale sign that Dr. Vernon says is proof positive that you are livin' la vida low-carb well. So what's up with the LDL? Is the particle size where it is supposed to be?

The answer is YES! Dr. Westman said that when he analyzed the LDL subset breakdown, he saw a clear majority of the LDL was the large, fluffy kind that you want to protect against cardiovascular problems and very few if any of the small, dense kind. The exact numbers were that 98% of the LDL was the good kind and a mere 2% were the dangerous kind. So, despite my seemingly astronomical LDL and total cholesterol numbers, they really are a non-factor in heart disease risk because the small LDL-P was a mere 30 out of nearly 1500 LDL particles. That's pretty amazing! And keep in mind my HDL "good" cholesterol is high like it needs to be, so that contributes to the total cholesterol number, too.

So if you've been to the doctor after being on a low-carb diet and you see numbers similar to my cholesterol, don't panic! Get your particle size tested so you can be armed with the facts about what to do in response.

Speaking candidly about this issue regarding cholesterol, Dr. Vernon said the way doctors evaluate cholesterol these days is based on little to no understanding of the differences in a patient who is on a low-carb diet.

"One of the problems with this issue is that physicians are educated on the outcomes of constant storage metabolism and have no information about the risks or lack of risks associated with low-carb," she explained. "I can tell you that I have several patients who have had no progression of cardiovascular disease after low-carbing for several years."

Since Dr. Vernon works directly with people following a low-carb regimen daily in her work with obese and diabetic patients, I am more apt to trust her empirical, anecdotal observations than I would the robotic response that most doctors are regurgitating to patients these days. Thank you Dr. Vernon for sharing your wisdom and keep up the great work on behalf of livin' la vida low-carb. Find a low-carb doctor in your area by visiting LowCarbDoctors.blogspot.com.

In July 2009, I returned to see my family doctor after a few years of avoiding him since he wanted to put me on a statin drug. I wanted to see if they would pull a blood sample and spin it for me to run an updated NMR LipoProfile test, but they said I would need to come in for a visit to see my physician first. I was not excited to pay for an office visit just to have my doctor authorize me to have a test run. This is one of the things that's wrong with healthcare in America today — patients who take control of their own health are forced to follow medical protocol. I love my doctor but this visit was unnecessary.

I brought my NMR LipoProfile test results from 2008 which showed an elevated LDL and total cholesterol number, but an extraordinarily low small LDL-P number of just 30. As soon as my doctor saw that number, I heard him mumble to himself, "That's impossible." With a big grin on my face that ran from ear to ear I'm sure and playing dumb I said, "What?" He went on to explain that he had never seen anyone with that low a small LDL particle size number and that it was simply spectacular. My doctor also said that he fully expected my LDL particles to be well over 2,000 with my cholesterol numbers as high as they were and I explained how LDL cholesterol numbers are different in people who eat low-carb. It was an educational experience for my doctor and he admitted he had changed his views somewhat since I had last seen him.

My doctor then went on to give me the lecture comparing LDL to spiders and snakes — there are poisonous ones and non-poisonous ones that he looks out for in people with high-LDL. And he said I have nothing to concern myself with regarding my "spiders and snakes" because they look to be harmless. He added that with the heart health issues that my late brother Kevin and my father have both had that I should get a CT heart scan done. I told him I had been looking for a place in our area to have one done as recommended by Dr. William Davis from the *Heart Scan Blog* (who provided the quote at the beginning of this chapter) and he gave me a prescription for a place about five miles from my house. Cool! I got this $99 test done soon to see what my calcium score was in August 2009. It came back clean as a whistle with a calcium score of zero — as in zilch, nada, nothing! So much for a high-fat, low-carb diet clogging your arteries, eh?

Incidentally, my family doctor started running the NMR LipoProfile test on his other patients a couple of years ago after I shared my experience taking the test previously. This is why I like seeing my personal physician because he is willing to learn from his patients which is the sign of an excellent doctor. It's the doctors and other medical professionals who remain closed-minded and think they have all the answers that do a disservice to their patients. At the end of my visit, my doc also knocked off 20% from the "brief visit" charge, so I paid less than $50 to see him which isn't half bad these days.

Hopefully now you know why most cholesterol tests that are run by your doctor are virtually meaningless and that there are better ways to measure heart health than LDL and total cholesterol. Coming up in the next life lesson I've learned from livin' la vida low-carb, we look at a substance that is quite literally in just about everything we eat these days — sugar and its evil twin high-fructose corn syrup!

LESSON #3
Sugar and high fructose corn syrup can be serious threats to health

"Sugar and HFCS are both half fructose. Fructose is the only highly addictive substance we feed children from birth. It is also likely to be the primary cause of heart disease, Type II diabetes and obesity."

— **David Gillespie,** author of *Sweet Poison: Why Sugar Makes Us Fat*
(SweetPoison.com.au)

In my 2005 book about my weight loss entitled *Livin' La Vida Low-Carb: My Journey from Flabby Fat to Sensationally Skinny in One Year,* I included an entire chapter on the subject of sugar entitled "Sugar Is Rat Poison." Of course, when I refer to "sugar," I'm not just talking about the white, granular stuff. There's an equally dastardly substance that has infiltrated our food supply since the early 1970s when I was born that has arguably been one of the major reasons why our modern-day society has become more obese, diabetic, and sicker than ever before! It's called high-fructose corn syrup, aka HFCS.

But not everyone agrees with my assertion that HFCS is bad. The President of the Corn Refiners Association Audrae Erickson disagrees with me. In June of 2005 Erickson stated that I mischaracterized HFCS as a unique contributor to obesity. She believes it is a natural home grown sweetener from the U.S. corn fields.

No doubt a product made in the USA is better received by the American public, but that doesn't necessarily make it healthy for you. Sugar is sugar no matter what you call it. And HFCS is a potent man-made sugar substance that is catastrophic to anyone who is trying to lose weight or maintain good health. To suggest otherwise is dangerous to the health of all consumers.

Erickson asserted that scientific experts have found that HFCS is "not a unique contributor to obesity." There are plenty of other studies that have found just the opposite to be true. They are easy to find in the literature but one must take a little time to do some research. According to Erickson HFCS has been proven beneficial to consumers through its use in many foods and beverages, including several products that are specifically made for people trying to control their weight.

I am appalled that anyone would suggest HFCS is healthy for you. The mere fact that it is found in foods and beverages does not necessarily mean it is not going to impact your blood sugar, weight, and health. That's like saying the alcohol found in beer is good for you because it is so prevalent in adult beverages. Just because it's in there doesn't mean your body needs it.

As for HFCS being included in products made for people trying to control their weight, that's not surprising since many of the low-fat foods are generally loaded with sugar and/or HFCS. While this sweetener may not have any fat in it, HFCS is certainly not healthy. Sugar in any form can cause you to rapidly gain weight in excessive amounts because it stimulates a massive rise in blood sugar and insulin — a double whammy!

But HFCS is a lot different than plain sugar. Actually, it is a highly refined, artificially-made product that transforms cornstarch into a sweet, thick and clear liquid that is sweeter than sugar and prevents the body from burning stored fat. This is NOT good when you are livin' la vida low-carb!

HFCS replaced sugar during the 1970s because it was cheaper to produce and the obesity problem has only gotten progressively worse ever since. Americans consume more than 63 pounds each of HFCS annually today compared with just a half-pound in 1970. Fifty-five percent of sweeteners used in food manufacturing in the 21st Century are made from corn.

The onset of HFCS goes back to around the time my generation was born in 1971 when manufacturers decided to stop using sucrose, aka table sugar, as the primary sweetening agent found in most soft drinks at the time and switched it over to fructose, a form of sugar extracted from fruit, instead. Sounds innocent enough, doesn't it? Not so fast.

Unfortunately, these days HFCS is in everything. Just read the ingredients label on just about any food item at your local grocery store and it's almost impossible to pick up very many foods at all without coming across this health menace. That's one of the major concerns science journalist Michael Pollan shared in his instant classic 2007 health book *The Omnivore's Dilemma: A Natural History of Four Meals*.

You may be wondering what's so bad about fructose compared with sucrose. There are several metabolic issues at work that should shed some light on this:

Fructose needs the liver to break it down

The process of metabolizing fructose uses up lots of energy molecules called Adenosine triphosphate, or ATP. When this happens, the body reacts by feeling really tired and repeating this strain on the liver has been found to cause fatty liver disease and could lead to metabolic syndrome. Additionally, the more fructose that is in your system, the greater risk you are putting on your body to deteriorate. And that's not a good thing at all!

Fructose needs sucrose to be absorbed properly

The abundance of fructose combined with the lack of sucrose in the modern diet means most people are putting a strain on their lower intestine to digest the fructose. This causes painful gas and abdominal issues, including bloating and diarrhea.

Fructose doesn't just add calories; it's harmful on its own

While most of the so-called health "experts" talk about sugary sodas as merely "empty calories," the fact is the fructose in them is what causes the most problems in the weight and health of those who consume it.

This is a scary thought for me personally because I used to consume the equivalent of 16-20 cans of Coca-Cola on a daily basis before I started livin' la vida low-carb. That's about 45g sugar each, all in the form of high fructose corn syrup, per can. So I was guzzling down — brace yourself — upwards of 900 grams of sugar (much of which came in the form of HFCS) just in my soda consumption before going on the Atkins diet. And we won't even talk about the sugar and HFCS that was in all those snack cakes I used to eat, too! Ouch!

I thank the good Lord above that I didn't do major damage to my body putting my body through HFCS shock treatment on a daily basis because the negative side effects of this sugar are difficult to ignore. Studies have already shown that fructose speeds up the process of becoming obese, but it gets even worse than that! Fructose is known to raise your triglycerides which also leads to obesity and metabolic syndrome. Uric acid is raised in the body and the risk of getting gout increases leading to inflammation of the arteries which rapidly begins clogging your arteries (see, it's not the fat you consume, but the sugar in the form of fructose that leads to inflammation which causes the cardiovascular problems most people experience).

There is also a form of fructose intolerance similar to lactose intolerance with milk-based products that may cause some people's bodies to experience severe cramping, gas, stomach pain, indigestion, and worse. If you thought you were suffering from a nervous stomach, then you may actually be the victim of intolerance to fructose!

In light of my horrendous consumption of 900+ grams of fructose just from sugary sodas before 2004, you might think you can get away with a lot less than that with no ill effects. But you would be wrong. The fact is all you need is as little as 60g fructose commonly found in one large soft drink from McDonald's or Super Big Gulp from 7-11 and the potential damage to your liver and the accumulation of dangerous visceral body fat will commence. Is there any wonder how my weight ever got to be over 400 pounds now?

The scary part about fructose is that it is not just in sugary sodas. Most people get hundreds of grams MORE of this stuff in their body when they eat foods like bread, cookies, cake, ketchup (yep, HFCS is in it, too!), snack cakes, and even fruit. You'll notice all of those foods just happen to be high-carb, too, so it's yet another reason why you should be livin' la vida low-carb.

But even those of us on the low-carb lifestyle should be mindful of the fructose that is put in barbecue sauce and other grilling condiments because of something known as advanced glycoslated end products, or AGEs. This one should be easy to remember because AGEs lead to advancement in aging. We already know a high-carb/high-sugar diet leads to age-related macular degeneration and a whole host of other health ailments, but this one should make you pay close attention.

AGEs are created when a chemical reaction happens to proteins as they are heated in combination with fructose sugars. Toasting or grilling leads to a process known as cartelization where the protein reacts to the fructose it comes into contact with to cause stiffening of the arteries and an increase in blood pressure. The AGEs also damage your kidneys, eyes, and essential organs. Our bodies will absorb 10 percent of the AGEs we consume — enough to cause some serious damage if you are not careful.

Try to avoid using sugary sauces when cooking meats, but also keep in mind that a lot of grilled meats have sugar injected into them. That's why getting the best quality of grass-fed beef, for example, is going to be the healthiest for your low-carb lifestyle. Just because it tastes good doesn't necessarily mean it's good for you. Visit EatWild.com to find a good supplier of grass-fed meats in your area.

Most egregious of all regarding fructose that comes from HFCS is the fact that the corn has more than likely been genetically modified (GMO). These GMO crops are a huge question mark as it relates to your health. There are absolutely zero long-term studies on the safety of consuming anything with GMO in them and God only knows what this is doing to our bodies. The highly-refined process of creating HFCS makes this potentially hazardous substance that much worse.

Hopefully now you understand a little better why our modern-day society is so full of heavy people who are sicker than they've ever been before. It's not a coincidence! The next time someone heralds the healthiness of HFCS, just remember it is a dangerous sugar that should be avoided if we are ever going to get this obesity problem under control.

It's not just the HFCS hawkers, though. Sugar Association president and CEO Andrew Briscoe has also said there is not a link between sugar and obesity as has been suggested by people like me. Instead, he blames obesity on people eating too many calories and not getting enough exercise. He made these comments at the 22nd Annual International Sweetener Symposium in 2005.

"Every major, comprehensive review of the total body of scientific literature continues to exonerate sugars intake as the causative factor in any lifestyle disease, including obesity," Briscoe contended. "We believe in calories in and calories out. Sugar is not a part of obesity issues."

That quote right there from the most powerful voice in the sugar industry is exactly why nearly two out of every three Americans are overweight or obese today. Pretending that this problem does not exist and that sugar does not play a factor in it is irresponsible.

Briscoe believes that sugar is a natural part of any healthy diet and he also contends that it does not matter how much sugar you consume, it will not harm your body in any way. At just 15 calories per teaspoon of sugar, how can something so innocent be so vilified? Thus, a national marketing campaign ensued in 2009 attempting to create this image in people's minds that sugar can and even should be consumed as part of a healthy lifestyle.

While sugar consumption per capita was at 102 pounds in 1972, that number had fallen to a net 45 pounds per person in 2002. In other words, the sugar industry is hurting and hurting badly. The greater focus people place on the role sugar has played in their health and obesity problems have been credited with this decline.

You can probably even give some of the credit to the late great Dr. Robert C. Atkins and other low-carb lifestyle advocates for educating consumers about how harmful sugar consumption and sugar addiction is to their bodies. Fellow blogger Connie Bennett (SugarShockBlog.com) wrote a book in 2006 entitled *SUGAR SHOCK: How Sweets and Simple Carbs Can Derail Your Life — And How You Can Get Back On Track!* which opened a lot of people's eyes to the negative effects sugar has on people's health. But none of this sits very well with the sugar lobby. And they will certainly not go down without a fight.

Ever since I first started writing at my blog about how sugar, not fat is what has led to the obesity problem in the United States, I have received numerous negative messages from people in the sugar industry telling me how wrong I am about their product because it is "all-natural" and completely safe for anyone to consume regularly.

If you walk up to the average man on the street and ask him if eating a lot of sugar is either good for you or bad for you, I am confident that nine out of every ten people would say it is bad for you. This universally-accepted notion must be rooted in something that is substantively true or else people would not feel so strongly about it.

Another point to ponder is the fact that eating a low-fat diet generally means you will consume a lot higher amount of sugar than you would on a low-carb program. The reason for this is so many low-fat foods contain added sugars and salt to mask the disgusting taste once you remove the fat from the original product. The trade-off is marketed as "healthier," but all of that extra sugar is not good for you either. This ever-present, never-publicized fact about the low-fat diet rears its ugly head yet again. The inseparable connection between low-fat and sugar needs to be illuminated for the entire world to see.

So, the root question I have to ask is this — Can sugar be part of a healthy lifestyle? With everything we know about sugar and its negative effect on our bodies, there is only one obvious answer to that question. No matter how much the sugar industry attempts to put forth the notion that sugar consumption has no bearing on the obesity problem, I think it is clear that sugar is, has always been, and will forever be unhealthy. If you are livin' la vida low-carb, then avoiding sugar and high fructose corn syrup (HFCS) is essential to controlling your weight.

According to a press release I received from the Vice President of Public Relations for the Washington, DC-based Sugar Association Melanie Miller in September 2008, the incredible "healing" properties of sugar were cited as a reason why people should not be shunning the granulated white stuff quite so quickly.

"We all know that sugar makes good foods taste better, helps breads rise, creates cookie's crunchiness or chewiness, and protects the safety of jams and jellies," Miller wrote in the release. "But, did you know the same preserving power sugar brings to jams and jellies can also help heal wounds?"

It seems the Sugar Association Is desperate to reshape the negative image that sugar has been getting.

In the press release, Miller stated that the properties that make sugar a great food preservative gives it "healing powers" to treat serious wounds and burn victims. According to Miller, sugar "absorbs the wound's moisture necessary for the growth of infectious bacteria" and it also "supplies the very nourishment damaged tissues require for healing and re-growth."

Okay, all of this is well and good if we are talking about using sugar for topical medicinal purposes. But why are they sending this press release out in 2008 when it's been over ten years since scientific research provided on this was published?

"Maybe Mary Poppins wasn't wrong when she said a spoonful of sugar helps the medicine go down," she concludes in the release. "Science is showing that it helps wounds heal, as well as preserve the safety of our foods."

It is hard to believe the Sugar Association would make such a claim. In fact, one of the up-and-coming sugar alternatives is the fiber-based sweetener oligofructose — aka chicory root — and it too has been shown in studies to heal wounds. So there's no real monopoly by sugar as a topical healer.

The Corn Refiners Association ran an aggressive marketing campaign in fall of 2008. You may have seen the ads on TV or on the internet, telling you that you are in for a sweet surprise about HFCS and encouraging you to visit their web site to get the facts. They state HFCS has no artificial ingredients and is nutritionally the same as table sugar. They further state HFCS has the same number of calories as table sugar.

This does not make me feel better about using HFCS. Stating that it is virtually equal to sugar does not make it so. In reality HFCS is much worse than sugar, if that's possible.

The sudden switch to fructose from sucrose in the 1970s brought on some rather devastating effects to the weight and health of modern-day life.

Pick up just about any product — even non-food products like cough syrup and toothpaste — and you'll likely see "high fructose corn syrup" or some corn derivative included in the ingredients listing somewhere. It's amazing how accepted this practice has become and most people are completely oblivious to it. There's even a book by Dr. Richard Johnson called *The Sugar Fix: The High-Fructose Fallout That Is Making You Fat and Sick* that talks about how HFCS has virtually taken over the food manufacturing industry these days and people are literally eating themselves sick.

No matter how you try to dress up sugar or high fructose corn syrup in slick packaging, it's still harmful to your health and weight. There is no doubt in my mind that sugar and high fructose corn syrup are both serious threats to your health and need to be avoided as much as humanly possible. Speaking of avoiding, this next lesson tells you why that low-fat, low-calorie diet you've heard about may not be as "healthy" as you bargained for!

LESSON #4
Low-fat, low-calorie diets do not have a monopoly on "healthy"

"Since losing 50 pounds over 25 years ago, the most important lesson I have learned is that low-fat and low-calorie has done nothing but perpetuate unsafe dieting with temporary results. Losing weight is about finding YOUR center, YOUR approach and applying it to YOUR lifestyle. Low-fat and low-calorie is misleading and is in my humble opinion the root of the obesity crisis."

— **Nicki Anderson**, author of *Nicki Anderson's Single Step Weight Loss Solution* (StopGainingStartLosing.com) and President of Reality Fitness (NickiAnderson.com)

I was browsing around the Internet one day doing my daily routine of looking for stuff to blog about and came across some science that explains why low-fat/low-calorie/portion-controlled diets do not produce permanent weight loss and improved health over the long-term as has often been shoved down our throats for nearly three decades despite dismal results. Although eating "low-fat" has become synonymous with being "healthy," nothing could be further from the truth. The calories in/calories out mantra is nothing more than a myth according to research released in January 2006.

The three-month study published in the January 2004 issue of *Archives of Internal Medicine* featured 34 overweight adults who were split up into one of three categories: 1) high-carb, low-fat diet with no exercise; 2) high-carb, low-fat diet with exercise; and 3) a control group that ate the same way they were already eating. At the conclusion of the study, the group that ate the high-carb, low-fat diet without any exercise lost an average of seven pounds, the high-carb, low-fat diet group that exercised four times a week on a stationary bike lost an average of 11 pounds, and the control group maintained their weight.

Lead researcher Dr. William Evans from the Nutrition, Metabolism and Exercise Laboratory at the University of Arkansas for Medical Sciences said the old adage of "calories in minus calories out" may not be a deciding factor in weight loss.

"Calories in, minus calories out, does not always determine the amount of weight loss," Dr. Evans explained.

In his study, Dr. Evans allowed the participants to eat as much as they wanted to eat and return any uneaten food to the researchers so they could determine the caloric intake of each participant. The study participants ended up eating an average of 2,400 calories during the study. And yet they still lost weight, even the ones that did not exercise.

Well, somebody stop the presses because I thought it was all about "calories in, calories out?" Isn't that what we have been told by health and fitness experts? And yet these study participants were consuming 2,400 calories and STILL shed weight off their bodies. Can you imagine how much MORE weight they could have lost had they eaten 2,400 calories and reduced their carbohydrate intake, too? That would have been a very telling sub-group for this study to observe and measure their weight loss as well.

Even with evidence like this in the scientific data, the calorie apologists will still claim you can't lose weight without cardiovascular exercise. As someone who has lost a significant amount of weight both with and without exercise, I have to disagree with that statement, though. While exercise is a great way to maintain your weight loss, the makeup of your diet plays a much greater role in burning stored body fat and weight than all the exercise in the world.

The problem is most "experts" who call for more and more exercise are also pushing upwards of 60 percent of their caloric intake in the form of carbohydrates. They claim that you need that for energy to fuel your workouts. There is no denying some people can eat a lot of carbs and still lose weight. But how your body reacts to all of those carbs is why so many people are unable to continue eating that way forever. Hunger, irritability, deprivation, cravings, and more will overcome so many people and bring them to their knees begging for the pain to go away (can you tell I was suffering on a low-fat, high-carb diet in the paVst?!).

Here are my criteria for what comprises a "healthy" weight loss diet:

1. Will I lose weight and keep it off eating this way forever?
2. Will eating this way prevent me from being constantly hungry?
3. Am I getting an adequate amount of healthy nutrients in my diet?

If you cannot answer YES to all three of those questions, then whatever "diet" plan you are on will not work to help you lose weight, get healthy, and stay healthy. For me, low-calorie diets were just not reasonable over the long haul and often left me so hungry and irritable that I couldn't even think straight. While I might have been eating four ounces of so-called "healthy" foods, I was always left begging for more and literally couldn't wait until the next meal. I felt so deprived that I was not satisfied with my lifestyle, despite the enormous weight loss I had accomplished when I shed 170 pounds on a low-fat diet in 1999.

Ever since I started the low-carb lifestyle, though, I have never run into this problem. I eat the amount of high-fat, low-carb foods that I want to eat without regard for restricting fat grams, calories, and definitely not unnecessarily cutting my portion sizes to teeny tiny meals. That's just not required when it comes to livin' la vida low-carb. Just watch the net carbs (total carbohydrates minus fiber mainly and some sugar alcohols if you must), eat to satiety, and let the miracle of low-carb do what it does in you.

There are many reasons why low-fat and low-calorie diets fail, but most of it has to do with the inadequate nutritional content in the foods that many people on those plans do eat. Just because a product packaging blares the words "fat-free" or "low-fat" on them doesn't mean you could or should eat them without any regard for the sugar and carbohydrate content in them. Oftentimes, there is even more sugar and salt in these foods just to make them taste somewhat familiar. That's just not natural or healthy!

And yet we so often hear just how "unhealthy" low-carb diets are. But what about switching that claim to the low-fat diets instead? Just how "healthy" are those low-fat, low-calorie diets we keep hearing that we need to be on anyway? Has there been any solid, long-term research conducted on those diets to confirm or reject their monopolistic claim of being what they say they are? I'm glad you asked that question because there is plenty of science to share — and it doesn't look too good for the low-fat advocates.

A study published in the January 4, 2006 issue of the prestigious *Journal of the American Medical Association* looked at 48,000 women who ate a low-fat, high-carb diet and found that they lost a measly 2 pounds over a seven-year span. WOW, two whole pounds in seven years?! Really? Man, makes you want to go out and start livin' la vida low-fat right away, doesn't it? Are you kidding me? NOT!

Lead researcher Dr. Barbara Howard heralded her study stating it proves that low-fat diets aren't the reason for the obesity epidemic getting worse.

"It will help people to understand that the weight gain we're seeing in this country is not caused by the lower-fat diets," Dr. Howard said.

I'm uncertain how a two-pound weight loss over seven years leads her to conclude this. The study really proves that a low-fat diet does not cause significant weight loss — and that's all it proves.

Dr. Michael Dansinger from the Tufts-New England Medical Center and a weight loss consultant for the hit NBC-TV weight loss reality show "The Biggest Loser" was not at all happy with the findings of Dr. Howard's study.

"This is like losing the Super Bowl but claiming a second place victory," Dansinger said. "The results are disappointing in the context of a country trying to battle obesity."

Dr. Dansinger is right on target with his comments. A lot of people take credit for making efforts in the battle against obesity, and yet the obesity rates keep going up and up. Real solutions to the obesity problem will result in a rapid decline of those rates and that means we need to look at methods other than the same old low-fat dogma we've been fed for years.

The women in the study cut their fat content down to 20 percent and ate more fruits, veggies and whole grains, including eating a lot more carbs. The low-fat dieters lost almost 5 pounds in their first year, but quickly gained back most of the weight. Meanwhile the control group maintained their weight over the entire seven years. Although the study was not specifically designed to observe weight loss but rather the effect of low-fat diets on heart disease and cancer, Dr. Howard felt there needed to be a response to the low-carb proponents who often link obesity with the low-fat diets recommended by doctors, health groups and even the government.

As someone who lost 170 pounds on a low-fat diet in 1999, I KNOW that you can lose weight by reducing your fat intake. But the problem comes in when you try to keep the weight off for good eating that way. It is a virtual impossibility because you are constantly hungry, feel deprived of the delicious foods you want to eat, and just feel like crap most of the time. At least I did. It was nice being somewhat skinnier than I was before (although that pudge in my abdomen just wouldn't go away), but I just couldn't keep it up and eventually gained all my weight back in rebellious fashion.

But there was an even more significant study that came out just one month later in the same medical journal that is arguably the most damning research results against low-fat diets ever published. In fact, you can mark down February 7, 2006 in the annals of history regarding health, diet, and nutrition as the date the unraveling of the three-decades-long low-fat diet dominance began. The published results of an eight-year study on the low-fat diet that day showed that there were zero health improvements in the risk of getting cancer and heart disease.

This is the same low-fat diet recommendation that we have heard from our doctors, government, and health experts since the early 1970s.

The eight-year study of 48,835 women published in the *Journal of the American Medical Association* in February 2006 found that the study participants failed to lose a measurable amount of weight on the low-fat diet. In fact, most of them even remained overweight which put them at an even greater risk for cardiovascular disease despite following their low-fat regimen. In other words, the low-fat diet was an utter and dismal failure.

While advocates of restricting fat for weight control, disease prevention, and good overall health have long received a free pass by much of the media, health officials and physicians in the US and around the world, studies like this one cannot be ignored and the ramifications of dismissing it rather than making changes in the way we think about health and diet could be devastating in the long-term. It is clear to everyone who has eyes to see that we must look at other nutritional approaches and stop monopolizing the public health message with an exclusive low-fat message. Doing the same thing over and over again expecting a different result is the very definition of insanity — and we've been nutritionally insane for decades!

The $415 million study that began in 1998 found there was no difference in the rate of breast cancer, colon cancer and heart disease among those eating a low-fat diet and those who did not. Low-fat supporters quickly defended these stunning results as not surprising because the study supposedly failed to look at the difference between eating good fats and bad fats.

Additionally, they claim that the low-fat dieters who participated in the research must not have cut their fat consumption enough to make a real difference in the disease rates. This makes no sense since the researchers had the ability to control the amount of fat the women consumed to a specified level. All they had to do was make it part of the study. It seems wrong for them to blame the test study participants and it makes you wonder if the researchers did this just because the study did not turn out the way they expected.

It truly is time for the low-fat advocates to admit that what's been told to us over the years has been incorrect. It's okay to tell people you were misled and that you sincerely thought you were sharing information that would help them be as healthy as possible.

But now that the truth has come out in a LONG-TERM study, it's time to set the record straight and open the door to new opportunities to educate the public about a wide variety of dietary plans that can and will help them lose weight, improve their health, and live a much longer and more fulfilling life.

The researchers admit that certain good fats like those found in olive oil and nuts are a healthy part of a preventative program against heart disease. Those are both excellent healthy foods to consume when you are livin' la vida low-carb!

American Heart Association President Dr. Robert Eckel released a statement soon after this study was published that these results will be misunderstood if they are not interpreted correctly.

"It would be easy to misinterpret the results of this study," he said.

What is the reason Dr. Eckel cannot simply embrace the results of the study? We deserve an explanation from our government and health leaders why a more thorough examination of all the potential ramifications to our health weren't studied sooner before recommending a low-fat diet to the American people.

Research or no research, I have always had my own personal doubts about low-fat, low-calorie diets. They do work to produce weight loss, but only for the people who are willing to put up with feeling hungry all the time and don't mind eating for the most part terrible-tasting foods. I lost a significant amount of weight on a low-fat diet a decade ago, but I literally could not continue to eat that way for the rest of my life.

I was starving for real foods that would satisfy me — namely fat and protein! That was not a healthy way to live, regardless of the weight loss I had achieved. And because you deprive your body of food when you are starving yourself on low-fat/low-calorie diets, your body goes into survival mode and holds on to every bite of food it can not knowing whether or not it will receive enough food to give you the energy you need.

While low-fat/low-calorie dieters are proud of the fact they count each and every fat gram and calorie in specific portions for their meals, they may not even realize how much they are confusing their own body with how they eat. No wonder people who get off of low-fat/low-calories diets rapidly gain back their weight and then some! That's exactly what happened to me in 1999 until I started my low-carb lifestyle on January 1, 2004.

There has been no direct correlation shown that simply cutting calories will produce any weight loss. None! But let's give the calorie-restriction argument merit for a moment and assume it does help with weight loss. Are there any other barriers to being successful on this kind of eating plan over the long haul? You bet there are!

Low-calorie diets are hard on you psychologically! It's darn difficult to continually give up all the foods you love and enjoy. No more unlimited quantities of potato chips, no French fries, no doughnuts or whatever your particular comfort food is. Wow, that's one of the most challenging things you will ever face. This alone makes a diet of this type nearly impossible to stick with over an extended period of time.

It's funny how people think low-carb is hard because you supposedly deprive your body of foods you love. While it is a challenge for some to give up these vices, it's not nearly as difficult as what you give up on low-fat/low-calorie diets. With low-carb you have plenty of choices, but those other diets leave you with hardly any choices at all. That can certainly work on your mind (where you might be asking yourself, "what the heck am I doing this to myself for?") and will soon derail your weight loss efforts. The low-carb lifestyle is different because you get to enjoy lots of great-tasting foods and never feel deprived.

This is why low-fat shouldn't be the only way recommended for people to lose weight and be healthy. Low-carb succeeds because it offers people who have tried and failed on low-fat, low-calorie diets a taste of better living. They can enjoy a much wider selection of foods to feel satisfied with. It really is a lifestyle change that people can make and feel good about. I have been livin' la vida low-carb since January 2004 and wouldn't have it any other way!

Of all the people I have had the privilege of interviewing for my popular Top 20 Fitness & Nutrition iTunes podcast called "The Livin' La Vida Low-Carb Show with Jimmy Moore" (TheLivinLowCarbShow.com), one of the most memorable ones will always be Mr. Low-Fat diet himself, Dr. Dean Ornish. Although he and I are about as diametrically opposite as you can get when it comes to dietary philosophies, he was nothing but respectful towards me and I him. But I couldn't resist challenging his insistence over and over again during our conversation that we "agree" with each other on some key points.

I will give Dr. Ornish credit that the ideals espoused in his 2008 book entitled *The Spectrum* are definitely a step forward in attempting to forge some common ground among those who advocate a low-fat or a low-carb diet. But it didn't take long after reading his book to see that what Dr. Ornish believed was on the healthy end of the "spectrum" of food choices was the same high-carb, low-fat vegetarian ones and the foods on the least healthy end were the more fatty, meat-based choices. In other words, not much had changed at all in the Ornish philosophy! It was just repackaged to appear more conciliatory towards other plans.

As you would imagine we did disagree over many issues during the interview, and I was unable to persuade him to answer questions about carbohydrate or fat intake. Another thing we disagreed on was whether more fiber eaten with carbohydrates would significantly slow the blood sugar rise and insulin response in the body. When I have attempted this my body is sent into a major sugar rush.

While Dr. Ornish has many supporters, some of them are actually moving forward and leaving behind the research Dr. Ornish relies on. One such researcher is Dr. David Ludwig who is a low-carb researcher interested in issues involving childhood obesity and health.

We also disagreed on a favorite author of mine, Gary Taubes and his brilliant book *Good Calories, Bad Calories*. It is an understatement that Dr. Ornish disagrees with me on this book, though I won't say all the negative things he had to say about it.

I did ask him that if low-carb was so unhealthy, why was I able to lose such a significant amount of weight and attain such good health? He would not answer this question.

That's fine that he declares his diet is the only one to be proven to "reverse heart disease" but I'm not buying it. I'm sure Dean Ornish will never want to do another interview with me again after this, but that's of no concern to me. I have to speak the truth and the truth is I couldn't remain silent. Whether he likes it or not, livin' la vida low-carb is mainstream now and here to stay. It's not low-carb versus low-fat — it's what works for the individual. His refusal to even acknowledge that a low-carb program will work for some gets to the very heart of the matter.

Even I am the first to admit that low-carb will not necessarily work for everyone, but it's an option that should at least be promoted by health groups and tried by people who have struggled on the over-recommended high-carb, low-fat diet as I did for most of my life before going on the Atkins diet in 2004. My mantra is for people to find the proven and effective plan that works for them, follow that plan exactly as prescribed by the author, and then keep doing that plan for the rest of their life. If that's an Ornish-styled low-fat diet and you're happy with it, then I say go for it. But if it's an Atkins-styled low-carb diet, then that should be something you should openly encourage people to follow, too.

What I've been talking about in this chapter comes down to one central issue that we must all ask ourselves regarding this idea of what is healthy. If low-carb diets are as effective as low-fat diets (and that's what the evidence has shown in multiple studies), then don't they deserve equal footing, equal treatment, and equal endorsement by our leaders? The time for talking about this is over. We've seen the research and it shows that low-carb is as good or better than low-fat diets for weight loss and health improvements for at least one year (and likely longer).

Livin' la vida low-carb doesn't have to be advocated but simply put on the table as a viable option for people to try if they need to lose weight and get healthy.

Sometimes you can start to feel like a lonely voice in the wilderness when you put yourself out there as an avid spokesperson for a nutritional approach like low-carb that is so universally mocked and scorned by the current health experts. But this reminds me of an old legend about the actions of a "good and just man" who was in a similar circumstance where he had a choice between doing what was right and taking a lot of heat for it or turning his back on the truth just to blend in with the crowd and be accepted.

Here's my own low-carb variation on how that story goes:

A good and just man began speaking with individuals within his sphere of influence one day trying to convince them one-by-one of the truth about livin' la vida low-carb. As much as he tried to capture their attention with all the latest research studies confirming this way of eating as incredibly effective for managing weight loss well, controlling blood sugar and insulin levels especially for diabetics, and warding off a whole host of preventable diseases, nobody would engage him in conversation. They just didn't show any interest at all in the truth.

Refusing to give up, this good and just man then started carrying around a picket sign that had "TRUTH" written on it in large letters. He stood ready to share the truth about low-carb living being the diet of our early ancestors thousands of years ago up until just a few decades ago when the low-fat, low-calorie, portion control mantra was thrust upon the world by a vocal minority who took it upon themselves to change the way people viewed "healthy" eating. The result has been a rampant outbreak of obesity and disease like we've never seen in the history of the world. But, again, NOBODY paid any attention to his sign nor did they care about hearing the truth.

Finally, he began going from street to street and from marketplace to marketplace shouting from the top of his lungs, "Men and women, stop eating all that sugar, starchy carbs, and junk food. What you are doing to your body is wrong. Don't you know those foods will make you sick, fat, and possibly even die?!"

The people in the street and at the marketplace laughed at this good and just man every single day — but he just kept on shouting the truth. One day, a curious person stopped the man and asked, "Dude, can't you see that your shouting at all of us is absolutely useless and ineffective?" Then he responded back, "Yes, I see that." The person then asked, "So, why do you continue with this day after day after day?"

That's when the good and just man made the most profound statement he had ever uttered. "When I first arrived on the scene, I was fully convinced that I could change the thinking that others had about low-carb. But now I continue shouting the truth because I don't want THEM to change ME."

The moral of this story: Speak out for the truth about low-carb lest your silence sends the wrong message to others. If you choose to remain silent regarding the truths of livin' la vida low-carb, then others may take your silence as an agreement with their outrageous positions like low-carb is a dangerous "fad" diet that will give you heart disease and eventually kill you. Obviously, that's not at all what you believe, but refusing to share the truth sends that message loud and clear — and could leave you vulnerable to the low-fat propaganda.

Even if you feel like that lonely voice in the wilderness espousing the low-carb lifestyle, you know the truth because you've embraced it, absorbed it, and lived it. Now go let your light shine if for no other reason than to remain grounded in that truth for the rest of your long and healthy life. And if just a few others happen to open their eyes to the truth along the way, then you can feel proud that they will be out there sharing the truth, solidifying their grip on it, and joining us in this journey to better health that tens of millions more need to participate in.

If you do not stand firm... you will not stand at all. Isaiah 7:9

It is clear to me that low-fat, low-calorie diets do not have a monopoly on "healthy." We'll be exploring this subject a little further in some upcoming chapters. Coming up next, we'll find out why the current health experts and the press don't have a clue about what livin' la vida low-carb is really all about.

LESSON #5
The media and health "experts" are dead wrong about low-carb

"For many years, I have researched the idea that a high fat (high saturated fat), diet is damaging to human health and causes heart disease — and almost any other disease you care to mention. It has become crystal clear to me that this, the diet-heart hypothesis, represents the pinnacle of human stupidity. A stunning triumph of dogma over fact. As with all idiotic and wrong hypotheses, however, there is a scientific brotherhood who toil endlessly to keep it alive. A brotherhood who attack anyone who dares the question their orthodoxy with all the weapons available to them. The usual form of attack can be boiled down to this. 'We are very clever, we are experts, we know much more about this than you — you dreadful non-expert. Just look at the number of letters after my name. I AM VERY IMPORTANT.' The media, unfortunately, when confronted by medical 'experts' are cowed into submission. As with any other sort of fanatic, you can't be an expert in heart disease, or nutrition, or dietary research, unless you sign up to the dogma that low-carb diets are bad for you. To an extent I don't blame the experts for creating their dogma, and sticking to it. That is what experts do. But I do blame the media for their craven acceptance of such an idiotic and damaging piece of scientific nonsense. Get some backbone guys, and do the research yourself."

— **Dr. Malcolm Kendrick**, M.D., UK physician and author of *The Great Cholesterol Con*

I've noticed a trend since I started blogging about livin' la vida low-carb beginning in April 2005. While there are negative articles against the Atkins diet and other low-carb programs here and there throughout the year, it seems the media and the current health experts like to orchestrate a huge negative splash to pour it on against low-carb every six months or so in an attempt to discredit this healthy and effective way of eating.

I've seen a lot of headlines over the past few years attempting to throw livin' la vida low-carb under the bus. But never have I ever responded to such an incredibly inept column like the one published in the *Augusta Free Press* in 2006 by a woman named Vee Jefferson. When I first saw it, my initial reaction was to ignore it and move on. But the more I thought about it and the more of my readers who kept asking me to respond to it, I changed my mind and decided to confront Jefferson's column directly. As a registered nurse for the past decade, she has been sharing with her ideas about health.

In her column entitled "Low-carb diets - some dangerous truths uncovered," Jefferson immediately laid the groundwork for her attack against the low-carb lifestyle by declaring it as "a very unhealthy way to lose weight." She added that it is "dangerous" for reasons that go far beyond the high-fat content and added calories.

The side effects of low-carb that generally come in the first few days of Induction and highlighted in studies are described by Jefferson as "signs of impending crises." She does not state what the crises actually are. The only state of crisis that I am aware of is the obesity and diabetes ones we are experiencing currently which is why so many people need to be livin' la vida low-carb now more than ever before! Jefferson's two biggest concerns about low-carb — she described them in her column as "the most important dangers" — are low blood sugar and low potassium which she believes are "the quick killers."

Low blood sugar and potassium are stabilized by low-carb living, not the other way around.

She did have ONE good thing to say about livin' la vida low-carb before attempting to "tear down" what she thinks is bad about it. Jefferson claims it is "a very good idea to limit carbohydrate intake," primarily sugar.

This confuses me. She supports low-carb eating, but not the lifestyle. How very odd.

"These are the diets that can kill if the dieter is not familiar with the dangers," *Jefferson wrote.*

Here is her list of reasons for NOT doing low-carb.

1. FIBER

"Low-carb dieters may not get enough fiber, which keeps bowel movements regular and reduces the risk of heart disease, some cancers and diabetes. Without eating carbohydrates from plant sources like fruits, vegetables, whole grains and beans - foods limited or banned on low-carbohydrate diet plans - it is difficult to get the daily recommended amount of fiber."

It is not difficult for me. From day one of my low-carb lifestyle which began back in January 2004 when I weighed 410 pounds, I have taken a fiber supplement in addition to the fiber I receive from the foods I eat, such as flax seeds and other fiber-based products. Some of my favorite low-carb bars, including GoLower nut bars (available from CarbSmart.com) as well as ChocoPerfection chocolate bars (ChocoPerfection.com) are loaded with more fiber than most of the fruits, veggies, whole grains and beans you can eat. Fiber is an integral part of a low-carb plan and stating otherwise is intentionally manipulating the truth about this amazing way of eating.

2. WATER WEIGHT LOSS

"The truth about low-carb dieting is that you do lose weight. The first bit of weight loss, however, is water weight."

A study published in the March 15, 2005 issue of the *Annals of Internal Medicine* by a research professor of biochemistry at the Temple University School of Medicine named Dr. Guenther Boden found that reducing carbohydrates in the diet produces a spontaneous reduction in calories and, thus, fat loss. This flies in the face of low-carb weight loss being all "water weight."

3. MUSCLE MASS LOSS

"As you progress on the [low-carb] diet, you will lose some fat, but you will also lose some muscle mass. And let's not forget that the heart is a muscle, too. The marketers of these low-carb diets tell you that you should consume extra protein to avoid losing muscle mass, but experts say that eating excess protein does not prevent this because there is a caloric deficit."

A study by Dr. Annsi Manninen published in the February 2006 issue of *Nutrition & Metabolism* found muscle mass is preserved on a low-carb diet, echoing the fantastic research conducted by Dr. Donald Layman from the University of Illinois at Urbana-Champaign who had previously noted that a low-carb/ high-protein diet burns fat, not muscle.

4. WEAKNESS AND LACK OF ENERGY

"When insulin levels are chronically too low, as they may be in very low-carb diets, catabolism (breakdown) of muscle protein increases, and protein (needed for muscle building) synthesis stops. Because this causes of (sic) quick muscle fatigue, the person generally exercises and moves less (often without realizing it), which is not good for caloric expenditure and basal metabolic rate (metabolism)."

Before I started livin' la vida low-carb, the constant rollercoaster ride I gave my blood sugar was leading me straight towards becoming a Type 2 diabetic. But when I removed sugar and other refined and starchy carbohydrates that turn to sugar in my body, for the first time in my life I was no longer enslaved by those foods that kept me in constant physical bondage. No more ups and downs with insulin working overtime to keep up. Low-carb living normalized and balanced that in my body for good and I've been healthier ever since.

While the first few weeks were difficult with the energy as my body was getting used to burning fat for fuel rather than carbs, ever since then I have been one of the most energetic people you will ever meet in your entire life. I am an avid exerciser getting in hours of volleyball and other competitive sports playing each week. Jefferson is again being misleading about the effect of low-carb on your body. You will want to exercise more because of the energy rush you get from being on it. Once you get past Induction, look out! Whoooooooosh comes the energy...I've got the power! It's gettin', it's gettin', it's gettin' kinda hectic (love that Snap song)!

5. KETOSIS IS DANGEROUS

"Ketosis is usually marketed to the consumer by low-carb diet advocates as being a good thing - a positive thing. I'm telling you now, it's not. I've actually read a very popular book on low-carb dieting - I'm not naming any names - where the writer actually encourages the readers to go out and buy ketone test strips so that they can have proof that their bodies have reached the desired state of fat burning."

It was Dr. Atkins and I proudly used ketone strips during my low-carb weight loss in 2004 to see if I was in ketosis or not. Seeing that pink or purple strip was a reminder of the good I was doing for my body on my way to losing 180 pounds.

"Ketosis, left unchecked, can lead to very serious consequences. Ketosis occurs when the amount of carbohydrates (the fuel required to make the body function) drops below a critical level."

Ketosis is not dangerous. Regarding carbohydrates, they are NOT the fuel of a low-carber. Fat is the fuel that we live off of which burns much more efficiently than carbohydrates.

"This forces the body to turn to protein and then to the body's fat stores to do the work carbohydrates are supposed to do. When protein is used in this manner, it releases nitrogen into the blood stream, placing a burden on the kidneys as they try to expel excessive urinary water due to the loss of sodium (salt). When fat is likewise used, the breakup releases fatty acids, or ketones, into the bloodstream, which causes a further burden on the kidneys. If ketosis continues for long periods of time, serious damage to the liver and kidneys may occur. Liver failure means absolute death, because doctors can do nothing to fix this. Kidney failure means dialysis, and may eventually lead to death as well."

Both my kidneys and liver are doing quite well despite being on low-carb for over five years now and counting. If the above dire consequences were typical I would be on dialysis by now!

6. LOW BLOOD SUGAR LEVELS

"When a person stays on a low-carb diet over a long period of time, one day they may notice that they are unusually weak. They may feel an overwhelming urge to lie down and may even feel dizzy and lightheaded. It's very important that you are aware of what is going on so that you will be able to treat yourself fast. You need sugar FAST!"

No you don't! I haven't had much sugar at all in a very long time. If I get dizzy, then it probably means I need to eat something, not jump to get sugar in my blood as soon as possible. That's just plain ridiculous advice! And actually that would only make the problem worse as an insulin rush would then be followed by the inevitable blood sugar crash soon thereafter — a ruthless rollercoaster ride.

"Now, since you're not diabetic, it's only important for you to raise your blood-sugar level fast. Any sugar is good. Drink a soda or some juice, eat some candy or anything you have that has a good bit of sugar in it. Then eat something starchy, like a sandwich or a potato, to maintain your blood sugar and lay off the diet now."

This advice is irresponsible and I suspect it is intentionally alarming to keep people from trying low-carb.

"What's the seriousness of very low blood sugar? You will eventually pass out, stop breathing, and die. If you're home alone, that means no one will be able to save you. If you're driving, it means you may have an accident and possibly hurt or kill someone else in the process."

This statement is misleading. Low-carb does not cause the kind of low blood sugar levels that are hyperbolized about here. What it does is bring balance to blood sugar where it was previously out of kilter. In five years I've never passed out, stopped breathing or died (unless I am typing this as a ghost!)

7. LOW POTASSIUM LEVELS

"Diets low in carbohydrates may also be low in potassium. Foods rich in potassium, but also rich in carbohydrates, such as potatoes, fruits and beans, are restricted or banned. Low potassium, also medically known as hypokalemia, is potentially fatal. There may be no symptoms at all, but the condition is still just as deadly."

Muscle pain, muscle cramps, seizures, and disturbed heart rhythm which could lead to death are all alleged symptoms of a lack of potassium in the diet. While it is true many foods high in potassium are also high in carbohydrates, that doesn't mean you can't get enough potassium in your diet from supplements. I took 300mg of potassium supplements in the early days of my low-carb plan to ward off the leg cramps and maintain adequate potassium levels in my body. This has never been an issue on my low-carb plan...ever!

"One thing I really want the person considering doing a low-carb diet to understand is how dangerous a muscle cramp can be. No pain, no gain, right?

Wrong! Your heart is a muscle! And what do you think happens if your heart starts to cramp?"

This seems rather dramatic and implies high-carb diets are healthier simply because they contain slightly more potassium. Low-fat diets are also low in many nutrients and minerals and the advice for that is to take a vitamin. Taking a potassium supplement is not difficult to implement.

The author of this column then went on to give some personal advice of her own.

- Always talk to your doctor before starting a diet and fitness regimen.

Sure, but be prepared to do your own research if your doctor does not support your decision to begin a low-carb diet. The latest studies are showing that low-carb is healthier than those in the medical profession once thought. Find a physician who will support your decision to start on a low-carb lifestyle change at LowCarbDoctors.blogspot.com.

- Eat a healthy, balanced diet and leave the fad diets alone.

Here we go again! What is a healthy diet? Most of us would agree that the low-fat diet is much more of fad diet than low-carb is. Many people could stand to benefit from reversing the negative effects that have happened to them as a direct result of following the low-fat nutritional approach by switching to a healthy low-carb lifestyle instead.

- If you are very overweight, inquire about the use of prescription diet pills with your doctor.

Natural weight loss is always better than taking drugs.

- Exercise regularly, at least three times per week, alternating between cardiovascular and muscle strengthening exercises.

While I am a fan of getting adequate exercise for stress relief, muscle tone, and endurance conditioning, most cardio exercise is absolutely useless for weight loss. It's better to do high intensity interval training and resistance workouts to produce the best fat loss results.

- Drink 8-10 glasses of water daily.

AT LEAST! I drank as much as two gallons daily when losing weight and still drink about a gallon per day now. Water breathes life into low-carb and works with the fiber you consume to flush the stored body fat out of your body.

- Make sure you get enough fiber.

Eating foods like the ones I previously mentioned as well as low-carb fiber-rich products will give you all the fiber you need to allow your bowel to shake, rattle, and roll!

- Sleep is important to reaching and maintaining a healthy weight. Get enough sleep every night. Eat within 20 minutes of waking (this revs up the metabolism for the day).

You won't hear me bemoan this advice. Quality sleep of 7-8 hours nightly is essential to your health on so many levels and eating breakfast is vital to starting your day off fueled up ready to take on the activities of your day.

- Make breakfast your biggest meal, instead of dinner. Eat five small meals throughout the day, instead of three large meals.

It's better for your blood sugar to eat your larger meals earlier in the day, but you don't have to keep constantly eating meals throughout the day. Fellow low-carb blogger and author of *The Primal Blueprint* Mark Sisson (MarksDaily Apple.com) recommends doing the exact opposite of frequent meals — try consuming meals that are high-fat, moderate-protein, and low-carb and only eating when you are hungry without worrying whether or not it is the appropriate "time" for your next meal.

- And try not to get on the scale too often. A healthy weight loss should be no more than 1-2 pounds per week. If you get on the scale and are disappointed or frustrated by your progress, it may cause you to back slide. Mostly measure your success by how good you feel and how your clothes fit, or better yet, don't fit!

While studies show weighing daily is a good way to keep the weight off for good, I encourage people to put the scale away for a few weeks if it is discouraging them. Ms. Jefferson is right about measuring your success in other ways rather than the scale such as measurements and how you feel. Finally something I agree with.

- But most importantly, if you do insist on starting on a low-carb diet, make sure you take a break from it at least every two weeks, by resuming a normal, healthy carbohydrate intake.

This is very bad advice that should not be followed at all. If you go back to eating carbs every two weeks, then your body will never get to experience the extended weight loss and health benefits that livin' la vida low-carb will afford you. And Ms. Jefferson knows this which is why she wants people to get off of low-carb so quickly after starting. What will happen is your weight will begin to stall unnecessarily as it keeps trying to begin burning stored fat again. But the carbs you've eaten will need to be burned off first while you try to get your insulin regulated again before fat-burning can commence. You're dooming your low-carb diet to fail if you take her recommendation.

Ms. Jefferson's column was a great lesson in why I am doing what I can to educate, encourage and inspire people about low-carb living.

But that's not the end of the story. After many of my blog readers wrote to her about her anti-low-carb column, the author penned a response to and about me entitled "On Blast by Jimmy Moore - the biggest loser ever!" where she accuses me of "blasting" her and "saying really nasty things about" her as well.

No, Ms. Jefferson, that is not what I did. All I did was simply point out the error in your opinions about livin' la vida low-carb because the information you were providing in your column was not grounded in any truth whatsoever. If an article is going to be about low-carb the author should at least inform themselves on the science of low-carb.

"My article was criticized because of its lack of case studies and reference materials," Jefferson wrote. "And while it is true that case studies and references can add more legitimacy to any written work, the truth in this case is that I wrote this article from pure experience, both personal and professional."

In her column she described me as the poster child for low-carb diets and said I have marketed myself as "the biggest loser" and my website is nothing more than marketing myself.

I've never called myself the "biggest loser" on my site, just one man whose life was radically changed for the better because of "Livin' La Vida Low-Carb." And I don't apologize for offering products and services on my blog that can help people who want to lose weight. As someone who has been morbidly obese and was able to overcome it after years of frustration, it is my duty and mission in life now to share with others that there is hope for a better day. If pointing them to some excellent, high-quality products that I believe in as part of that, then so be it.

Nobody is forcing my wonderful readers to come to my blog or anywhere else for that matter. They choose to do it because they find value in what is being presented whether they buy anything or not. Many of them do buy my books and frequent those companies who sponsor my projects as a show of gratitude for what I do.

I make no bones about what I do at my blog: providing quality daily information to help people who want and need to lose weight by researching current news as well as products and services that will serve them well in their journey. Sure I make a little bit of money along the way, but I've invested literally thousands of hours to earn those dollars. There is nothing wrong with being compensated for my work.

My expertise does not come from a nursing or medical degree; it comes from losing triple digits and keeping it off for years. I plan on livin' la vida low-carb for many years to come, so everyone might as well get used to hearing the name Jimmy Moore defending this healthy low-carb way of eating. It has worked, is working, and will continue to work until the good Lord decides to take me home. The scientific evidence continues to mount in favor of this amazing lifestyle change.

"Jimmy...dude...really, I've written only one article on this subject. I'm not the queen of anti-low-carb dieting. I'm not the 2006 anti-fad diet guru either. But I will gladly accept my new title of anti-low-carb pinhead of the year (given to me by Jimmy himself), if I save just one life. So now Jimmy, you really should take a Vee break and get on with your life already."

You're just the latest low-carb antagonist. There are many more where you came from who have used some of the same old tired, erroneous arguments against low-carb and I've called them out as well. If you are going to write on a subject like low-carb, the least you can do is a little homework on the plan.

"I never take for granted that the world is ignorant. I never take for granted that my readers are ignorant. But I do believe in educating people about the things that I have learned about, and I would never write an article about anything that I haven't researched or learned through experience. And in this day of computer savvy surfers, anyone with access to the Internet can do the same."

I don't ever suggest my readers are "ignorant." It is possible to educate people without insulting them. The low-fat, low-calorie, portion-control diets that have dominated our society for decades are clearly not working, so people are perusing any web site and resource they can find that will finally tell them the truth. That's what my "Livin' La Vida Low-Carb" brand is all about.

Sure, there are tens of thousands of anti-Atkins, hate-filled sites about low-carb on the Internet about the so-called "dangers of low-carb dieting" that are bought and paid for primarily by anti-meat, radical vegan groups. But sites like mine and many others are sharing the unbridled truth about livin' la vida low-carb to those who are willing to listen and absorb it. It takes guts to do low-carb because you are bucking the trend, but tens of millions of us are doing it with great results happening to our weight and health.

Kathy Goodwin, a psychologist, has also given her opinion on the subject of the continuing popularity of the Atkins/low-carb approach.

"Many do feel an attachment to Atkins and other low-carb plans because a great number truly do lose weight," she exclaimed. "If the indicator of a successful diet is initial weight loss alone, and not permanent fat loss achieved in a healthy way, then my hat's off to Atkins! Unfortunately, this and many other fad diets will not serve your long term health or your long-term success at weight control."

The reason people feel an "attachment" to low-carb is precisely because it has worked when everything else has previously failed. The Atkins diet is the best weight loss method around today for a whole lot of people despite the constant criticisms about how it's supposedly so unhealthy. If it were so unhealthy our hospitals would be filled with droves of low-carb dieters who have irreparably damaged their health.

No longer do I deal with such personal struggles related to my obesity such as high blood pressure, difficulty breathing, tight-fitting and constantly ripped clothes, chronic back pain, wheezing, lack of energy, uncomfortable seating at movie theaters and on airplanes, profuse sweating, overeating junk food, constantly feeling hungry, lack of adequate sleep...all of this because of low-carb not in spite of It. Low-carb diets were what produced these results for me, five years and counting.

"Do you honestly feel that a low-carb plan is something you can stick with for the rest of your life?" Goodwin asks. "If not, then it's just temporary like the rest of the fads. No more chocolate cake, mashed potatoes, French fries, spaghetti, pancakes, apple pie or other favorites. Forever. Even Atkins admits that if you go back to a higher carb diet again, the pounds will return."

Actually, yes, I do envision low-carb as a diet I can stick with for the rest of my life. It's the diet that's right for me and I plan on doing it forever and ever amen! That's the most important aspect of any effective diet program, regardless of which one you choose. Many people like me are discovering that livin' la vida low-carb gives them exactly the kinds of foods they want without ever feeling deprived. That laundry list of foods you displayed shouldn't be a part of any "healthy diet," whether you are on low-carb, low-fat, low-calorie or whatever. All of those foods are unhealthy and likely to cause weight gain if you add them back to your diet.

Goodwin contends the mechanism behind what makes low-carb living work is about the lack of food choices which leads to lower calorie consumption.

"The Atkins diet essentially eliminates several foods and food groups like fruits, cereals, breads, grains, starches, baked goods, dairy products, starchy vegetables, and sweets. The basic weight loss formula is: calories burned must exceed calories consumed. Easily done when the majority of the foods on a typical day's menu are eliminated. There's nothing revolutionary about this regimen."

Again, this shows that Ms. Goodwin is absolutely clueless about what true low-carb living is all about. The Atkins diet does not eliminate ANY food groups as is so commonly misstated by those who seek to tear down this wonderful way of eating. As an active low-carber for the past five years, I can tell you I have eaten plenty of non-starchy, green leafy veggies, low-glycemic fruits such as blueberries, strawberries, and melons, great-tasting low-carb and even zero-carb breads, yummy low-carb baked goods, and oh-so-delicious sugar-free, low-carb sweets that leave me wondering why I ever ate sugary desserts in the first place! If you need some low-carb variety in your meals, then simply pick up any of the outstanding bestselling low-carb cookbooks from my friend and avid low-carber Dana Carpender (HoldTheToast.com) who wrote the foreword to this book. I eat about 2400 calories daily with a wide variety of delicious and nutritious foods as part of my low-carb lifestyle. Nothing is "eliminated" and I have greater flexibility in my food choices now than I ever did when I ate all those nasty-tasting low-fat foods.

Losing a whole person like I did convinces you that this way of eating indeed is revolutionary like nothing that has ever been tried before. I don't mind sharing with others the miracle that has happened in my life as a result of the Atkins diet because I will never be the same again.

What's amazing is how people routinely go around talking about how the Atkins/low-carb way of eating is going to fade away into obscurity when the reality is that this way of eating has been around since the very beginning of time (How do you think cavemen ate? It sure wasn't tofu and bean sprouts!) Guess what? Low-carb is gonna be here long after the proponents of low-fat dieting vanish from the limelight. Science will keep on proving livin' la vida low-carb is an excellent way to not only lose weight but get healthy, too. It always has and it always will.

"The idea that a high-carb diet is responsible for obesity and illness (a concept supported by low-carb plans) is completely contradicted by many population-based studies," she said, "For instance, in Japan, carbohydrates compose the overwhelming majority of daily caloric intake. High-carb foods like grains, rice, and vegetables are daily staples of Japanese life, and intake of high protein, high fat animal products is minimal. In contrast to the reported 'evils' of carbohydrates touted by low-carb plans, Japan has some of the lowest rates of obesity, heart disease, cancer and diabetes in the world. Enough said."

Consuming carbohydrate from sugar, processed foods, starchy vegetables like potatoes, and white flour leads directly to obesity, heart disease, cancer and diabetes, among many other health conditions. Add to that the constant swings in your blood sugar with the impact it has on your body and it's a recipe for disease disaster. So what if people living in other countries want to eat that way. They will eventually have to suffer the consequences of their dietary choices. But most of my fellow low-carbers will attest to the fact that they have never felt more in control of their body than when they are on a low-carb plan.

That's the kind of freedom from the dietary bondage that livin' la vida low-carb brings those who have been enslaved by carbs. 'Nuff said!

"If these plans [low-carb] worked in the long run, the release of new diet books wouldn't even be necessary. The followers would have actually been capable of maintaining weight loss by eliminating high-carbohydrate foods for over 25 years. Their long term weight loss success stories would have spread worldwide as the cure to obesity. Paradoxically, as more and more diets appear, the weight loss industry continues to get richer, and America continues to grow fatter."

There are currently many more low-fat diet books than low-carb, so by that logic, low-fat books would not be necessary either. I agree it is disgusting that the weight loss empire has grown as large as it has, but you can't put the onus for that on low-carb diets like Atkins. Low-carb is not necessarily for everyone, but it is an excellent choice for people who are tired of being told they have to eat low-fat, lower their calorie intake and cut their portions. I'm here to tell you the truth: You do not! Take it from a man who used to weigh over 400 pounds and was able to dig himself out of that rotten existence to become an athletic and energetic man enthusiastic about life and is now sharing the amazing health benefits of livin' la vida low-carb with the world.

Another columnist, Laura Donnely wrote about the subject of diet and the Atkins low-carb diet was discussed.

"Look at the success of the ghastly Atkins diet: How any intelligent human being could think that a diet recommending crumbled fried pork rinds as a substitute for bread crumbs is logical is beyond me, but this diet did appeal to lots of menfolk. And everyone I know who tried this diet has gained the weight back. Again, let me preach: Everything in moderation."

I decided this was just a wee bit over the top for my blood, so I wrote a letter to the editor to the *East Hampton Star* responding to Ms. Donnelly's article. I introduced myself and informed her about the Atkins diet and all it had done for me. Now she would know that not everyone who had tried the diet had gained weight back again.

I highly encourage you to submit a letter to the editor about your low-carb story whenever you see a misleading article about low-carb dieting in the newspaper and simply share your experiences following a low-carb regimen.

Speaking of letters to the editor, I noticed something rather odd in September 2005 that probably happens a lot more often than newspaper editors want to admit. I first noticed it in the Niagara Falls, New York *Gazette* newspaper where they printed a letter to the editor allegedly from a local man named Nate Odell who claimed he wrote the following just weeks after the Atkins Nutritionals company had filed for bankruptcy (they have since emerged from bankruptcy proceedings and are thriving as one of the top-selling health bar and shake brands in 2009):

'Old Abe' was right after all: "You can't fool all the people all the time." And the company founded by diet guru Robert Atkins, after subverting America's best nutritional consensus, wound up in bankruptcy court Aug. 1.

The Atkins high-protein diet craze peaked in early 2004, when over 9 percent of United States' adults subscribed to such diet, according to market research firm NPD Group. That figure declined gradually to 2.2 percent last month after a consumer advocacy group released a medical examiner's report showing that Atkins was overweight and suffered of heart disease.

Over the past three decades, a dozen expert panels reviewing thousands of diet and health studies concluded that Americans should replace meat and dairy products in their diet with vegetables, fresh fruits, and whole grains. None reached the opposite conclusion.

As consumers, we need to be constantly vigilant for entrepreneurs who exploit our obsession with physical appearance to promote their profit-driven agendas. The price we pay, beyond an inflated food bill, is life-long chronic afflictions and a curtailed life span. Let's hope that this lesson does not come too late for victims of the Atkins diet.

This letter sounded very familiar to me when I read it and I quickly discovered it was virtually the EXACT SAME LETTER with very few changes that appeared in another New York state newspaper I had read — *The Binghamton Press & Sun-Bulletin* — in early August 2005 supposedly written by an Angola, New York man named Vance Williams who wrote at the time:

Old Abe was right after all: "You can't fool all the people all the time." And the company founded by diet guru Robert Atkins, after subverting America's best nutritional consensus, wound up in bankruptcy court.

The Atkins high-protein diet craze peaked in early 2004, when over 9 percent of U.S. adults subscribed to such a diet. That figure declined gradually to 2.2 percent last month after a consumer advocacy group released a medical examiner's report showing that Atkins was overweight and suffered from heart disease.

As consumers, we need to be constantly vigilant for entrepreneurs who exploit our obsession with physical appearance to promote their profit-driven agendas. The price we pay, beyond an inflated food bill, is life-long chronic afflictions and a curtailed life span.

This strange coincidence seemed very unusual to me with two different men, two different newspapers but virtually identical information. I decided to do a little further research on this.

When I typed in "Old Abe" and "Atkins" as a keyword search in Google, I found this same letter had also been printed in many other newspapers under different names:

- *Ithaca Times* published on August 24, 2005 written by Ian Baum from Ithaca, New York

- *News & Record* published in August 2005 written by Glenn Gustafson from Greensboro, New York

- *San Francisco Chronicle* published on August 3, 2005 written by Mike Singer from San Francisco, California

- *Columbia Daily Tribune* published on August 6, 2005 written by Carl Dix from Columbia, Missouri

- *Anchorage Daily News* published on August 10, 2005 written by Amos Dotson from Anchorage, Alaska

- *The Monitor* published on August 17, 2005 written by Bill Motter from McAllen, Texas

And these examples are just from the first page of the Google search that I found! This innocent-looking letter from a concerned citizen had apparently been copied, pasted, and then printed in well over 100 newspapers and was still getting printed in newspapers for months thereafter. I know when I have written a letter to the editor in my local newspaper they always ask me if I was the original author of the letter since they do not print form letters that have appeared in other media formats.

One would think that this same protocol would have been in this case as well.

Also, I think it is especially telling that this letter was printed in so many different places all within just a few days of each other. Letters to the editor can take as much as a week or more to get confirmed and approved to run in the newspapers. So how did all of these people from all over the U.S. get the same letter to be printed virtually simultaneously?

But even if the newspaper staffers did ask the people sending them these letters if it was their original writing and they claimed it was, all they had to do was a quick Google search of keywords like I did and they would have found this same letter had already been printed over and over again since the Atkins Nutritionals bankruptcy announcement on August 1, 2005.

Where is the journalistic integrity? How could this exact same anti-Atkins letter make the newspaper rounds and nobody else notice it happening? If you wanted to see a shining example of why I attempt to combat the lies that permeate from the media about the low-carb lifestyle, then this is it!

As long as I have the ability to write, I will continue to challenge the media to lay aside their personal opinions about low-carb. And by all means newspaper editors, stop printing this same form letter!

To follow up on this low-carb Lettergate scandal, I personally sent an e-mail to each of the newspapers that printed that anti-Atkins letter explaining how they were duped by a bogus letter that many people claimed as their own. I heard back from just four of those newspapers.

Jim Robertson from the *Columbia Daily Tribune* wrote me back with this intriguing and encouraging response:

Thanks for the heads-up. We do have a system of verification for letter-writers. I'll have to investigate to see how this one got through. It reminds me of the anti-meat letters we get occasionally from "local" writers who provide a local street address and a toll-free telephone number. We've become pretty adept at intercepting those. Feel free to submit your own letter exposing the anti-Atkins writer. We have a 250 word limit and require name, address and a telephone number where we can reach you for verification. Thanks again.

Since he gave me permission to write a response, I decided to submit the following for consideration:

Dear Editor,

A letter to the editor recently published in your newspaper looked extremely familiar to me when I read it. It detailed how the recent bankruptcy of Atkins Nutritionals, Inc. proves that low-carb is just another fad diet on its way out and supposedly dangerous to those who use it to lose weight.

As a former 410-pound man who successfully lost 180 pounds in 2004 thanks to the Atkins diet, I could not disagree with that characterization more.

This way of eating has been and continues to be the easiest and best way for me to control my weight so that I will never again allow myself to get that morbidly obese again. Livin' la vida low-carb literally saved my life.

The letter from a local resident sounded very sincere and undoubtedly the person who submitted it claimed the words were his own. However, did you know this exact same letter has also appeared in over 100 other newspapers throughout the United States over the past six weeks?

All you have to do is a quick Google search of "Old Abe" and "Atkins" to find all of the other newspapers who were also duped into printing this bogus letter.

Isn't it odd that an anti-Atkins letter just miraculously showed up within days of each other in all of these newspapers? The radical behind-the-scenes agenda to undermine and destroy the healthy low-carb lifestyle by those who oppose it has never been clearer to me.

I got a call on my cell phone within hours of sending that letter to them confirming they got my letter and asking my permission to print it — which of course was a yes!

Another response I received from a newspaper editor came from Don Sorchych at the Cave Creek, Arizona-based *Sonoran News*. Here was his pithy response to my charge that he had been duped:

The operative word is "knowingly."

Short and sweet. While that is technically true, I'm sure he and the other editors who let this one slide through could have done a little more research to make sure they were completely "in the know." I also submitted a response to be printed in their newspaper, but it never got posted.

I received yet another response from Carroll Wilson at the Wichita, Texas-based newspaper *Times Record News*:

If we printed it and you want to respond, send a letter of no more than 350 words to me.

And so I did. Finally, I heard back from the reader's representative for *The San Francisco Chronicle* who said he wanted to write a story about this bogus letter scandal:

Jimmy,

Just back from vacation and scurrying to get caught up. Saw your e-mail. Definitely looks like what the politicos call "Astroturfing." I'm looking into this. I'll see what I can learn and will discuss verification procedures with the editorial page editor.

Am curious to know if you've learned anything about the origin of this "letter" and the author's motivation.

By the way, I might write a column on this so I assume that what you tell me is for the record (and you can assume the same).

Thanks for bringing this up.

Dick Rogers
Readers' Representative

San Francisco Chronicle

Here was my response:

Hey Dick,

THANKS for writing and being willing to print the truth about this mysterious letter. While I have not been successful at tracking down the origination of this letter to the editor, I certainly have my suspicions.

As someone on the frontlines of the battle over the low-carb lifestyle, I can tell you the enemies of this way of eating are many. Whether it is the anti-meat PETA fanatics or bread and potato industry groups, I really couldn't tell you.

But a coordinated letter-writing campaign that was as organized and orchestrated as this had to be from an established group just waiting to pounce on the opportunity to strike. When Atkins Nutritionals, Inc. filed for bankruptcy on August 1, they smelled blood and attacked. These letters have been showing up ever since.

What's interesting is that Atkins Nutritionals, Inc. and the low-carb lifestyle don't have anything to do with one another. One is a business that had had to deal with economic reality and make some difficult choices. The other is a way of life for people like me because it has helped us lose weight and keep it off for good.

I lost 180 pounds on low-carb in 2004 and have kept it off by continuing to eat this way. It goes against everything we've always heard about good nutrition our entire lives, but it is the only thing that has ever worked for me over the long haul.

If you would like to speak with me further with any questions about this subject, then I'd be happy to speak with you anytime. THANKS again for writing back!

It would be great if the origin of that letter could be discovered and "Livin' La Vida Low-Carb" is credited with breaking the story first! We may never really know for sure where this letter started, but maybe the perpetrators will pause before trying to pull something like this off again.

The media tends to get quiet for a while, but inevitably start back talking negatively about low-carb again eventually. Take the column in the *Times & Democrat* newspaper by journalist Teresa Hatchell in her piece on low-carb entitled "Well-balanced diet makes common sense."

For the past few years, people throughout America have been touting the benefits of low-carb diets as if consuming as few carbohydrates as possible is the magic answer to controlling their weight.

It's not just people in America, but around the world to the tune of tens of millions of happily devoted followers.

I have watched many relatives and friends "suffer" through week after week of low-carb dieting.

The only suffering would be done by people who don't like the delicious benefits of eating high-quality cuts of meats and cheeses while enjoying other fat and protein-packed foods like eggs, nuts, seeds, butter, cream, sugar-free chocolate, coconut oil, spinach leaves, green beans, cauliflower, blueberries, melons, etc. I've never been so excited about eating this healthy before starting low-carb, so there must be something about it to keep people like me so devoted. Also you can't eat most of these delicious kinds of foods on a high-carb, low-fat diet!

And, sure enough, they lose a good bit of weight initially.

You bet your sweet bippy you lose LOTS of weight on low-carb right away! I lost 30 pounds in my first month on Atkins and 40 more pounds in the second month back in 2004! The weight does come pouring off of you on this way of eating, that's for sure.

Eventually, they quit losing weight and have to "shock" their metabolisms by eating carbs for a few weeks, only to resume the monotonous diet again.

Regardless of the diet you choose, there will be a point where your weight will stall. But this is no reason to give up and quit. I went 10 weeks in a row in 2004 during my 180-pound weight los without a single pound coming off that scale, but I put my head down and kept chugging along. The weight loss I had up until that point proved to me that this plan worked and my body was just going through an adjustment. Giving up will never lead to success.

Carbohydrates are the main source of energy in our diets, with fats second.

Your body absolutely needs fat and protein, but it most definitely does not need carbohydrates thanks to a beautiful metabolic mechanism known as glu-coneogenesis (more on this fancy schmancy word coming up in a few more chapters) where the body can produce its own carbs to fuel the body. Ketone bodies are what are original ancestors survived on and these were produced naturally by their very low-carb, high-fat, moderate-protein diets. If carbs are the "main source of energy," then how in the world did they survive? Try telling that to low-carb Canadian researcher Dr. Jay Wortman (DrJayWortman.com) who studied the original diet of the Namgis First Nation group of Alert Bay in Canada and featured it a 2008 documentary film that appeared on CBC Newsworld's "The Lens" entitled *My Big Fat Diet* (MyBigFatDiet.net).

So, if you want to lose weight, reducing carb intake is a good way to do it.

Not just good but extremely effective. In fact, many recent studies have shown low-carb to be the best of all the diets for weight loss in head-to-head com-parisons.

However, cutting them out as much as possible is neither sensible nor practi-cal, as you will also be cutting out important nutrients.

As I've stated before, I've never eaten so healthy in all of my life than what I have these past five years on low-carb. It is the MOST sensible and practical way I have even eaten in my entire life and I'll never go back to a high-carb diet again!

Nutritionists stress that it is unwise to embark on a drastic reduction of carbo-hydrates all at once.

Well, that's not surprising since most nutritionists have been taught that a high-carb, low-fat diet is healthy. I've had my differences of opinion with these well-meaning folks many times at my blog. In a way, I don't blame them for thinking low-carb is bad. But I wish they would do their own research and find out how awesome this healthy lifestyle change really is. Just ask registered dietitian Diane Kress, author of the 2009 book release *The Metabolism Miracle* about how important switching to a low-carbohydrate nutritional approach has been for her and her clients with Metabolism B. And my life proves it again and again every single day!

If you introduce the new eating pattern gradually, you will not encounter the mood swings or hunger pangs that accompany drastic diets.

I disagree. If you are going to start livin' la vida low-carb (and it's highly rec-ommended, especially for people who are insulin resistant, diabetic, and/or have a lot of weight to lose), then eliminating sugar, white flour, starchy carbs, and refined carbs from your diet immediately is priority one. It shouldn't be a gradual decrease because you need to make the transition from your poor habits to better ones. Once you get off of your addiction to sugar/carbs, you'll feel so much better than you ever have before! Believe it!

Besides, such diets usually result in frustration and failure.

Not if you are committed to them from the beginning and realize those first few days are the toughest. Get on your chosen low-carb plan, push through the temporary pain in week one, and you will notice something incredible happen to you — a sudden boost of energy, stabilized blood sugars, mental clarity — and, oh yeah, LOTS OF WEIGHT LOSS, baby! It's impossible to get frustrated and fail when you have all that happening for you.

Maintaining a balanced diet, with a slight reduction of carbs and fats, and cutting out fat- and carb-laden snack foods is a much more common-sense approach to losing weight and maintaining a healthy weight.

If losing weight and keeping it off only took common sense then there'd be a whole lot less fat people walking around this planet these days. Unfortunately, there is such subjectivity when it comes to a "healthy diet" that people have become unnecessarily confused about what they should be eating. Do what works for you, I always say, but that may mean substantially lowering your carbs while someone else may need to reduce their fat intake. There is no one-size-fits-all diet that works for everyone.

And even my own local newspaper couldn't resist publishing an anti-Atkins column! The *Spartanburg Herald-Journal* in South Carolina charged General Assignment Writer Teresa Killian with writing an article in 2005 entitled "Low-Carb Atkins diet on the run" featuring lots of dissenting voices regarding the Atkins diet.

She quoted the local owner of the Krispy Kreme franchise in Spartanburg who exclaimed *"the low-carb craze pretty much fizzled, and now we are selling more doughnuts than ever. The Atkins diet, I think they're the ones feeling the pinch now."*

With obesity rates continuing to rise at unprecedented rates, a doughnut shop owner can take great pride in knowing he is contributing directly to the problem whether he cares or not. Doughnuts are still one of the worst possible foods you can eat because they are loaded with both sugar and white flour. There will come a time when people realize that Dr. Atkins was right, but I'm afraid many more people will have to get heart disease and die prematurely from being overweight and obese before they finally wake up.

Killian continued her column by looking at a local bread store which claimed their sales were up and she quoted a registered dietitian who said of Atkins, *"That's not a diet we ever advocated because of the lack of balance"* because it allegedly cuts out so many nutritious foods.

On Atkins I get to eat plenty of delicious and healthy fruits, vegetables, nuts and more as part of my eating program. This whole idea that Atkins is lacking in nutrition is unfounded. If you read *Dr. Atkins' New Diet Revolution*, then you will see all of the great foods you can enjoy during the various phases of following the Atkins diet. While the Induction phase is the most restrictive regarding carbohydrate restriction, you only stay there for two weeks. Most of the time, the majority of people enjoy in excess of 50 grams of carbs per day which is a lot more than you think once you start livin' la vida low-carb.

One woman in the story testified that she had never tried the Atkins diet because she "couldn't live without potatoes." But of the people Killian interviewed for her story who had tried the Atkins approach, none of them lasted for more than a few weeks on it. They complained that it was too hard to follow for more than a couple of weeks or so.

If you can survive the first two weeks of Atkins, then the rest of the experience is a breeze by comparison. I won't lie to you, though, that first two weeks is pretty tough. But that's your body going through the necessary changes it needs to make to purge your system of the toxic impurities that have caused you to become overweight or obese. For me, it was definitely the sugar. I was addicted to sugar and my body felt the withdrawal when I first started livin' la vida low-carb. It was a literal hell for me. But once that short-term phase was over, I noticed that I felt much better than I ever had and that feeling continued as my weight dropped and dropped while my energy level began to skyrocket!

Quoting the NPD Group's market research showing that just 2 percent of adults were on low-carb as of 2005 statistics, Killian said this movement was apparently "waning." However, the statistic she quoted is well off the 12-15 percent numbers that another survey from Opinion Dynamics Corp. that year showed about low-carb's continued popularity. Regardless of whose numbers you believe, the fact is that millions upon millions of Americans are still choosing the low-carb lifestyle to get their weight under control.

About the only positive comment about low-carb in this story is when Killian noted that Dr. Arthur Agatston's *South Beach Diet* was still a *New York Times* bestseller. She didn't mention this in her story, but Dr. Atkins was recognized by online retail giant Amazon.com as their all-time bestselling health author. Despite the negative coverage regarding his diet, the books by Dr. Atkins still sell extremely well to this day because people are looking for dependable low-carb answers about losing weight.

A food industry analyst in the story said the Atkins diet had been losing popularity since February 2004 because it has simply "ran its course." Killian even added in her story that Atkins went from "fad to fade like so many others before it," comparing the diet to the Scarsdale and cabbage soup diets. Well, if Atkins is a fad diet, why has been around for nearly four decades and is still going strong? How many other diets can claim this kind of track record for success? I fully intend on eating this way for the rest of my life whether health experts or the media likes it or not.

Thanks to my improved health, I believe that will likely be a lot longer than it would have been had I remained obese! Sadly, Killian quotes nutritionists and health experts at the end of her story who recommended eating smaller portions and watching your fat and calorie intake while exercising more. That's the same old message we've been hearing forever and ever. Livin' la vida low-carb is so much more exciting, fulfilling and long-lasting than any low-fat diet!

While she did mention the glycemic index at the very end of her column, Killian did not bring up even one success story of someone who had been on the Atkins diet. Incidentally, I contacted her about my low-carb weight loss success and did hear back from her about doing a follow-up story on my Atkins success story. The piece entitled "Once you've had a taste of the low-carb life you'll never be the same" was published on August 31, 2005.

I appreciated Teresa Killian writing such a beautiful and brief description of my Atkins low-carb weight loss success story. Issuing a challenge to her after writing a negative story about the Atkins diet following their bankruptcy announcement, Killian stepped up to the plate and delivered a grand slam! The way she weaved the various elements about my low-carb experience into a compelling story made me very proud of this piece. In fact, my wife suggested I get it professionally framed for hanging on our wall and it's proudly displayed in our living room to this very day.

If only all the other members of the media and the current health experts could admit that they've gotten it all wrong about livin' la vida low-carb. I know I'm dreaming, but the breaking point will come someday soon. Many of these experts have long held that people should simply eat in moderation and make it a balanced diet. But what does that mean exactly, and is it better than low-carb? That's the lesson we'll explore in the next chapter.

LESSON #6
"Moderation" and a "balanced" diet aren't better than low-carb

"Instead of 'balanced' I recommend aiming for 'nutritionally complete'. This is not at all difficult to achieve while reducing carbs. It turns out that most sugary and starchy foods don't have boatloads of nutrients, while many low-carb foods such as eggs, broccoli, and avocados do. Once upon a time, someone figured out that a blood transfusion was just the thing to help people who had lost a lot of blood. But the advice 'give fresh blood, but not too much' turned out to be inadequate as a general rule. We are at that place with nutritional advice. If only more people would catch on."

— **Laura Dolson**, popular low-carb blogger as Low-carb Diets Guide at About.com (LowCarbDiets.About.com)

Don't you just hate it when you hear somebody make a statement like the following?

"Just eat in moderation and you'll lose all the weight you want."

This is a very simplistic nutritional message. Although I believe diversity in the various diet plans allows for compatibility with your specific lifestyle needs and challenges, many nutritionists and diet gurus say this kind of dietary variety just confuses the public.

I don't feel confused. What it does for me is provide people with a myriad of ways to lose weight since we don't all do well on a "one-size-fits-all" diet plan. If we did, then everybody would be on that plan and there wouldn't be a need to have so many diets to begin with. But the grim reality of the situation is that people should find the proven plan that works for them, follow that plan exactly, and then keep on doing it forever to maintain their weight and health. As strongly as I support low-carb living for me, I am not so shortsighted to realize that it may not necessarily be for everyone. Unfortunately, many advocates of a low-fat diet do not afford this same courtesy to people who choose a low-carbohydrate nutritional approach.

But there is a common theme among the self-proclaimed health leaders that food choice alone does not make a person healthy or unhealthy. I could not disagree more. Food choice is precisely why most people have become overweight or obese in the first place. They chose to consume too much sugar, fast food, junk food, and the like over and over and over again every single day of their lives. Those choices are precisely why two out of every three Americans are overweight or obese today.

At the same time, food choice is the exact reason why people like me who have overcome their obesity problem have been as successful as they were. When I started out livin' la vida low-carb in January 2004 at a robust 410 pounds, making the conscious decision to stop eating sugar, white flour, and other excessive and unnecessary carbohydrates in my diet as part of my new healthy lifestyle, that move alone was the beginning of a dramatic change in me that made me healthier in the end when I shed 180 pounds. You can't tell me that my food choices were not an instrumental part of my eventual success.

Sure, your genes, how you live your life, the type of diet, and your level of physical activity can all play somewhat of a factor in determining what happens with your weight. And yet your lifestyle choices can make the biggest difference in controlling your weight when you make the decision to stop eating the wrong foods. A pitiful diet consisting of McDonalds, Dairy Queen, and Krispy Kreme all day every day will not put you on the road to becoming skinny and in tip-top health!

A common complaint about low-carb diets is when the current health experts tell people it is unhealthy to completely eliminate a whole category of food. (They say this about low-carb, but virtually never talk about how vegetarians and vegans eliminate meat entirely from their diets — but I digress!) Livin' la vida low-carb doesn't eliminate any foods. Most low-carbers eat between 20-60g carbohydrates daily when they are attempting to lose weight. This isn't "eliminating completely" the consumption of carbs. It's simply bringing the intake of this macronutrient down to a level that will enable stored body fat to be removed from the body while stabilizing blood sugar and insulin levels. What's so wrong with that?

But nothing gets me more than the concept to "eat in moderation." That advice to me is just plain silly. When do you know when you've gotten enough of something? How much sugar is needed for my diet to be "in moderation?" How about white flour, processed foods, and starchy veggies? People need direction about how to eat because most of us haven't got a clue about what is healthy and what is not.

Since there is such a glut of advice out there for people to know how to eat healthy, then how can we ever expect them to know what is right for them? The answer is elementary, my dear Watson. If you want to lose weight and keep it off for good, then find a plan that fits within your lifestyle, follow that plan faithfully even when it gets tough, continue to execute the dictates of that plan until you reach your goal, and then keep on doing that plan as your permanent lifestyle change until the day you take your final breath. There's no need to make this any more complicated than it needs to be.

Does this mean you will never be able to eat something you shouldn't? Oh heavens no. But if you have the right perspective about what you need to be doing to control your weight rather than vaguely trying to "eat in moderation" all the time, then and only then will you find the pathway to lasting weight loss and greatly improved health. There's no better way to live than to be in control of your own health.

If you've read a popular magazine or even been to see your doctor while carrying around a few extra pounds, then I know you have heard these not-so-subtle recommendations about what you need to do in order to start doing something about your weight. Doctors try not to offend anyone and offer generalizations about diet and health that are not truly helpful in the end.

But maybe we need to start offending a few people with obesity rates continuing to go up and up. Why can't doctors just come out and say something like this: "You know, Jimmy, I'm looking at your charts and I must say I am very concerned about what I see regarding your current state of health. If you continue to go down your current path as you have for the past few years, then you are headed straight for a situation you don't want to be in. But I have good news for you. If you decide to take back control of your life by implementing a program with a proven track record for weight loss and improved health, then I think you will not only overcome the difficulties that will most certainly come but you will also experience life like never before!"

Wow, talk about inspiring your patient to achieve greatness! Had I heard that speech ten or twenty years ago, then I wouldn't have had to suffer through all those extra years of carrying around excess weight like I did. While I longed to hear words to that effect from my doctor, unfortunately it never happened. Doctors may be reticent to say this kind of thing for fear of litigation.

Case in point: Dr. Terry Bennett, a 66-year old Rochester, New Hampshire physician who graduated from Harvard Medical School, came under investigation by the New Hampshire Board of Medicine in August 2005 because one of his patients was offended by one of his infamous "obesity lectures for women" where he urged her to lose weight for her health and for her long-term well-being. Bennett regularly warns his patients that obesity can and will very likely lead to such debilitating conditions such as high blood pressure, diabetes, acid reflux, heart attack and stroke.

"I told a fat woman she was obese," Bennett said in a news report about the investigation. "I tried to get her attention. I told her, 'You need to get on a program, join a group of like-minded people and peel off the weight that is going to kill you."

While it might have been a little blunt for Bennett to share his opinion about his patient's condition the way that he did, there is absolutely nothing wrong with a doctor expressing his medical assessment that one of his patients is obese and should probably do something about it. While it may anger her to hear her doctor tell her something she didn't like, instead of suing her doctor she would be better served to use that anger to motivate herself to finally do something about a very real problem. If we cannot rely on our own doctors to tell us the truth about our physical health, then who is going to do it?

I remember substitute teaching at a local middle school just a few months before I started livin' la vida low-carb and this pudgy little boy waited until my back was turned to class as I wrote some instructions on the chalkboard to exclaim very loudly, "Mr. Moore is fffffffaaaat!" Predictably, the entire class burst into raucous laughter and even I laughed to try to keep from crying about the truth in that statement. Those words rang in my head haunting me for months afterward and got me to seriously assess my weight and health.

Should I have sought legal action against that 12-year old child for stating the obvious to me? Heck no. In fact, that kid did me a BIG favor by shaking me into reality about my morbid obesity and very likely rescued me from a heart attack or worse — an early grave. How people respond to criticism about their weight will determine whether they will be successful at losing their weight permanently or not.

Ironically, everything that Bennett told this woman about her health actually came to pass since he told her she was obese. Not only has she gained additional weight, but now she has become diabetic, developed acid reflux and experienced frequent chest pains. Bennett did the gentlemanly thing when he found out she was offended and penned a personal apology letter.

"That should have been the end of it," Bennett said.

Actually, though, it was only just the beginning. The New Hampshire Attorney General's Administrative Prosecution Unit was dispatched to investigate and bring resolution to the complaint. They recommended Bennett attend a medical education course for patient sensitivity training and admit wrongdoing. Not surprisingly, Bennett refused.

"I've made many errors in my lifetime. Telling someone the truth is not one of them," Bennett said.

You go boy! There is nothing for Bennett to apologize for because he has done absolutely nothing wrong. Nevertheless, this issue was not laid to rest. A public hearing was scheduled about what to do with Bennett. But what is there to talk about? What did Bennett do that is so wrong that his stellar career is now being jeopardized?

Wake up lady! Your health is going to pot and you will very likely die a premature death if you don't get your weight and health under control as soon as possible! I wish more medical professionals would be willing to be that blunt about obesity. Then maybe we could get more people to get off their duff and take some personal responsibility for a change.

Bennett's attorney says this whole fiasco is (quoting Shakespeare) "much ado about nothing" and Bennett will not "roll over on this, he is going to fight."

"If the board wants to get into policing how doctors talk to their patients, they are going to be very busy."

Expressing his concern that one of his patients was angered by his comments, Bennett said this incident is very disturbing and that his only motive was to help her change her life for the better. Many of Bennett's patients have rallied around him in support of his methodology by signing a petition and testified at a public hearing that he had helped them get back on the road to healthy living with his honest feedback.

"Is he a fortune teller? No," said one of Bennett's patients. "He was a man trying to do his job. Whether I wanted to hear it or not, he was telling me the truth."

There's something missing in this story and that is the fact that this woman who was so offended by Bennett's comments about her obesity is the one who put herself in that position to begin with. Was it Bennett's fault that she had become obese? Absolutely not! We each have to take responsibility for our own actions and stop blaming anyone and everyone else for our short-comings.

Getting back to this issue of health advice, don't you just love that word "balance?" Be sure you eat a healthy, balanced diet. What the heck is that anyway? Who determines how much of what you should eat is balanced? Do we need to include sugar, white flour, starchy foods, and processed foods to "balance" out our diets? I sure don't think so and I know I am much better off having eliminated these foods from my diet as much as possible.

One of my blog readers told me he lost over 80 pounds on the Atkins diet in eight months back in 2003 and has been able to maintain his weight by continuing to do so ever since. He made an interesting comment regarding this topic I'd like to share with you:

"Like yourself I find the hypocrisy in the medical profession when it comes to 'low-carb' simply amazing because when you examine most diet plans, they usually recommend that you eat a controlled portion of meat, fresh vegetables and fruits. Isn't this basically a 'low-carb' diet?"

Excellent point! Contrary to popular belief, livin' la vida low-carb does include fruits and vegetables along with the meat that is so often heavily associated with this way of eating. People on a low-carb diet have never eaten a more "balanced" diet in their lives with fresh real whole foods rich in nutrients that nourish their bodies with essential vitamins and minerals for healthy nutrition. In fact, noted low-carb researcher and biochemistry professor at SUNY Downstate in Brooklyn, New York Dr. Richard Feinman (NMSociety.org) did a survey of 3,000 real low-carb dieters on the popular Active Low-Carber forum (Forum.LowCarber.org) in 2006 and found that their vegetable intake DOUBLED once they started on a low-carb plan.

Anyone who tells you the low-carb lifestyle is unhealthy because it isn't "balanced" obviously hasn't paid much attention to what it is really all about. Do your own research on low-carb diets and don't rely on what you've heard people say about it.

Some have suggested that perhaps we need to rename "low-carb" something else so people will get it. It really doesn't matter what you call it, the critics are still going to jump all over it if it even closely resembles "low-carb." It's who these people are and what they do. That's why I refuse to back down from using the term "low-carb" in describing my diet because I think people need to know what it really means to follow the healthy low-carb lifestyle, not what the media wants them to believe it means. Can you imagine what it would be like if we had to share about "low-carb" without explicitly using that term?

You know, I've found the [BLANK] lifestyle to be one of the easiest and best ways to keep the weight off permanently and live healthier than I ever have before. Since I started my [BLANK] diet in January 2004, eating all the wonderful [BLANK] foods that are available to you when you are [BLANK]ing makes this way of eating far superior to any other weight loss plan out there for me and tens of millions more. I'm so glad I'm livin' la vida [BLANK]. What's wrong with this picture?!?!?! What the [BLANK] is going on?

I have just demonstrated for you the current state of affairs as it relates to "low-carb" in the post-Atkins era. It seems that everyone who used to champion anything and everything related to low-carb is jumping ship from using that term anymore. Some of the loudest voices in the wonderful world of low-carb no longer want to be affiliated with that term. The latest low-carb books by well-known authors no longer use the phrase "low-carb" in the title (the book you are holding right now is one of the few released in recent years that proudly proclaims "low-carb" in the title). Additionally, you've got companies in the food industry shying away from using "low-carb" in their name or on the packaging and marketing of their products, although the products themselves haven't changed a bit.

Why are the biggest low-carb personalities and companies that made a name for themselves using the term "low-carb" all of a sudden sidestepping it completely and avoiding using it like it's some kind of disease or something? Is it just a wee bit strange to anyone else why this is happening when much of the success they have had can be attributed directly to their affiliation with "low-carb" in recent years?

Some people might be wondering, "Jimmy, what's the big deal? I don't care what we call it as long as I'm able to keep my weight under control and improve my health with this way of eating. Does it really matter that it has to be called 'low-carb'?" In my opinion, the answer to that question is a loud and un-equivocated YES! Absolutely it matters that we keep calling it "low-carb." Let's examine for a moment five of the popular new terms being thrown out there to replace "low-carb" and why they are inadequate for describing this way of eating:

1. Low-glycemic

I would venture to say that most people on the street don't even know what the glycemic index or even the glycemic load is all about (most people still don't even know what the low-carb lifestyle is all about, but that's another story!). This is a tricky concept to explain to people and it's not as cut and dry as "low-carb." I know this is a phrase that a lot of companies are hedging their bets on, but I don't see it sticking in the United States (currently 93% of Americans don't even look for GI information on the foods they buy) like it has in Europe.

2. Diabetic-friendly

What if I'm not diabetic (and I'm not!)? How does this improve the term "low-carb" in the least? Diabetics know that sugar-free, low-carb products are good choices for them, so why alienate the low-carb consumer by using a phrase with "diabetic" in it? I don't get this one either.

3. Controlled-carb

Actually, I have used this phrase myself because it does serve a good purpose when explaining what my lifestyle change is all about. While you certainly eat "low-carb" (between 20-60g carbs daily) when you are losing weight, most low-carbers transition to more of a "controlled-carb" approach (60-100g carbs daily) once they are ready to maintain. I suppose by comparison to the 900-1000g+ carbs I used to eat on a daily basis before I started livin' la vida low-carb, it's all pretty "low-carb" by comparison.

4. Carb-restricted/Carb-conscious

Similar to "controlled-carb," this phrase was no doubt created to remove any negative stigma from the "low" part of "low-carb." The media and those who oppose this way of eating take that "low" and change it to "NO" to make it "NO carb" which is absolutely silly. Nobody ever talks about eating ZERO carbs and yet that's the common belief about this way of eating. But using the term "carb-restricted" or even "carb-conscious" attempts to change this perception and it's a good attempt. I still don't think people know what you are referring to with this phrase, though.

5. Nutrient-dense

Of the five replacement phrases for "low-carb," I actually like this one the best because it insinuates that the foods you eat are healthy and give you all the essential nutrients you need to consume. That perfectly describes the kind of foods consumed on the low-carb lifestyle. But is this phrase going to translate to the average person on the street? I'm afraid not.

So what do we need to call it then? Is there really a need to change the term "low-carb" at all? My 180-pound weight loss was a God-given miracle in my life. I think it goes without saying what an incredible difference it has made in my life. I am a new man because of it and nobody will ever be able to take this accomplishment away from me.

I'm not ashamed to use that phrase one bit. While others have purposely backed away from using "low-carb," I have actively embraced it with every ounce of resolve within me because it is the plan that made me healthy and fit for the first time in my adult life and it is what will keep me in the best health possible for the rest of my life. Why would I call it something different now?

Perhaps I am being naive about my decision to continue using the term "low-carb," but I don't think so. If it weren't for "low-carb" being a part of my life, had

I not learned more about what "low-carb" living is all about, and if the principles of "low-carb" could not be communicated to the masses of overweight and obese people who need to understand what it is, then where would I be today? I'd be 400, maybe 500+ pounds with high blood pressure, high cholesterol, breathing problems, or quite possibly, six feet under due to complications from morbid obesity!

I don't mean to put it so bluntly and sound so grim, but defining the term "low-carb" and helping others understand clearly what that actually means is why I started the whole "Livin' La Vida Low-Carb" concept to begin with. For all those critics of the term "low-carb," let me ask you something. If "low-carb" is no longer viable, then please explain to me why my blog, podcast show, forum, YouTube videos, books, and so much more which all prominently use the phrase "low-carb" continue to attract new people every single day? What could possibly be bringing so many people to these "low-carb" projects if it isn't the subject of "low-carb" itself? I believe it's a bit too premature for us to be abandoning and sidestepping "low-carb" just because we think it has run its course. People are still looking for information about "low-carb" and I'm happy to give it to them.

The term "low-carb" is NOT going to stop being used by me anytime soon because I refuse to allow the media and the current health experts to erroneously redefine that cherished term to the people who want to know more about it. I stand proudly in defense of the term "low-carb" and will gladly share what it means to me in the presence of anyone who desires to learn more about what it is. And I'll always give 'em the truth about low-carb! Let others hem and haw about what to call "low-carb" but as for me I will not run away from it!

By the way, the next time you hear someone throw out the excuse to you that your low-carb diet is just too unbalanced to be healthy, just look at that person straight in the face, smile, nod and say, "thanks for sharing your concerns, but I'm livin' la vida low-carb, baby!" Then let your weight loss and improved health speak for itself. Coming up in the next lesson, you'll find out why it is the high-carb, low-fat diets that are actually keeping us so fat and sick.

LESSON #7
High-carb, low-fat diets are keeping us fat and sick

"From the 1830s to the 1960s, the conventional wisdom had it that carbohydrates are uniquely fattening. Then the medical community, backed by the U.S. government, decides that a healthy diet, by definition, is low in fat and high in carbs. And that's what we started eating. Since then, the number of obese and diabetic Americans has skyrocketed. It would be nice to think this is just a coincidence, but human biology argues against it."

— **Gary Taubes**, award-winning science journalist and bestselling author of *Good Calories, Bad Calories*

Oftentimes we hear critics of livin' la vida low-carb asking those of us who support it to provide evidence that a high-fat, low-carb diet is healthy. But what nobody ever seems to say back to these people is how the entire American population proves that the high-carb, low-fat diet is such a dismal failure. We've been encouraged to eat that way for decades now and yet obesity and disease is still running rampant. What's wrong with this picture?

Let's examine just a few areas of health where the science has shown a high-carb, low-fat diet causes great harm to your body:

1. HDL "good" cholesterol drops and triglycerides skyrocket

Lead researcher Dr. Anwar T. Merchant, assistant professor in the Department of Clinical Epidemiology & Biostatistics at the Hamilton, ON-based McMaster University and a member of the Population Health Research Institute, and his fellow researchers observed the diet and lipid profile of 619 Canadians of

Native American, South Asian, Chinese and European descent to determine if the differences in cholesterol and other blood fat levels could possibly be tied to diet.

However, unlike previous studies that had exclusively looked at the role of dietary fat, Dr. Merchant and his colleagues decided to see if carbohydrate consumption had something to do with the disparity among the different ethnic groups. South Asian participants eat more carbohydrates and had the lowest levels of HDL cholesterol in their blood. Conversely, the Chinese participants ate the least amount of carbohydrates and they exhibited the highest levels of HDL cholesterol.

Dr. Merchant noticed that when fat was removed from the diet and replaced with an equal number of carbohydrate calories, both the LDL and HDL cholesterol levels drop while triglycerides go way up. Even when adjustments are made for age, ethnicity, body mass index and alcohol intake, the carbohydrate connection to lower HDL levels was undeniable. The high-carb group saw an average level of 1.08 mmol/L while the low-carb group experienced an HDL level of 1.21 mmol/L.

The researchers found that each additional 100 grams of carbohydrates consumed daily led to a 0.15 mmol/L drop in HDL cholesterol and a corresponding rise in triglycerides. The primary culprits named in the study for higher carbohydrate intake include sugary soft drinks, fruit juices and junk food snacks with extra sugar and carbohydrates.

"Reducing the frequency of intake of sugar-containing soft drinks, juices and snacks may be beneficial," the researchers concluded.

This study was published in the January 2007 issue of *American Journal of Clinical Nutrition.*

Despite the fact that low-fat diet activist Dr. Dean Ornish described HDL cholesterol in his first podcast interview with me in 2006 as "garbage trucks" to get rid of the junk (fat) that you put in your body, the fact is that higher HDL cholesterol and lower triglycerides is a very good thing. It's also an excellent indicator whether or not you are actually livin' la vida low-carb correctly because, as previously noted, your HDL will be over 50 and triglycerides below 100.

We have seen from other research that lower HDL levels put you at a greater risk for heart disease; thus, we can infer that higher levels of HDL actually protects against heart disease. Plus, respected low-carb nutrition researcher Dr. Jeff Volek from the University of Connecticut has asserted that examining the triglyceride/HDL ratio is a much better marker than total cholesterol and LDL levels for protecting against heart disease.

I don't know about you, but I trust the findings of a researcher like Dr. Volek who has poured his entire life into this subject over a blatantly inaccurate 30-second television ad that blares across my screen 20,000 times a night pushing a statin drug. Anyone who is confused about why LDL, HDL, and triglyceride levels are important or simply wants to educate themselves further on the role of cholesterol in the body can easily find out the truth in a book by British health advocate Dr. Malcolm Kendrick called *The Great Cholesterol Con*.

2. "Fatty liver" disease from eating carbs, not saturated fat

For those of you who are not familiar with what this is, a "fatty liver" is known in medical circles as Non-Alcoholic Steatosis, aka non-alcoholic fatty liver disease (NAFLD), which can then lead to a much more serious medical problem called cirrhosis which is the precursor to liver failure. If your liver shuts down, then you need a transplant ASAP or you will die.

Currently, nearly one-fourth of Americans are believed to have a "fatty liver" and it occurs most often in males who are obese and/or diabetic. It is estimated that by the year 2020 non-alcoholic liver failure will be the #1 reason for liver transplants in the United States. But the sad part is liver donations are in short supply which makes them very expensive to obtain. Plus there may not be enough to meet the rising demand.

This possible life-threatening health issue needs to be taken more seriously if we are going to prevent certain catastrophe from happening in a little more than a decade from now. What's amazing is the fact that a "fatty liver" is actually made worse not by the consumption of the much-vilified saturated fat (no, contrary to popular belief, a "fatty liver" is not created by fat consumption), but rather with something even more devious and dangerous to your health — carbohydrates!

Specifically, I'm referring to those starchy high-carb foods like those cereals being touted for weight loss and other such "healthy" whole grain products that have been heavily marketed to the public as being good for you. Even the popular and convenient cereal bars you see on store shelves as the perfect breakfast on the go food are destructive to your health no matter what their manufacturers tell you is good about them in their advertising.

Interestingly, a study by the Johns Hopkins University School of Medicine found that the traditional high-carb, low-fat diet recommendation for obese patients suffering from a "fatty liver" actually increases their risk of liver inflammation seven-fold compared to obese patients placed on low-carb, high-fat diets which were actually found to be "protective" and even reversed the progression of the "fatty liver." This is a major finding!

These "fatty" deposits on the liver can indeed be improved by simply lowering the insulin levels in the body. How do you do that? By lowering your consumption of refined carbohydrates like you do when you are livin' la vida low-carb. Cut out the sugar, refined carbohydrates, and bleached flour from your diet. In fact, any foods containing added sugars and even those healthy whole grains should be removed from your diet as well. Don't get fooled into thinking you can have them just because they are promoted as "healthy." Clearly, they are not! Another study published in the February 2007 issue of *Digestive Diseases and Sciences* by researchers out of Duke University concluded a low-carb diet led to "histologic improvement of fatty liver disease."

It's a good idea to eat a low-carb diet and make sure you get adequate protein with every meal you consume throughout the day. Consult with your physician or dietitian about what amount would be best for you in treating your "fatty liver." So, to anyone who has concerns about causing damage to your liver with a low-carb diet because you have a "fatty liver," I think the better question you should be asking yourself is how much damage is that high-carb, low-fat diet doing to your already compromised liver?

3. Low-fat dairy leads to infertility

We've all heard that we should eat an adequate amount of dairy in our diet, but that we should choose the low-fat or fat-free versions of milk, cheese, and yogurt to provide the most healthy food for our bodies. If you are a woman in those precious few childbearing years, thought, that widely-accepted dietary advice is just about the worst thing you could ever follow if you want to have a baby, according to a Harvard study.

Lead researcher Dr. Jorge Chavarro, research fellow in the Department of Nutrition at Harvard School of Public Health, and his team observed 18,555 married, premenopausal women ages 24-42 with no history of infertility attempting to get pregnant over an eight — year period (1991-1999). This group of study participants was a subset of the larger group of 116,000 women that were part of The Nurses' Health Study II.

Dr. Chavarro monitored very closely the dietary intake of dairy foods by the women in the study, including the types and frequency of consumption, over the eight years. The women were also asked to provide information about the regularity of their period, if there were any problems with ovulation, and how their attempts to conceive a child were going.

A total of 438 women in the study experienced difficulty trying to have a baby during the study and Dr. Chavarro noticed that most of these women ate more than two portions of low-fat dairy foods daily. In fact, he quantified that women who eat that amount or higher of low-fat dairy every single day are 85 percent more likely to experience infertility compared with those women who eat it less often than once a week.

Interestingly, the researchers found something even more remarkable considering the dietary recommendations that rule the day in our society — those women who ate full-fat dairy foods, including whole milk and even ice cream, on a daily basis saw their risk of being infertile caused by ovulation problems drop by 25 percent compared to those who only ate full-fat dairy once a week. You read that right — Consuming full-fat dairy drops the risk of infertility by twenty-five percent!

What does the lack of dietary fat from the dairy products consumed by women have to do with their risk for infertility? Plenty! The researchers believe there is a fat-soluble substance in the full-fat dairy foods that works to improve the function of the ovaries. Thus, when that fat-soluble substance gets taken out during the conversion to 2% or non-fat skim milk, the health benefits dissipate as well.

Additionally, the processing of full-fat milk to skim milk (yes, removing fat from milk makes it a processed food) requires the addition of whey protein to the milk to give it a more "natural" taste and color. However, whey protein has been found to produce testosterone-like effects in lab rats and may be the culprit with the infertility found in women consuming low-fat dairy.

The results of this stunning Harvard study appeared in the February 28, 2007 issue of the scientific journal *Reproductive Health*.

This study is more proof that cutting your fat intake way down low is harmful for fertility especially. I decided to check out the government food pyramid (MyPyramid.gov) just to see what the current health experts are advising our government had to say about dairy intake. Under the "Milk Group" page you see that they highly recommend that the "milk group choices should be fat-free or low-fat."

Check this out (see if you can find the common theme):

- Include milk as a beverage...Choose fat-free or low-fat milk.
- If you usually drink whole milk, switch...to fat-free milk.
- Try reduced fat (2%), then low-fat (1%), and finally fat-free (skim).
- If you drink cappuccinos or lattes — ask for...fat-free (skim) milk.
- Add fat-free or low-fat milk...to oatmeal and hot cereals.
- Use fat-free or low-fat milk when making...cream soups.
- Have fat-free or low-fat yogurt as a snack.
- Make a dip for fruits or vegetables from yogurt.
- Make fruit-yogurt smoothies in the blender.
- Make chocolate...pudding with fat-free or low-fat milk.
- Top cut-up fruit with flavored yogurt for a quick dessert.
- Top casseroles...or vegetables with shredded low-fat cheese.
- Top a baked potato with fat-free or low-fat yogurt.

Why all the intense focus on "fat-free or low-fat" options? Clearly these heavily-publicized dietary recommendations are creating a lot of unhappy young couples who are trying to bring a little bundle of joy into the world that they can call their own. On what basis are they pushing these nasty foods that are actually working against women who want to conceive a child all in the name of "better health?"

I remember from my personal low-fat diet experience in 1999 how un-appealing those low-fat foods really are. The worst ones to me had to be the fat-free cheeses and skim milk. The cheese didn't even seem like real food. Describing it as a cardboard box texture is being much too kind. The skim milk seemed like white colored water. Getting low-fat 2% was as close as I could get to skim!

However, one thing I continued to do even after I stopped my low-fat diet and started gaining my weight back was to keep drinking 2% milk instead of whole thinking it was somehow a "healthy" alternative. When I started livin' la vida low-carb, though, I didn't drink regular milk anymore (because the lactose in it is nothing more than a sugar) and switched to Hood's Carb Countdown (now called Calorie Countdown) milk instead.

Yet, I kept on buying 2% milk for my wife Christine. We have been desperately trying to have a baby since we said "I do" to each other in August 1995. But, unfortunately, the good Lord has not chosen to bless us with a little munchkin just yet and we trust that will happen in His perfect timing. But after reading this study, I couldn't help but think what role the 2% milk Christine has been consuming over the course of our marriage may have had on our inability to conceive children. I don't know if it has anything to do with it or not, but it makes you stop and wonder.

I know one thing we immediately started doing after I read this study — buying whole milk for Christine again! In fact, we try to find real full-fat raw milk (RealMilk.com) at our local Whole Foods store, which is legal in our home state of South Carolina to purchase, whenever we can. There have been previous studies that hinted at the possibility of problems with infertility linked to dairy foods, but hardly any of them have been on humans like this one was. That's why Dr. Chavarro wanted to see what impact the fat content in the dairy foods consumed in a woman's diet can play regarding the prospect for motherhood.

Their conclusion? *"High intake of low-fat dairy foods may increase the risk of anovulatory infertility whereas intake of high-fat dairy foods may decrease this risk."*

Eating lots of low-fat dairy increases infertility while eating lots of high-fat dairy decreases infertility. If you are a woman trying to have a baby, Dr. Chavarro recommended what I did to Christine's dairy intake.

"Consider changing low-fat dairy foods for high-fat dairy foods; for instance, by swapping skimmed milk for whole milk and eating ice cream, not low-fat yogurt," he stated.

Now that's a switch seeing a recommendation to consume the high-fat version of a food instead of the low-fat one. How many tens or even hundreds of thousands of women have been left without an answer to their infertility problem while our government has kept on peddling the very reason they never got to be a mother? How very sad.

4. Ineffective weight loss approach for high insulin levels

When I was in Nashville, Tennessee in 2007 for the American Society of Bariatric Physicians (ASBP.org) obesity conference, there was a presentation made by researcher Dr. Jeff Volek from the University of Connecticut who said we've had it all wrong for years attempting to deal with the obesity problem. He said we have long been focused too heavily on obesity itself rather than looking at the symptoms which is why the high-carb, low-fat, low-calorie diets have failed to put a dent in the rising rates of people who are overweight and obese. Instead, Dr. Volek said the primary focus should be on dealing with hyperinsulinemia (excessive production of insulin) to treat obesity and the resulting illnesses that come from that. Dr. Volek makes a brilliant point that science now basically confirms is true.

Lead researcher Dr. Cara B. Ebbeling, assistant professor of Pediatrics at Harvard Medical School and the co-director of obesity research at the Boston, MA-based Children's Hospital, and her research team observed 73 obese adults between the ages of 18-35 for a six-month intervention period followed by one year of follow-up. The purpose of the study was to look at insulin production in the study participants and how dietary changes would impact it. The researchers basically wanted to know why a low-fat diet works for some, but doesn't necessarily work for everyone. Dr. Ebbeling said conventional wisdom always had an answer for this.

"The usual explanation is that some people are more motivated than others," she noted.

However, the results of her research found that it goes much deeper than mere willpower and is actually tied to controlling insulin secretion levels with a specific kind of diet. The study participants were split in half and put on one of two protein-neutral diets with varying fat/protein/carbohydrate ratios:

HIGH-CARB/LOW-FAT DIET — fat/protein/carb ratio of 20/25/55

LOWER-CARB/MODERATE-FAT DIET — fat/protein/carb ratio of 35/25/40

The study began by measuring each study participant's insulin levels 30 minutes after being administered 75 grams of glucose and tracked their progress at 6, 12, and 18 months. So, what were the results?

Interestingly, the difference in weight loss between the two groups was identical, which matches what most studies have found in recent years comparing low-fat to low-carb diets for weight loss. But, the study participants with "above-average insulin levels" actually lost five times more weight on the lower-carb/moderate-fat diet after 18 months (12.8 pounds) compared with the high-carb/low-fat diet (2.6). In fact, the body fat percentage comparison was equally impressive — down 2.6 percent vs. down .9 percent, respectively. Wow, now that was quite a difference!

It wasn't just good for their weight loss, though. The lower-carb/moderate-fat diet group also raised their HDL "good" cholesterol as well as lowering triglycerides better than the high-carb/low-fat diet group. However, LDL cholesterol improvements were better on the high-carb/low-fat diet (something previous research has confirmed time and time again). The conclusion of the researchers is that people who struggle to lose weight on a traditional low-fat diet may want to start livin' la vida low-carb to better manage their weight and health.

Well, hallelujah! I've been touting that message for years because it has always been my contention that a low-fat diet has monopolized dietary recommendations by our government and the current health "experts" for far too long. Dr. Ebelling's study adds even more fuel to the fire of my argument that both low-fat and low-carb should be recommended alongside each other as equally healthy ways to deal with obesity and health problems. Why are we still begging for this to happen when the science is clearly showing what has been obvious all along?

The results of Dr. Ebelling's study appeared in the May 16, 2007 issue of *Journal of the American Medical Association*.

I wonder how many people even realize they may have hyperinsulinemia these days. Most people probably wouldn't have a clue what that means which is why diabetes has become such an epidemic along with obesity. If we can help people control their insulin production, something livin' la vida low-carb has shown to do time and time again, then perhaps we can reduce obesity and diabetes. But it is going to take a serious movement to move the mountains of complacency that have built up for decades.

I challenge groups like the American Heart Association (AHA) and the American Diabetes Association (ADA) to take a good look at studies like this one and try to defend their current positions on a healthy diet in light of what the science is showing us. And the same goes for the United States Department of Agriculture (USDA) and the Food & Drug Administration (FDA). I suppose you'd like to see people like Jimmy Moore just go away, but I won't be leaving anytime soon. I'd love to go to Capitol Hill before Congress and share what livin' la vida low-carb has done to change my life for the better.

5. Fruits and veggies are ineffective against breast cancer.

The high-carb, low-fat fruits and vegetables diet recommended by the current health experts took a major blow in the largest study of its kind when it found that women who showed early signs of breast cancer who ate this way did not have a lower risk of breast cancer recurrence compared to women who followed a diet consisting of five servings a day of fruits and vegetables.

The study published in the July 18, 2007 issue of *Journal of the American Medical Association* substantiates the growing evidence against high-carb, low-fat diets even more.

Lead researcher Dr. John P. Pierce, professor at the University of California San Diego Cancer Center in the Family & Preventive Medicine Cancer Prevention & Control Program, and his fellow researchers observed 3,088 American women (between the ages of 18-70) who were previously diagnosed with the early stages of breast cancer and split them into two groups:

INTERVENTION GROUP — 1537 of the study participants were randomly assigned to receive a telephone counseling program supplemented with cooking classes and newsletters that promoted daily targets of 5 vegetable servings plus 16 oz of vegetable juice; 3 fruit servings; 30g of fiber; and 15% to 20% of energy intake from fat.

OR

COMPARISON GROUP — 1551 of the study participants followed a written form of the "5-A-Day" dietary guidelines.

The intervention group ate twice as many fruits and vegetables as the comparison group over the course of the study that took place in seven different cities. Each of the women was observed from 6-11 years. What did the researchers find? The Intervention group increased their servings of vegetables by 65 percent, fruits by 25 percent, fiber by 30 percent, while lowering their fat intake by 13 percent. These changes were confirmed by blood tests among those in that group.

There were a total of 518 recurrences of breast cancer over the average 7.3 years of follow-up among both groups. But the difference between the two groups was insignificant:

INTERVENTION GROUP — 256 women (16.7 percent)
COMPARISON GROUP — 262 women (16.9 percent)

Similarly, there were 315 deaths with eight out of ten of them due directly to the breast cancer, but there was little statistical difference between the two groups:

INTERVENTION GROUP — 155 women (10.1 percent)
COMPARISON GROUP — 160 women (10.3 percent)

"I think we believed that by eating real food and nutrient-dense food, we were going to come up with a different outcome, but we didn't," she explained.

Perhaps rather than being upset, Dr. Stefanick, why not learn from the empirical knowledge you have gleaned from this research to realize that perhaps the old adage of "eat lots of fruits and vegetables" was just plain bad advice? It's okay to admit that even if it goes against everything you ever believed about a healthy diet. Dr. Pierce was a bit more pragmatic in his response to the results explaining there is a "threshold effect" when it comes to your intake of fruits and veggies.

"I look at it the other way," he stated. "We're telling women they don't have to go overboard here. They can have a good quality of life without worrying about their dietary pattern all the time."

A voice of reason in the scientific community at last! This obsession with requiring people to eat unlimited amounts of fruits and vegetables as if it is the great cure-all has been annoying at best. I've always contended that kind of dietary advice is a copout, mainly because what most people consider their veggie intake is primarily potatoes and more specifically, fried potatoes with ketchup (another food considered a "vegetable" by many people) and their fruit intake consists of the high-sugar ones like bananas and oranges — not very healthy at all.

The researchers said the recommended vegetables are the nutrient-dense, non-starchy dark leafy greens, sweet potatoes and carrots and not the popular nutritionally bankrupt ones like iceberg lettuce and the extremely high-carb white potatoes. One area of study that may be pursued further is whether consuming a diet low in fruits and vegetables as a young person results in lower breast cancer risk. An overwhelming preponderance of evidence is building that a high-carb, low-fat diet may even be responsible for such cancers as brain cancer, pancreatic cancer, esophageal cancer, kidney cancer, breast cancer, and prostate cancer among others. We'll explore cancer and the carbohydrate connection in a later chapter of this book because I think it's both prudent and desirable to arm yourself nutritionally to keep this terrible disease at bay.

6. Eating potatoes increases your chances of getting Type 2 diabetes.

Researchers at the prestigious Harvard Medical School led by Thomas L. Halton released a 20-year study of about 85,000 American women ages 34-59 with no history of chronic disease which found that higher consumption of potatoes increased their risk of developing Type II diabetes. By the end of the study, there were close to 4,500 new cases of Type II diabetes among the study participants. Of even greater concern to the researchers was the fact that obese women, who are already putting themselves at a greater risk for developing diabetes because of their weight, may be especially adversely affected by eating large amounts of high-carb potatoes.

The results of this eye-opening study were published in the February 2006 issue of *American Journal of Clinical Nutrition*.

For far too long society has tried to convince us that potatoes are healthy by dressing them up as goofy cartoon characters and even through a freak of science genetically modifying them to create a low-carb version. But the fact remains that potatoes are decidedly unhealthy for you because of the excessive carbohydrates that are contained in them and what that does to your body. Eating a potato is tantamount to eating a big slice of chocolate cake metabolically speaking! They both cause a rise in your blood sugar followed by a rapid drop requiring more and more carbohydrates to start the ruthless cycle all over again. I got off that rollercoaster ride once and for all when I started my low-carb lifestyle and I don't miss it one bit. Stabilizing your blood sugar and keeping it under control is one sure-fire way of doing your part to prevent diabetes from becoming a part of your life.

But potatoes are relatively cheap and people sometimes buy whatever they can afford because it saves them money, especially when the economy becomes squeezed like it is right now. Yet one of the lessons I have learned from my low-carb experience is that people must make better choices for themselves about the kind of foods they put in their mouth — even if it is a little more expensive in the short-term. Sure potatoes are inexpensive compared with certain healthier choices, but what price can you put on your long-term health?

If avoiding potatoes can keep obesity, diabetes, and other such diseases from becoming a part of my life and draining my future income with unnecessary medical bills brought on by my predictable declining health, then by golly that's what I'm gonna do for myself. The fact is we do not NEED potatoes in our diet and the world would be a lot healthier place if people would stop consuming them forever. Of course, this will never happen in my lifetime, but it would make a noticeable difference if a good many people started doing this as soon as possible.

The study found that the high glycemic index of potatoes caused huge spikes in the participants' blood sugar which caused damage to the pancreatic cells that produce insulin, the key ingredient in metabolizing blood sugar. Additionally, the researchers explained that those who are carrying around excess weight and do not exercise are already prone to becoming insulin resistant where body cells lose their sensitivity to insulin and it eventually leads to diabetes. Dr. Halton states that potatoes hurry up this process which leads to a more rapid onset of diabetes. Therefore, it is a good suggestion for the obese to stop eating potato-based products such as French fries, potato chips, etc. to improve their chances of warding off diabetes, the researchers recommended.

The risk for diabetes increased 14 percent for those study participants who ate the most potatoes and rose by 21 percent for those who chose to eat French fries as part of their diet. Interestingly, the researchers noted that the women in their study generally ate potatoes and white flour products in lieu of whole grain foods such as high-fiber vegetables, fruits and beans. Halton concluded that the diabetes risk would most likely be modestly cut if they just started eating whole grains instead.

I have talked about this before and I'll keep saying it. People in general and especially Americans eat way too much sugar, white flour, starchy foods and processed foods. We don't need this JUNK in our diets. I know it feels good and is dirt cheap to eat this way, but look at what we are doing to our health as a nation. If we want the children of today to live a long and healthy life themselves, then we need to be the examples for them to lead the way on eating healthy and living right. This madness must come to an end!

The stigma that has been placed on livin' la vida low-carb is unprecedented in the history of mankind. What are these people so afraid of about the low-carb lifestyle? If it gives hope for even one person out there who can find a permanent way to lose weight and keep it off forever while obtaining optimal health, then isn't it worth getting the word out about what it is?

As someone who once weighed 410 pounds and knows the pain of feeling hopeless regarding weight loss and being healthy, the answer to that question is yes! It is so worth it! Don't ever let anyone tell you that you shouldn't try the low-carb life if everything else you've tried has let you down. You just start low-carbin' for yourself and watch the unbelievable results begin happening for you, too! And don't you dare ever look back or start listening to the naysayers who will only try to drag you down.

This is your day. Now is the time. There's nothing that is going to hold you back from becoming the thin and healthy person that you so deeply desire to be. Throw away the excuses and just do It! Make today the first day of the rest of your long and healthy life. Because today you are gonna start livin' la vida low-carb. Go for it!

We were all saddened to hear in the Summer 2008 of the untimely death of NBC-TV's "Meet the Press" host Tim Russert as a result of his first heart attack. So, how did a 58-year old man die from a heart attack when he was doing all of the things his doctor said he should to prevent it? Should we be concerned about what doctors are telling us about how to ward off cardiovascular disease so that we don't become the next victim of what befell Tim Russert?

I do have some things to say about Tim Russert's death that just have to be said. Isn't it interesting that Tim Russert did everything his doctor wanted him to perfectly and yet his very first heart attack was a fatal one? I don't think that's a coincidence either and it happens every single day without a blink of an eye from anyone.

Check out Tim Russert's lipid profile at the time of his death:

LDL — 68
HDL — 37 (up from the lower 20's)
Total Cholesterol — 105

Most doctors would look at those numbers and say, "See how healthy this person is because we lowered his cholesterol." And they would be proud of putting someone like Tim Russert on a statin drug to artificially make this happen. But what good did it do him in the end? He's gone now because of that advice and yet there's no outrage about it. Worry, concern, perplexity, stunned disbelief, yes — but nobody is angry that this preventable death was made worse by the use of all the traditional means for improving heart health.

According to Russert's doctor, he didn't have Type 2 diabetes nor did he have any blood sugar issues at all. His A1C was in the normal range and as I noted previously his cholesterol was considered very healthy. For all intents and purposes according to the modern day medical conventional wisdom, he was the epitome of perfect health. And yet he tragically died before his time. We now know posthumously that Russert had coronary heart disease that he was being treated for, but his doctor apparently didn't know how severe it was.

How could this be since he was ostensibly eating a high-carb, low-fat diet and taking a statin drug? But even if his doctor did know it was extremely serious, what else would he have recommended to Russert? Higher doses of his statin drug? Even less fat in his diet? More exercise? In the end, all of these seemingly good strategies from the conventional wisdom point of view would have very likely done nothing to prevent this from happening.

His doctor put him on blood pressure lowering medication as well as a cholesterol-lowering statin drug to see if that would help. And Russert even rode an exercise bike to try to lose weight, although it didn't seem to work. There's no doubt the calcified plaque buildup in the arteries leading to his heart was getting bigger and bigger over the years until his heart couldn't take it any longer. We know that too low LDL can lead to depression, suicide and death. We also know that HDL "good" cholesterol (Russert's was very low — not good) and triglycerides (something Russert dealt with having too high over the last few years of his life) are better indicators of heart health than LDL and total cholesterol. And it's a high-carb, low-fat diet that leads to lower HDL and higher triglycerides. No doubt this is precisely the kind of diet Russert's doctor had him on.

This cholesterol issue is one I am quite passionate about as I noted in an earlier chapter because the modern means for dealing with it is simply exacerbating the problem. The medical community has the blinders on and they refuse to take them off long enough to see the harm they are doing to patient after patient they put on these risky prescription drugs for a purpose that is futile and fatal in the end like it was for Tim Russert. It's time to break all those years of cholesterol indoctrination. There will be confusion and concern in your mind at times, but that's okay. My pithy response to anyone who challenges me on cholesterol is simply prove to me that it's unhealthy.

Hopefully you know now that consuming a diet lower in carbs, higher in fat, and with moderate protein at every meal is what is going to work best for improving your heart health over the course of your life. If only Tim Russert had been given this information instead of the antiquated traditional low-fat, high-carb diet advice he had received, then maybe his fatal heart attack could have been averted. Perhaps this event will begin a serious discussion of heart health treatment in this country so that others can benefit from the healthy low-carb lifestyle, too. We can only hope.

One of the major criticisms of livin' la vida low-carb is that it is a dangerous "fad" diet that is just a kooky flash-in-the-pan weight loss program. But in the next lesson, you'll learn very quickly that low-carb is not even close to being a fad diet as we take a look at some of the most recent ones to come on the scene.

LESSON #8
Low-carb is not even close to being a fad diet

"Low-carb diets are not fad diets. In fact, low-carb diets should not even be considered diets as everyone should be eating low-carb. If you suffer from obesity, heart disease, type 2 diabetes, reflux esophagitis (heartburn), any inflammatory condition such as fibromyalgia, rheumatoid arthritis, lupus; if you are pregnant and are at risk for gestational diabetes, pregnancy induced high blood pressure, pre-eclampsia/eclampsia; suffer from allergies, asthma, psoriasis, or eczema; then you need to be limiting your carb intake. Low-carb diets are not fad diets but a way everyone should be eating to remain healthy for the rest of their lives."

— **Dr. James E. Carlson**, M.D., author of *GENOCIDE! How Your Doctor's Dietary Ignorance Will Kill You*

Whenever you read a media account about the low-carb lifestyle these days, it's usually described with the "f" word. No, not THAT "f" word! I'm talking about the word "fad." I just have to scratch my head whenever I hear how low-carb is a fad, when it has and continues to be the healthy living choice of tens of millions of Americans, and it is here to stay.

Speaking of "fad" diets, there are some truly outrageous and genuinely wacky and quacky weight loss methods that people have tried to lose weight over the years.

The Cabbage Soup Diet
Consisting of 6 large green onions, 2 green peppers, 1-2 cans diced tomatoes, 1 bunch celery, 1 package Lipton Onion Soup Mix, optional buillion cubes and 1 head of cabbage. The diet recommends you eat this soup whenever you are

hungry, and as much as you want. Otherwise, follow a strict menu of fruits and raw vegetables.

The Grapefruit Diet
Eat a ½ grapefruit with every meal. And the point is?

Scarsdale Diet Plan
A precursor to the low-carb theory in the '70s, the Scarsdale diet involved a lot of low-carb food staples, except for ½ grapefruit eaten every morning.

The Coffee Diet
A new coffee brand, Java-Fit, promises to help people lose weight while drinking its herbal-infused java. The only side effect is you can never get any sleep. HA!

The Apple-Cider Vinegar diet
Drink a cup of warm water with a teaspoon of apple vinegar before each meal. Expect many trips to the bathroom with this one. Gotta go, gotta go, gotta go right now.

The Myrtle Beach Diet
It features some vaguely scientific discussion of carbohydrates. And it is advertised with lots pictures of attractive people. Sex sells but it doesn't cause weight loss.

Weightlossforidiots.com
Discusses metabolism rates and features a picture of a cartoon woman saying "I'm a certified idiot." Couldn't have said it better myself!

While most of these obvious "fad" diets are about as useless as buying a lottery ticket, many people are still so desperate that they'll try anything (admit it, you've probably tried one or more of theseW in your life, haven't you?). That's why I encourage anyone who wants to lose weight to use common sense along with reading up on what makes a weight loss program successful. This strategy is exactly what attracted me to the healthy low-carb lifestyle and why I am still on it over five years after starting. I plan on being on this way of eating for the rest of my life so I will never have to put up with weighing over 400 pounds ever again!

So, what exactly is so crazy about the Atkins diet that people want to describe it as a "fad" diet? I know, I know, we've all heard the excuses about how it contains too much fat and too many calories.

I am offering an open invitation to anyone who would like to clearly and specifically explain why the low-carb approach to losing weight is crazy. Can you make the case for the low-fat, low-calorie lifestyle over the high-fat, low-carb one? Is anyone willing to defend the low-fat diet plan when it has now been proven to fail so many people for so many years?

Think about how much our diet is already transforming into a low-carb one, albeit ever-so-slowly, and realize that someday we'll look back on this abysmal low-fat era as one that was mired in gross misinformation and hyperbole about what healthy eating is about. And there's no denying the success that people like me and many others have experienced by livin' la vida low-carb. What will the people who recommend low-fat diets do with the ever-increasing population of us who have lost a whole lot of weight and kept it off on low-carb over the long-term? Will people living a low-carb lifestyle actually be the ones to have the last laugh? I certainly think so.

But in the meantime there are plenty more truly "fad" diets we can focus on that are much more extreme than any of the low-carb plans out there. Let's take a look at just a few of them:

The "No-Diet" Diet

Have you heard about the anti-diet book called *The "No-Diet" Diet* that claims because there are so many fad diets on the market today recommending you do this or that to lose weight and none of them seem to work, why don't you just eat a "sensible" meal plan and exercise so that everything will be okay? Don't you just love how simple and easy they make that sound? Newsflash: If it were that easy, then we wouldn't have an obesity crisis and fad diets wouldn't exist because everybody would be doing this! Okay, thanks for indulging me in a brief moment of outrage due to my sadness from being fat for most of my life. I'm glad I got that out of my system.

But seriously, think about it for a moment. Haven't we always been told that we just need to eat right and move our bodies more to make our weight fall into line with "normal" people? Of course, what they mean by "sensible" eating is a low-fat, low-calorie, portion-controlled diet consisting of foods that you would rather not eat if you didn't have to. Is that really how you want to live the rest of your life? If so, then yippy skippy for you. But not for me and the tens of millions of people who have found solace in the healthy low-carb lifestyle full of a buffet of scrumptious delicacies that will tickle your taste buds and put a smile on your face while the pounds melt away.

But don't mention livin' la vida low-carb to these no-diet advocates because they'll rail you so fast you won't even know what hit you! Describing the Atkins diet and other low-carb programs as "fads", they claim that books like *French Women Don't Get Fat* have been the ultimate "death knell" to low-carb. The "no-diet" diet says people should stop obsessing about what foods they eat and just eat whatever they want in "small portions" while using your two feet to get you from Point A to Point B. But how will you have the energy to walk around everywhere when you're so hungry from limiting your food intake to these small portions?

Eating healthy does not mean you have to give up eating all the wonderful foods you can and should enjoy when you are livin' la vida low-carb. And if you feel like eating more delicious low-carb foods than you ever have on any "diet" program you've ever been on before, then go for it! That's exactly what I did when I was in the midst of losing my weight in 2004 on the low-carb lifestyle. I ate as much as I wanted of the low-carb foods I decided to put in my mouth. As long as I stayed within my carb limit (which was around 25-30g carbs daily for me) and ate to satiety, the weight came off and I never got hungry.

Anybody who tells you that you must limit your food portions is un-informed. Now, is it a good idea to gorge yourself at every single meal, regardless of the carbohydrate content of the foods you are consuming? Of course not. Your food choices and the amount of food you eat will gradually come down naturally on its own. But I can still put away a lot of food when I want to — keeping it low-carb, of course.

I used to be a 410-pound behemoth monster! I didn't get that way without having an appetite. While I'm just a shadow of the man I used to be, the way I got there was by carefully selecting foods that I could eat without gaining weight. This isn't difficult to do as long as you know how many carbs you are putting in your mouth. That's it! You definitely don't have to portion control or count the calories of what you eat if you don't want to. I'm tired of that advice from the current health experts. If I listened to their advice, then I probably would have given up on low-carb a long time ago from food deprivation. Thankfully, I have just ignored their recommendations and just started livin' la vida low-carb for myself. That's what has helped me keep the weight off for the past five years.

Real low-carbers know that there's so much more to low-carb than just bacon and cheese (although I personally like both bacon and cheese as part of my healthy low-carb eating program). Low-carb is not the only way to lose and maintain your weight, but it's certainly an enjoyable healthy way. Many people have tried their entire lives to lose weight and keep it off and nothing has worked for them, and for them perhaps livin' la vida low-carb is the lifestyle change they've been looking for.

BodyTogs

Have you heard of using body weights called BodyTogs to shed the pounds? They are the invention of a bariatric doctor named Dr. Ayaz Virji and he wrote a book about it called *The Skinny Book* which outlines his plan for helping people lose weight and keep it off. But Dr. Virji apparently didn't think the diet principles in his book were enough so he created these BodyTogs for people to wear so they can get the benefits of exercising without having to participate in organized exercise.

So, by wearing these body weights that are "scientifically proven" (something mentioned quite a few times at the BodyTogs web site!) you will burn more calories and fat than you would have if you didn't wear them. In fact, Dr. Virji contends that wearing his BodyTogs for 10 hours doing no organized exercise is just as effective as running for 90 minutes on the treadmill. Dr. Virji thinks he is on to a revolutionary new way to help people lose weight with his invention.

"It's a medically sophisticated fitness device, but not a medical device. It's a first in its class weight loss product that is scientifically proven," he proudly proclaims.

I'm naturally skeptical of wearing weights in order to lose weight. That just seems so odd to me.

So how do these BodyTogs allegedly work? According to Dr. Virji, being overweight is not bad for you, but rather the fat in your body which leads to inflammation and cholesterol build-up. Because the body's metabolism slows down as people lose weight, Dr. Virji explains, overweight and obese people need to add the weight they lose back on their body to continue to burn calories at the same rate they did when they were heavier.

"It's almost like fooling the body to enhance caloric burn," Dr. Virji notes. "You get the exercise without the inflammation and cholesterol of fat."

You wear them on your arms and legs underneath your clothing and Dr. Virji says they are comfortable to wear and will give you the all the benefits of working out without working out. That sounds a lot like those diet pills that claim they'll help you lose weight without making any lifestyle changes. By Dr. Virji's own admission, you'll lose a whopping one pound of fat per month, but he believes you should supplement wearing his body weights with a "sensible weight management program."

"They're intended to enhance what you're doing, not replace what you're doing," Dr. Virji explained.

Just as the dirty little secret of diet pills is that you need to reduce your calories and exercise to make them work, Dr. Virji clearly states that his Body-Togs aren't good enough on their own to help you lose weight and keep it off. Exercise, like eating, needs to be a permanent lifestyle change. That's what happened for me when I changed the way I ate and I started on an exercise routine that I could sustain. The daily discipline of eating the right kinds of foods and moving my body to make it sweat while getting my heart rate up was essential to succeeding at losing weight, getting healthy, and remaining that to this day.

The Astro Diet

A celebrity psychic says the secret to weight loss success depends on your astrological sign. It's all detailed in a book called *Maria Shaw's Astro Diet* and I'm not kidding! She sincerely believes people should look to their zodiac sign and act accordingly to reach their desired weight and overcome obstacles to keeping their weight under control. As an accomplished author, this is Shaw's first book on dieting. She claims that there are certain times when it is best for people to try to lose weight, times when people should not try to lose weight, and times when people should just maintain their weight. In fact, Shaw said there are even "bad years" for trying to lose weight depending on your sign.

"Everybody has good years and bad years for losing weight," she said. "My last bad year was 1994. It's here again this year. I've gained 10 pounds already so I really have to watch it."

I guess that means 2004 was a "good year" for this Capricorn to lose weight since I did so well that year!

Shaw admits she is not a nutritionist or dietitian, and she includes testimonies of people who supposedly lost weight on her diet plan and gives instructions and predictions to dieters. She believes knowledge is power and that people should know when to expect progress and when to prepare for pitfalls.

"Timing is everything. Knowing when you'll lose weight and when you give in to temptation will help you to stick to your diet program," she opined.

This is news to me, and I'm skeptical. My own belief in the supernatural is limited to believing in the good sense and knowledge that God gave me is all I'll eve need to lose weight and keep it off. I will continue to pray that God would be gracious to me in my efforts to continue on with the weight loss path and give thanks for the miracle performed in me through the healthy low -carb lifestyle. This is a program built on sound science that makes more sense to me.

Shaw said she is now experimenting with her "gain year" to see if she can buck the trend and may write another book about it.

"With free will you can change anything. I'm working on proving that theory this year as I attempt to shed pounds in my weight-gain year," she revealed. "I want to prove free will is stronger. Even if you know it's your weight gain year you can fight it. If I'm successful I plan to write a sequel."

If astrology sounds logical to you as a diet aid, then this book is for you. If you need something a little more based on science then I invite you try Livin' La Vida Low-Carb!

Ear Stapling

Add to the ever-growing list of fad diets the latest to come along in the genre of weight loss gimmicks: Ear stapling! You heard me right. People are all excited about having their ear stapled in a 10-minute procedure with the hopes of finding a way to curb their appetite and lose weight. I'm not joking! This is a real product from a company called Staple Trim, which serves customers eager to have a staple put in their ear every single day in the hopes the fat will melt away. According to the marketing of this product, the staple releases endorphins into your body which, in turn, keeps you so content that you don't feel like you have to eat while stress is relieved. Other alleged benefits include improvements in sleep, constipation and even headaches.

Well, I can tell you why all of this is happening. Because you've got a freakin' staple in your ear and it hurts like the dickens! Wanna know the best way to cure any pain in your body? Make a bigger pain in another part of your body! When we were still kids, my brother Kevin used to stomp on my toe when I would complain about my head hurting. When I asked him why he did that, his reply was, "I bet your head doesn't hurt anymore!" And you know what? He was right! I wonder if this applies to the ear staple, too.

These ear stapling clinicians don't even need a license to shoot a staple through your ear. Yikes! Who can you complain to if something goes wrong? Double yikes! At $55 a pop every three months, many people will conclude that this is something worth trying to help them lose weight. As I have said many times before, when you are overweight or obese and think you have tried anything and everything to lose the weight, then you become hopelessly desperate to try anything that will work. I don't know if shooting a staple in your ear helps you lose weight or not, but I do know that it won't teach you anything about eating better or improving the bad habits that got you fat to begin with. The sure sign of a weight loss fad is when it expects you to do something strange to yourself and then leaves you hanging about what other important changes you need to make to keep the weight loss permanent. Keep that hole out of your ears and head!

Slim Café Weight Loss Coffee

One day my wife Christine says "Hey Jimmy, come check this out" regarding a television commercial she saw about a weight loss product called Slim Café. Apparently it is a fortified "diet" coffee that supposedly helps you shed the pounds to the tune of "a pound a week." Their slogan claims that Slim Café "tastes great" and will help you "lose weight." Okay, but how? What's in this stuff that makes people lose weight? Does it really taste good? What's the deal? According to the Slim Café web site, this Las Vegas, NV-based company actually guarantees you will lose weight by drinking their product three times a day. But they do offer a money back guarantee if you don't lose 4-8 pounds drinking their coffee and they will even pay people $1 for every pound they lose while using Slim Café for weight loss.

At a hefty $40 for just 28 ounces of this product, Slim Café is just the latest in a long line of products that are promising consumers will attain weight loss without making them adjust their lifestyle.

Let's imagine I'm a man who weighs 350 pounds and I need to lose 125 pounds. Obviously I've got some bad eating habits which have led me to reach the weight I am. I see this infomercial for Slim Café weight loss coffee on TV and think, "Hey, I can do that!" So I pull out my credit card and break the bank stocking up on this stuff thinking it alone is gonna help me lose weight. I start drinking my Slim Café coffee for breakfast with my normal half-dozen doughnuts and even dip them in my coffee, then I wash down my Big Mac with large French fries meal at lunch with another glass of Slim Café, and finally at dinner I down my third cup of Slim Café after a hearty meat and potatoes meal topped off with hot fudge cake a la mode! Let me ask you: Will I really lose weight this way?

The truth of the matter is that it doesn't matter what products you are eating or drinking to lose weight unless you are also willing to make the necessary changes in your current lifestyle to facilitate weight loss. Drinking a product like Slim Café as part of a lifestyle filled with overeating carbs and calories is not going to make any difference whatsoever in that person's weight. None whatsoever! What the makers of Slim Café don't want you to know is that, like diet pills and other weight loss schemes, in addition to drinking their product, you will also need to eat a vastly different diet than what got you fat to begin with in order to see the pounds come off of your body. Whether you choose a low-fat, low-calorie, or low-carb dietary approach, changing your current eating habits immediately will help you lose weight whether you start drinking Slim Café or not.

100-Calorie Snack Foods

It's been happening right under our noses in such a subtle way that most people can't even remember when it started. But the emergence of the "100-Calorie Food" fad has arrived in full force. The extreme measures being taken by food and beverage manufacturers to jump on this bandwagon became all too clear to me when I noticed one of the most recognized brands in the world repackaging and marketing their product with the words "100 Calories" blared across the front — Coca-Cola! When I first saw this in the grocery store, it made me stop in my tracks to do a double-take and the wheels started spinning in my head. Okay, I can drink this itty bitty can of Coke and "only" consume 100 calories or I can drink an unlimited amount of diet soda and still not even come close to 100 calories!

Just because a product has 100 calories does not make it healthy. In fact most of these products are simply 100 calories of sugar and carbs.

While the calories may have been cut down in these foods, you still get a ton of carbohydrates from the sugar and white flour they put in them. Eating these products will only make you think you are eating better, but it's very clear you're not. Calories are important, but the quality of the calories is much more important. The "100-Calorie" fad will hopefully pass quickly.

The Lip Balm Diet

While surfing the Internet one day, I saw the following ad from a company called Desoriente and it stopped me in my tracks:

Are You Obese?
Don't Work out, Don't Diet, Just Use
Lip Balm and Lose Weight Easily!

If you are overweight or obese and believe that rubbing a lip balm on your kisser is going to help you "lose weight easily" better than any kind of diet and exercise plan, then I've got a bridge in Brooklyn, New York that I'd like to sell you! These people are dead serious about their product and even offer a 60-day money back guarantee. The lip balm sells for $20 a stick of it!

Desoriente claims their product will give you "the benefit of appetite suppression while keeping your lips smooth, supple and healthy." Sigh. If only it were as easy as putting on lip balm. So how does this lip balm supposedly stimulate "appetite suppression?"

According to their web site, people gain weight from "over eating and unhealthy snacking." To combat this, Desoriente offers a proprietary blend of nine oils and extracts in their lip balm which contains smells that "suppress the feeling" of hunger. They claim application of the lip balm causes the oils to be "absorbed by the nasal cavity and olfactory system" to "lessen the feeling of hunger within seconds."

To me, the more "natural weight loss" method is one that encourages you to eat less because your body tells you it is satisfied (ostensibly from the fat and protein you are eating) and let that be the way to suppress your appetite so you don't overeat and snack in between meals. It's called satiety and it can be stimulated naturally.

Carb Blockers

Why do people try to make livin' la vida low-carb more complicated than it needs to be? There are some people following a low-carb diet for weight loss who think they have to start taking a pill called a "carb blocker." I'd never even heard of a "carb blocker" when I was losing my weight on low-carb in 2004, but it reminds me of all those so-called "fat blockers" that have been made popular since the low-fat diet was popular in the 1980s. In essence, these products are supposed to prevent the absorption of fat into the bloodstream which will allegedly help you lose weight. With the "carb blockers," they do the same thing except with carbohydrates.

Let me tell you, though, I lost 180 pounds and have kept it off without ever having to use a "carb blocker." The marketers of these pills will say you need to take a "carb blocker" pill because restricting your carbs as much as you do on the Atkins or South Beach diets causes you to become unnecessarily tired and easily fatigued until the body gets used to the lower amount of carbs. However this is what is supposed to happen when you begin the low-carb lifestyle. Most of us who started a low-carb program were used to eating 600, 700, or even as many as 1200 grams of carbohydrates in a day! When you bring that number down to 20g as part of the Induction phase of Atkins or 0g as part of the Induction phase on South Beach, your body cannot help but react to the change.

Even still, this change is absolutely necessary to get the body to begin burning stored fat as part of the process of getting ketosis to work its magic. Until you get into ketosis on your low-carb plan, you will not lose weight. Is this process a hard thing to go through? For some people, the answer is yes. I thought I was gonna die the first day I was on the Atkins diet, but something incredibly amazing happened. After just a few sho rt days, those negative feelings went away and I have felt fantastic ever since. I'm no longer addicted to the sugar and carbohydrates that were ruining my health! There is no dietary need for carbohydrates (which I'll explain in a later chapter), but the premise of a "carb blocker" is all wrong.

Marketers of these pills recommend people need to start taking a carb blocker to help them get away with eating a few more carbs than they are supposed to have during the weight loss phase of their low-carb lifestyle. But it doesn't work that way! If you want to see the results that come with being on low-carb, then you need to do low-carb exactly as it is written in the particular program you are on. Dr. Atkins didn't talk about taking a "carb blocker." And neither does Dr. Agatston or Drs. Mike and Mary Dan Eades in their *Protein Power* books. I was once offered a very lucrative five-digit sponsorship deal to promote a carb blocker at my blog, but I refused on principle. While some may say carb blockers are just another option for weight loss, the truth of the matter is you can lose all the weight you need without ever having to take one of these useless pills.

The OTC Weight Loss Pill "Alli"

The Food & Drug Administration (FDA) made it official in 2007 and gave the rubber stamp to sell the prescription weight loss drug orlistat under the new name "Alli." No, it's not pronounced like Muhammed Ali (AH-LEE), but rather like the word "ally" (AL-EYE) as in someone who is on your side. You've probably seen television commercials with country singer Wynonna Judd. The irony in that name is that the FDA is certainly no "Alli" to anyone desiring weight loss with their approval of this drug.

While they don't encourage children under the age of 18 to take this drug (but who are we kidding, parents will be buying this drug for their overweight kids left and right!), it is absolutely open game for adults willing to combine it with a low-fat, low-calorie, portion control diet and exercise program. That's right, just in case you missed the fine print from the FDA about this latest cure-all for obesity, the secret is you still have to diet! But don't you dare even think about livin' la vida low-carb while taking the 60mg capsules of "Alli" right before each of your three daily meals because it only works for people who eat little to no fat in their diet.

In addition to not absorbing dietary fat (which can be dangerous on a number of levels that you don't even want me to get into!), this drug may very well prevent you from absorbing some of the most essential nutrients in the foods you eat. Therefore, they recommend you take a multivitamin before you go to bed. While opponents of low-carb always chastise us for promoting vitamin supplementation on our very natural and healthy way of eating, here's the FDA telling people they need to eat a low-fat diet and take supplements if they decide to start using the "Alli" OTC weight loss pill. And this is the weak over-the-counter version of the drug — can you imagine what the full-strength one is like? Like most drugs, "Alli" is not without some really nasty side effects. Try this on for size: loose stools, excess gas, fatty stools, possible uncontrollable bowel movements, flatulence with discharge, abdominal pain, and a general sense of poop-poopy-doop 24 hours a day, 7 days a week, non-stop fun between you and the porcelain goddess!

Seriously, though, orlistat is NOT for everyone (I don't think it's for ANYONE, but that's just my take on it!). People who have had an organ transplant shouldn't take it because of drug interactions and neither should people on blood thinners, who are diabetic, have a thyroid problem, binge eating disorder, bulimia nervosa, or malabsorption syndromes. The FDA says people with these conditions should consult with their physician before using this over-the-counter drug.

Maybe I'm thinking too hard about this, but why make a drug OTC if there are very real dangers to a large segment of the population with all those ailments listed above? The end result will be more obesity and a lot more tummy aches. Come on over to livin' la vida low-carb and enjoy what REAL healthy living is like. No drugs, no forced diet plans, no disgusting foods to put up with — just delicious and nutritious whole foods that help produce amazing positive results in your weight and health. Why would you choose any other way?

An Obesity Vaccine

The long-awaited good news that overweight and obese people have been expecting to happen for years may have finally arrived. But don't hold your breath thinking it will involve any permanent lifestyle changes in your diet or physical activity levels either. Instead, scientists think they may have developed the be-all, end-all holy grail for weight loss: an obesity vaccine.

Lead researcher Dr. Kim D. Janda, a professor of chemistry at the Scripps Research Institute, injected lab rats with a vaccine which targets the ghrelin levels to help stabilize weight. Dr. Janda's vaccine supposedly reduces the levels of ghrelin in the body so you don't get as hungry and, thus, lose weight. But the rats in his study continued to eat just as much food as the control rats and yet they still saw "about a 20 or 30 percent reduction in weight" because of this obesity vaccine.

"We have enabled the immune system to recognize a molecule that it ordinarily won't recognize," Dr. Janda noted.

However, it is worth noting that the mice were fed an unpalatable low-carb, low-fat diet and Dr. Janda wonders how effective the vaccine would be on what tends to be a high-carb, high-fat American diet.

"Whether active immunization against ghrelin would help prevent the development of obesity caused by...high-fat 'Western' diets or would facilitate weight loss once obesity is established" is unknown, the researcher concluded.

Vaccine or not, I do believe anyone starving themselves on such a diet would no doubt lose weight and feel like they've been run over by a truck in the process!

"The study shows our vaccine slows weight gain and decreases stored fat in rats," Dr. Janda explained. *"While food intake was unchanged in all testing groups, those who were given the most effective vaccines gained the least amount of weight. To have an impact on appetite and weight gain, ghrelin first has to move from the bloodstream into the brain-where, over long periods, it stimulates the retention of a level of stored energy as fat. Our study is the first published evidence proving that preventing ghrelin from reaching the central nervous system can produce a desired reduction in weight gain."*

Other researchers and companies have been busy working on a ghrelin-attacking vaccine for the past few years and human testing is already underway. Dr. Janda said he's not ready to try his vaccine in humans yet, but will be trying various formulations in larger animals very soon with the hopes that human testing can begin in the coming years.

"We want to do real basic work and make sure we do all our homework before we look at it in humans," he stressed. *"We could do it quickly, but it's prudent to know exactly what's going on."*

They are currently looking for a major pharmaceutical company to come on board to help market and develop a usable obesity vaccine. It is uncertain at this point if one shot or multiple shots would be needed to bring about weight loss. Of course, they are also working on making the vaccine into an oral medicine that may be available for doctors to write as a prescription.

How long have we been told about the great weight loss pills that are supposed to revolutionize the pharmaceutical industry and help the millions of overweight and obese people lose weight?!

WHEN WILL THE MADNESS FINALLY END! If you are fat, then stop waiting on science to make you a pill to lose weight. It is time for you to find an eating and exercise routine that you can stick with for the rest of your life and execute it. Why are we making weight loss so difficult? While this research is promising for people who struggle with their weight, Dr. Janda is quick to point out this is not the ultimate answer for the obesity problem.

"What we are saying — and what our study confirms — is that this looks like a serious workable solution to the problem," Dr. Janda stated. "And while much more research is needed to understand the full therapeutic potential of immunopharmacotherapy in combating obesity, these initial results are extremely positive. Right now it appears that active vaccination against ghrelin is one avenue that can slow weight gain and fat build-up in the body."

Interestingly, Dr. Janda was working on a vaccine against drug addiction when they stumbled upon this area of research regarding obesity and shifted gears.

"While there were numerous possible hormones involved in obesity that could be targeted, we decided that ghrelin would be a good starting point to examine such a hypothesis," Dr. Janda said.

Currently there are three active vaccines being used in the lab rats: Ghr1, Ghr2, and Ghr3. Ghr1 and Ghr3 have been the most effective in the tests so far compared with Ghr2 and the control models. The Janda study was supported by the National Institute of Diabetes, Digestive, and Kidney Disorders and The Skaggs Institute for Chemical Biology.

After reading this chapter, how many of you STILL think low-carb is a "fad" diet? Coming up next, we will see that the evidence building for low-carb diets is absolutely undeniable within research circles and that mainstream acceptance of the scientific data is imminent. This lesson should give you hope that your low-carb dietary choices are backed by a solid foundation of data that proves it is the healthy way of eating you know that it is.

LESSON #9
The evidence building for low-carb diets is undeniable

"The belief that 'dietary fat increases LDL cholesterol and therefore causes heart disease' led to enormous resistance to accepting studies showing benefits of low-carbohydrate diets. The science supporting low-carb diets as a healthy lifestyle and as a treatment for many medical problems is now well-established."

— **Dr. Eric C. Westman**, M.D., Director, Lifestyle Medicine Clinic and noted low-carbohydrate diet researcher at Duke University Medical Center

Our generation is at one of the most critical moments in the history of health the world has ever seen. Preventable diseases arc running amok and much of the blame can be placed on the flawed nutritional advice people have been following from those who are supposed to be authority figures when it comes to diet and disease. Despite all of their best efforts to convince us that eating higher amounts of "healthy" whole grains, lowering our fat intake, and cutting back on calories is the optimum diet, where has it gotten us? Fatter and sicker than ever before!

As of research released in 2006, the combined total number of people who have Type 2 diabetes or are considered pre-diabetic based on their insulin resistance reached an unbelievable 73.3 million Americans and the number has no doubt grown exponentially from there in just the past few years. That's already over one-third of the U.S. population and it doesn't even include those who are walking around with the disease and don't even know it yet. All of this is taking a toll on the American healthcare system to the tune of $132 billion annually based on added medical expenses and missed time from work in

2002 alone. Can you see why the healthcare problems in America are more of a nutritional education problem than an access or spending issue as the politicians in Washington, DC believe? We are reaching the breaking point where something dramatic needs to happen very soon with the way diabetes is treated and educate people on what they can do to control this awful disease before it is too late.

If you've ever been on a low-carb diet, then you have undoubtedly run into one or more of the following statements before:

"The Atkins Diet is dangerous for your heart!"
"If you eat all that fat on low-carb, you'll have a heart attack!"
"Who cares about weight loss, you're destroying your health!"

For those of us on the low-carb lifestyle, hearing statements like this has become just another one of the many challenges we face while on the journey to attaining amazing weight loss success and vastly improved health. After losing 180 pounds on the Atkins diet in 2004 and keeping it off ever since, would you believe I still have people challenging me to this very day about the so-called "dangers" of eating low-carb because of the alleged health problems it is supposed to induce in my body? My simple, yet honest response to these people is — when am I supposed to get all these health problems from low-carb? When?!

This kind of hyperbole about low-carb living has gone on long enough and quite frankly those who are still engaged in spreading such vitriolic hatred towards this diet are beginning to look quite foolish in the process. Whether the low-fat apologists like it or not, there is PLENTY of research coming out in support of livin' la vida low-carb that warrants an entire chapter of this book. And here it is. This by no means is a comprehensive list of all the low-carb diet studies that have been published in recent years (we could fill volumes of books with an unabridged listing of all the studies), but I have included some of the more notable and recent ones that have been released in the 21st Century supporting carbohydrate-restriction for a variety of health concerns.

Type 2 diabetes clinically "cured" by low-carb diet

A six-month study published in the December 19, 2008 issue of the scientific journal *Nutrition and Metabolism* by lead researcher Dr. Eric Westman from the Duke Lifestyle Medicine Clinic in Durham, North Carolina placed 84 predominantly obese women with a mean age of 52 who have Type 2 diabetes on a randomized version of one of two diets:

LCKD: A low-carb ketogenic diet with 20g carbs or less daily
LGRC: A low-glycemic, reduced-calorie diet with a 500 calorie deficit

The LCKD group (38 patients) followed the principles of the Atkins diet as outlined in *Dr. Atkins New Diet Revolution* by the late, great Dr. Robert C. Atkins while the LGRC group (46 patients) was instructed on *The GI Diet* by Rick Gallop. The study participants on the low-carb ketogenic diet were allowed to eat as many calories as they would like of meat and eggs while restricting their carbohydrate intake to 20g daily consisting of limited amounts of hard cheeses, soft cheeses, salad vegetables, and non-starchy vegetables. Meanwhile, the low-GI patients were told to reduce their calories by 500 from the amount they would consume to maintain their weight in order to produce a calorie deficit and 55 percent of their daily calories were required to come from low-glycemic index carbs.

Participants in both of these groups showed up at regular meetings with dietitians to discuss their diet with doctor's supervision, were provided glucose-lowering nutritional supplements to go along with their eating plan, and given an exercise routine to follow (30 minutes, three times a week) for a period of 24 weeks. At the end of the study, blood tests were run to measure their hemoglobin A1c (HgA1c) levels, a key health marker used to determine how well blood sugar is controlled in diabetic patients in the previous few months.

Interestingly, only 58.3 percent of the participants in both groups completed the study — the biggest complaints were refusal to do the diet as written, difficulty adhering to the diet, and time constraints. For those who did stay in the study, the low-carb ketogenic diet group participants consumed an average of 49g total carbohydrates daily compared with 149g total carbohydrates eaten by the low-glycemic diet group.

The LCKD group showed greater improvements in their HgA1c levels than the LGRC group did. In fact, diabetes medications were either reduced or completely eliminated in 95 percent of the low-carb diet participants compared with just 62 percent who ate a calorie-restricted low-glycemic index diet. The HDL "good" cholesterol in the LCKD group increased 5.6 compared to zero for the LGRC group. And the HgA1c levels dropped sharply from 8.8 percent down to 7.3 percent in the low-carb group while there was little statistical change in the low-glycemic diet group dipping down from 8.3 percent to 7.8 percent. Finally, despite the fact that the low-carb study participants ate 215 more calories per day than their low-glycemic counterparts (1,335 compared with 1,550), there was greater weight loss in the low-carb group (averaged an 11-pound reduction) versus the low-glycemic (averaged just under a 7-pound drop).

Dr. Westman, who is no stranger to conducting quality research on low-carb diets and their impact on diabetes, concluded that the answer to treating diabetes is a "simple" one that has long been overlooked and ignored by physicians treating diabetic patients.

"If you cut out the carbohydrates, your blood sugar goes down, and you lose weight which lowers your blood sugar even further," he said. *"It's a one-two punch."*

For far too long, the diabetes problem has been getting worse while the low-carb answer has been virtually ignored. Although he admits following a low-carb diet may not be easy, Dr. Westman explains this is a "therapeutic diet" essential for people who are "sick" with diabetes.

"These lifestyle approaches all have an intensive behavioral component," he added. *"In our program, people come in every two weeks to get reinforcements and reminders. We've treated hundreds of patients this way now at Duke and what we see clinically and in our research shows that it works."*

The study was funded by The Robert C. Atkins Foundation (AtkinsFoundation. org), but they were not involved in the planning, design or conduct of the study and had no involvement in the interpretation of the data or the preparation and approval of the manuscript. While many diabetes educators these days are catching on to the need for lowering glycemic carbohydrates for blood sugar control, Dr. Westman has shown there is an even greater improvement by eliminating even these supposedly "healthy" carbs as well.

"Low glycemic diets are good, but our work shows a no-glycemic diet is even better at improving blood sugar control," he noted. *"We found you can get a three-fold improvement in Type 2 diabetes as evidenced by a standard test of the amount of sugar in the blood. That's an important distinction because as a physician who is faced with the choice of drugs or diet, I want a strong diet that's shown to improve Type 2 diabetes and minimize medication use."*

Interestingly, when the researchers analyzed the changes in blood glucose control that occurred during the study, they found it probably had very little to do with the weight loss and more likely a result of the diet composition.

"This supports the concept that weight change and glycemic control are not serially linked but rather may be the result of the same pathophysiologic process, such as abnormal insulin metabolism," the researchers explained.

Although there are many people who regularly begin a low-carb diet on their own and call it the "Atkins diet," Dr. Westman warns diabetics against starting such a dietary regimen without the express supervision of a trained medical professional. You can find a doctor who specializes in low-carb diets by visiting my "List of Low-Carb Doctors" blog (LowCarbDoctors.blogspot.com).

Noted low-carb medical practitioner and researcher Dr. Mary C. Vernon from Lawrence, Kansas says scientific research is showing the way of eating promoted by Dr. Atkins may be exactly what is needed to effectively take on the diabetes dilemma.

"Sadly, confusion generated in the media over the past couple of years by competing business interests has misled Americans and caregivers," Dr. Vernon said. "As a result many have turned away from what is likely the most effective means to not only control diabetes with fewer medical interventions and reduced medications, but actually reverse the course of the epidemic: The Atkins Diet."

Dr. Vernon has presented her findings at the annual meetings of the American Diabetes Association as well as the American Society of Bariatric Physicians.

Low-carb weight loss is more than "water" weight

A study funded by the National Institutes of Health and the American Diabetes Association and published in the March 15, 2005 issue of the *Annals of Internal Medicine* concluded that livin' la vida low-carb does indeed lead to fast weight loss results and the weight loss is not water weight, a change in the dieter's metabolism or attributed to being bored with the diet as so many of the opponents of low-carb often declare to scare people away from beginning a low-carb plan.

Lead researcher Dr. Guenther Boden, a diabetes expert and Research Professor of Biochemistry at the Temple University School of Medicine, observed ten obese patients who have Type 2 diabetes when he put them on the Atkins diet. The first week of the study allowed the participants to eat the way they normally would and then the next two weeks they were required to limit their carbohydrate intake to 20g per day with full access to unlimited amounts of protein and fat. Dr. Boden was astounded to find that the patients in the study actually ate less calories "spontaneously" and yet they also burned fat (in other words, not just "water" weight loss) without experiencing a change in their metabolism.

"When carbohydrates were restricted, study subjects spontaneously reduced their caloric intake to a level appropriate for their height, did not compensate by eating more protein or fat, and lost weight," Dr. Boden noted. "We concluded that excessive overeating had been fueled by carbohydrates."

How about that? Eating carbohydrates leads to overeating, according to Dr. Boden. That runs directly counter to what other conventional health experts have said boldly proclaiming that people who restrict their carbohydrate intake are prone to binge eating. It also flies in the face of low-carb weight loss being all "water" weight. Because eight out of every ten diabetics are either overweight or obese and prone to developing various health conditions including heart disease and stroke, Dr. Boden believed a study needed to be done to see why livin' la vida low-carb works so well to help obese people with diabetes lose weight fast and bring about changes in their overall body fat, appetite and blood sugar levels.

This was the first-ever controlled study of the Atkins diet that measured the exact number of calories consumed and spent by the study participants while they remained at the research facility. Other low-carb diet studies have relied heavily on the study participants to be honest about their eating habits when they went home. Dr. Boden believes this one component about his study provides his research with more credibility and makes it less prone to manipulation from inaccuracies. That's why the results were so surprising to him.

"When we took away the carbohydrates, the patients spontaneously reduced their daily energy consumption by 1,000 calories a day," Dr. Boden revealed. "Although they could have, they did not compensate by eating more proteins and fats and they weren't bored with the food choices. In fact, they loved the diet. The carbohydrates were clearly stimulating their excessive appetites."

They reduced their caloric intake by one thousand calories (from 3100 to 2100 daily) when they started livin' la vida low-carb! In other words, they didn't need to go on a low-calorie diet watching and measuring every morsel of food they wanted to put in their mouth. They simply ate low-carb and allowed the natural process of satiety from the protein and fats they were consuming to make them feel satisfied and get away with eating less in the process. Interestingly, they did not eat more protein or fats when they had the opportunity, but rather they simply ate the same amount of those macronutrients sans the carbs. The result? They weren't as hungry and they actually ate less food and calories overall. In the end, they made better food choices than they were previously making.

But it was very evident to Dr. Boden that carbohydrates driving insulin levels upward were indeed the root cause of the hungry appetites his diabetic patients were experiencing and the low-carb lifestyle actually took care of that problem. Meanwhile, they simultaneously "loved the diet." Besides eating less calories and losing weight, the study participants also saw dramatic improvements in their blood glucose levels, their insulin sensitivity, a reduction in triglycerides of 35 percent and in total cholesterol of 10 percent in the very short study span. Weight loss and health improvements happened in just two weeks!

The high-fat, low-carb Inuit diet is healthy

Lead researcher Dr. Eric Dewailly, professor of Social and Preventive Medicine at Laval University, and his colleagues observed the health of nearly 1,000 Inuit people living in the northern section of Quebec where the diet consists primarily of wild game and very little carbohydrates. What the researchers found was truly remarkable in terms of comparing this decidedly low-carb way of eating to what most people consider a "healthy" diet. Despite the fact that they ate a rather high-protein, high-fat diet, Dr. Dewailly said this kind of nutritional approach actually protects against both heart disease and cancer. Did you hear that? Here is a scientific researcher extolling the virtues of consuming meat as a hunter-gatherer by stating the fact that it has been found to be an extremely healthy way to eat.

This research confirms what most low-carbers already knew — there are plenty of benefits to heart health when you are livin' la vida low-carb!

"The traditional Inuit diet is fats and proteins, no sugar at all," Dr. Dewailly explained. "It is probably one of the healthiest diets you can have. The human body is built for that."

WHOA, did he just say that the low-carb lifestyle that consists of lots of fat and protein with "no sugar at all" is the "healthiest" diet?! Yep, he sure did and that's not just his opinion either. He's backing it up with scientific proof that deserves to be front-page health news around the world. It coincides with other studies clearly showing a high-fat, low-carb diet is one of the best diets you could ever go on to protect against heart disease.

But there was scant mention of Dr. Dewailly's study anywhere in the media when it came out in December 2006 which is not surprising since most of the media and current health experts don't ever want to acknowledge an increase in fat and protein combined with a low-carb diet is actually good for you. If they let that cat out of the bag, then their little agenda to suppress the truth about what constitutes living healthy would have to stop.

But the evidence is piling up and this research doesn't lie.

"The study shows that [high-protein, high-fat, low-carb diets] still have huge benefit and protection," Dewailly added.

He explained that the Inuit people get selenium from eating whale skin which makes prostate cancer virtually nonexistent as well as most other cancers. But you can't discount the fact that a sugar-free diet protects against pancreatic cancer while a low-carb diet has been found to prevent esophageal cancer (we'll be discussing the mountain of research out there regarding the low-carb/ cancer connection in a later chapter). Again, where is the news coverage of these revolutionary scientific studies on carbohydrate-restricted diets?

Additionally, Dr. Dewailly argues that it's the consumption of healthy portions of high-protein, high-fat meats that keep the hearts of the Inuit people as healthy as a horse. The Inuit diet has long been the evidence that proves livin' la vida low-carb is indeed a sustainable way of eating over the long-term since it promotes the consumption of wild game and fish while openly shunning such modern nutritional garbage as high-carb, sugary junk foods and snacks. Unfortunately, though, these new modern foods to the Inuit people are tempting younger generations of Inuits to consume them which is causing severe havoc on their health.

But there is hope for the younger Inuit population in Canada if they simply return to their native diet. Eating the kind of low-carb, high-fat diet that they have traditionally consumed has actually been found to improve mental health as well as maintain normal weight and health indicators. The Inuit people should reject the cultural influences on their way of life from their neighbors to the South — the United States — and forge ahead with their tried and true native high-protein, high-fat diet.

Long-term low-carb heart health concerns unwarranted

"There have been no long-term studies showing low-carb is safe!"

That's what we keep hearing all the time from so many opponents of low-carb diets who have thrown that assertion out there in the open arena of ideas to attempt to silence advocates of low-carb. But now they're going to have to come up with another excuse because there's a long-term study that was paid for by the National Institutes of Health and appeared in the November 9, 2006 issue of the *New England Journal of Medicine*.

Dr. Thomas Halton, a former doctoral student in the Department of Nutrition at the Harvard School of Public Health, along with direction from lead researcher and associate professor of nutrition and epidemiology Dr. Frank Hu, conducted a 20-year study on the heart health effects of low-carb diet programs such as the Atkins diet. This is the first such study on the long-term effects of low-carbohydrate diets to be released to the public and it is quite revealing. The research team observed information from the past two decades of 82,802 women participating in the Nurses' Health Study which began in 1976 and tracked their diet and health with periodic questionnaires. The researchers tabulated each woman's overall diet score based on the amount of fat, protein, and carbohydrates they consumed as a percentage of their total caloric intake.

Scores ranged from 0 to 30, with 0 indicating low-fat, low-protein, but very high-carb while 30 was designated for high-fat, high-protein, and very low-carb. The lower the number meant the study subject was following a low-fat diet and was labeled with "low-fat-diet score." Conversely the higher the number translated into the study participant being on a low-carb diet and the score was described as the "low-carbohydrate-diet score." Dr. Halton wanted an even further breakdown of the low-carbohydrate-diet score, so he split them into two subgroups:

1. Carbohydrate/animal protein/animal fat intake
2. Carbohydrate/vegetable protein/vegetable fat intake

Over the 20-year study, the researchers found a little more than 2 percent of the study participants (1,994) had documented cases of coronary heart disease. However, the most amazing statistic among those who developed heart disease was the fact that the low-carbohydrate diet score participants were not a major part of those numbers. In fact, Halton had fully expected the risk of heart disease to go up among those who ate the low-carb/high-fat diet, but...

"It didn't, which was a little eye-opening," he said.

Additionally, none of the scores were manipulated or modified to account for physical activity levels, body-mass index, or the presence or absence of high blood pressure, high cholesterol, or diabetes. Even with these conditions present, the low-carbohydrate diet score group did not have an increased risk for coronary heart disease. Interestingly, Dr. Halton and his associates said neither the total amount of fat nor the total amount of carbohydrates increased the risk of coronary heart disease.

But, they did notice the kind of fat and carbs can certainly be better for you. For example, vegetable fat consumption led to a reduced risk of heart disease while excessive refined carbohydrate consumption typical of a low-fat diet was the strong culprit in those who did develop heart problems. The researchers believe it was the high glycemic load of foods like refined sugars and carbohydrates consumed by the low-fat diet score group that quickly elevated their blood sugar levels and actually led to a doubling of their risk of cardiovascular problems.

The American low-fat diet movement for the past three decades is one of the major reasons why the rate of heart disease among this group has specifically skyrocketed, Dr. Halton revealed.

"The way Americans are going low-fat is very unhealthy," he told Reuters. "They have a very high glycemic load. They're taking sugar. They're taking white bread. They're taking white rice and pasta. That certainly isn't the answer."

Noteworthy, too, was the conclusion by the researchers that when vegetable sources for both fat and protein were selected instead of animal sources, those in the low-carbohydrate-diet score group experienced another 30 percent lower risk of coronary heart disease.

"They had a 30 percent reduction in the risk of heart disease over 20 years, which I find shocking," Dr. Halton said.

Halton stated that this study should ease the concerns of those who are worried that low-carb diets are increasing the risks for heart disease because the evidence shows they are no worse than the low-fat diets.

"This study suggests that neither a low-fat dietary pattern nor a typical low-carbohydrate dietary pattern is ideal with regards to risk of CHD; both have similar risks. However, if a diet moderately lower in carbohydrates is followed, with a focus on vegetable sources of fat and protein, there may be a benefit for heart disease."

On the question that people will have about the gender of the study participants all being female, Halton contended "the pathology of heart disease is not all that different in men and women" so it was not a concern to him. Finally, Halton said he'd like to see a long-term study which proves low-carb lowers the overall risk of coronary heart disease. I would personally like to see a long-term study which proves anything positive about a low-fat diet.

My goal all along has never been to say low-fat is necessarily wrong and that low-carb is right, but to simply allow people to have all the evidence so they can make up their minds which one they want to do for the sake of their own weight and health. Too often we have heard from anti-low-carb voices when they portend low-carb might be good for weight loss, but you'll be harming your health in the process. This is untrue.

We now know those concerns were greatly exaggerated and quite possibly turned off millions of would-be low-carb success stories from even trying this healthy diet all because of needless fear mongering. I think it's interesting what Dr. Hu said regarding Dr. Halton's study because it illustrates just how prevailing the stereotype of the Atkins/low-carb diet approach has become, even seeping into the mindset of those working in research laboratories.

"This study doesn't mean that you should load your plate with steak and bacon," he remarked.

I wonder what gives him the idea that eating a low-carbohydrate diet is about loading up solely on animal-based foods like steak and bacon. Could it be because that's been the most oft-repeated rumor spread by those in the media and current health experts about the low-carb lifestyle since it rose to widespread popularity? Anyone who has read any of the many books about low-carb, including *Dr. Atkins' New Diet Revolution*, knows it is so much more than meat. Those of us in the real world of livin' la vida low-carb know that we can eat a very flavorful variety of not just meats, but cheeses, eggs, low-glycemic fruits, and non-starchy vegetables. You can see for yourself exactly what I eat on a daily basis by looking at my low-carb menus blog (LowCarb-Menu.blogspot.com).

Check this out, though! Dr. Hu said even if people on a low-carb diet do eat more animal-based sources of fat and protein, he concluded "the adverse effects of animal products might be counterbalanced by reducing refined carbohydrates."

This highly-respected Harvard health professor just said there is nothing wrong with eating animal products as part of a healthy diet if combined with a low refined-carb diet. Is this the beginning of the rebirth of a dietary revolution? Studies like this are exactly why I keep telling people to just ignore those who seek to tear them down just because they are livin' la vida low-carb. Keep smiling, doing what you know you are supposed to do, and one day you will have the last laugh. Science is catching up to us and fast!

Dr. Halton says he is ready for the darts that will be hurled at him because of this study because he knows it "goes against a lot of what people think is common wisdom for nutrition." This isn't just some passing headline news that's here today, gone tomorrow. The ramifications of a long-term study like this putting low-carb in a favorable light has the potential to unravel a lot of the dietary science we have put up with for far too long. Government and health leaders need to take notice of this study and broadcast it to every man, woman and child in the United States of America.

This isn't a game; it's the future of this country. Will we continue to wallow in the obsolete theories of our past which have been the foundation of what we believe about diet and health? Or do we learn from our mistakes, admit we were wrong, and begin moving forward with educating the public that there are other ways to bring about improvements in weight and health? That's the clear and unadulterated choice we have before us in the here and now. Which direction will our nation's health leaders choose to go down?

Acne can be cleared with a low-carb diet

How many of us grew up hearing the advice from well-meaning people to stop eating chocolate and fried foods to help cure our acne when we were teenagers? I know I did and I even tried doing it (with very little success!) thinking that made sense. But now researchers out of Australia conducted a study that found it wasn't the fat that was making all those zits pop up on our faces, but rather the overabundance of sugary, processed, high-carb foods instead!

Lead researcher Dr. Neil Mann, associate professor of Nutrition and Food Science at RMIT University in Melbourne, Australia, observed 50 teenage boys with a moderate to severe acne problem over a three-month period to see what impact diet would have on their skin condition.

The study participants were randomly divided into two groups:

HIGH-CARB: Typical teenage diet of refined carbs/processed foods.
LOW-CARB: Healthier diet with more low-GI whole foods.

Obviously, the LOW-CARB group ate more foods that took time for the body to digest and, thus, they did not experience the wild swings in their blood sugar which dramatically raises insulin levels that is typical of a HIGH-CARB diet. In fact, most of the carbohydrates that would normally be consumed in a teenager's diet were replaced with high-quality sources of protein such as red meat and fish in the LOW-CARB group. At the end of the study, Dr. Mann found the acne among those in the LOW-CARB group had "improved dramatically, by more than half." You read that right — the LOW-CARB group reduced their breakouts by more than 50 percent! WOW!

"This new evidence suggests that a more natural diet, comprised of minimally processed foods, may serve as a defense against acne," he explained.

Dr. Mann said he was surprised by the incredible improvements that the LOW-CARB group saw that were seemingly based solely on their diet, something many dermatologists and health experts have long claimed has no effect on acne. But he believes the high levels of insulin generated by the typical HIGH-CARB diet that most teenagers eat is the root cause behind their facial breakouts. Lowering the carbohydrate intake of the study participants resulted in a reduction of the insulin levels and a correlating improvement in the production of pimples.

"It's as clear as day," Dr. Mann boasted of the faces in the LOW-CARB group.

He said it is natural for teenagers to develop zits as their bodies go through the typical changes associated with that period in their life.

"When you go through puberty you produce a lot of growth hormone that actually makes you insulin resistant temporarily," he revealed. "With chronically high levels of insulin you're going to get blockages in the pores and extra oil building up under the skin."

Not surprisingly, the typical HIGH-CARB diet makes the problem that much worse which is why putting them on a LOW-CARB diet is an excellent, all-natural way to help bring about drastic improvements in the complexion of adolescents.

"We're convinced the results show that if people do suffer from acne badly this sort of dietary change is going to help them a great deal," Dr. Mann concluded.

Further studies will undoubtedly be conducted in the future to test this theory regarding the correlation between insulin levels and acne even more which could make for yet another fascinating positive side effect of livin' la vida low-carb. For more information on this topic, you might want to check out a 2006 book written by *Paleo Diet* author Dr. Loren Cordain entitled *The Dietary Cure For Acne* (DietaryAcneCure.com). In fact, Dr. Cordain has published a series of scientific papers outlining the central role diet plays in causing acne, so check it out.

Low-carb is a reasonable alternative to low-fat diets

In a study published in the March 2007 issue of *American Journal of Clinical Nutrition*, lead researcher Dr. Kevin C. Maki, investigator at the Chicago, IL-based Radiant Research, wanted to see if lowering the glycemic load and increasing the protein content of the study participants' diet would provide any advantages when it comes to weight loss (a theory already substantiated by previous research). Also, the researchers were looking at body fat composition and cardio-vascular risk among the overweight and obese adults participating. Observing 86 study participants over an initial 12-week period and then for an additional 24 weeks thereafter, Dr. Maki split them into one of two dietary groups:

RGL—A reduced-glycemic load diet group

OR

LFPC—A traditional low-fat, portion-controlled diet group

The RGL group was specifically told to eat until they were satisfied, maintain a low-carb dietary intake for the first two weeks (simulating the Induction phase of the Atkins diet), and then to start adding low-glycemic index carbohydrate afterwards. They were not required to count a single calorie (something I've never done on my low-carb plan) and were permitted to eat as much as they wanted during the study. The LFPC group was the control for this study and was told to lower their fat intake and portion sizes aiming for an energy deficit of 500-800 calories/day. The total calories would vary by individual based on their activity level and food intake. But it was basically a low-fat, low-calorie, portion-controlled diet.

At the end of 12 weeks, the RGL group had lost nearly twice as much weight (10.8 pounds) as the LFPC group (5.5 pounds). Additionally, the RGL group lost more than double the amount of fat (4.2 pounds) as the LFPC group (2 pounds). As significant as these three-month comparison totals were, they became statistically less important at the end of 36 weeks. Weight loss as well as body fat composition after the six-month study concluded remained virtually the same as it was at the end of week 12. However, the researchers did note that the positive change in HDL cholesterol among the RGL group was twice that of the LFPC group. Dr. Maki concluded that the low-carb RGL diet is "a reasonable alternative to a low-fat, portion-controlled eating plan for weight management."

Atkins diet best for weight loss, health improvements

Lead researcher Dr. Christopher D. Gardner, from the Stanford, CA-based Stanford Prevention Research Center and Associate Professor in the Department of Medicine at the Stanford University Medical School, and his fellow researchers conducted a one-year randomized trial called "A TO Z: A Comparative Weight Loss Study." Recognizing the severity of the obesity epidemic that has become what they describe as "the single most significant nutrition-related health issue of the new millennium," Dr. Gardner wanted to know in his study if the monopolistic low-fat dietary recommendations that have been coming directly from government and health agencies for decades really were better for weight loss and improvements in various health outcomes than some of the other popular weight loss methods to come out in recent years, including the lower-carb Zone and Atkins diets, for example.

Observing 311 women who were overweight or obese at baseline with a body mass index of 27-40, non-diabetic, pre-menopausal, and willing to participate in the 12-month study, the researchers divided up the study participants into one of four diet groups:

ATKINS—(20g carbs daily for 2-3 months, 50g daily thereafter)
ZONE—(40-30-30 ratio of carbs to protein to fat)
LEARN—(55-60% carb intake, less than 10% saturated fat)
ORNISH—(No more than 10% calories from fat)

Additional recommendations for each study group regarding exercise, supplements, and other behavioral strategies for being successful on each plan as prescribed by the various diet books used were also provided to the study participants. Dr. Gardner said each of the study participants were also given eight weeks of intensive education from a nutritionist about their respective diet plan and then left on their own for the remaining ten months of the study.

While the primary outcome studied was weight loss, the researchers were also interested in some of the secondary health outcomes such as differences in cholesterol, including LDL, HDL, and triglycerides, body fat percentage, waist-to-hip ratio, fasting insulin and glucose levels, and blood pressure. Each of the study participants were measured for their progress on their specified diet plan at the beginning of the study, after two months, after six months, and then at the end of the 12-month study.

Interestingly, although the percentage of study participants who were able to stay on their specified diet plan was not statistically different, it was the AT-KINS group that led the pack for retaining the most dieters for the duration of the study among the four study groups:

ATKINS—88 percent
ZONE—77 percent
LEARN—76 percent
ORNISH—78 percent

So, what did Dr. Gardner and his team find at the end of the study? Weight loss among the ATKINS group was statistically higher as compared with the other diet groups, including triple the weight loss of the ZONE group, nearly twice as much weight loss as the LEARN group, and more than double the weight loss of the ORNISH group. Statistically speaking, there was very little difference in the weight loss between the ZONE, LEARN, and ORNISH groups.

While most people expected the ATKINS group to produce higher weight loss, the unexpected aspect of Dr. Gardner's study is what happened to the health of the individuals who followed the popular low-carb dietary plan as compared to the others. One of the frequent criticisms of the high-fat, low-carbohydrate nutritional approach is the assertion that it can lead to certain health complications, including the loss of muscle mass rather than body fat, a rise in blood pressure, and other such heart health risks. But this study confirms most of those arguments are all for naught.

The body mass index of the ATKINS group at the end of the study had been reduced by more than three times as much as the ZONE group and twice as much as the ORNISH group. At the same time, the body fat percentage loss for the ATKINS group after 12 months was three times higher than the LEARN and ZONE groups and twice as high as the ORNISH group. This echoes what previous research found regarding body fat loss on a low-carb diet.

As for cholesterol, LDL remained relatively stable among all groups except for the ORNISH group which saw a noticeable drop, but it was the HDL "good" cholesterol and triglycerides numbers that were dramatically different. The ORNISH group saw HDL remain exactly the same after 12-months (not good!) while the ZONE and LEARN groups saw equally modest increases in HDL. But it was the ATKINS group's rise in HDL that was more than double that of ZONE and LEARN while their triglycerides fell twice as much as ORNISH and LEARN groups and seven times as much as the ZONE group. Increased HDL above 50 and significantly decreased triglycerides below 100 are two of the best tell-tale signs that someone is following their low-carb plan correctly. You can't fake your way doing low-carb without these tests finding you out!

While the waist-to-hip ratio and blood glucose levels were not statistically different among all groups (although the ATKINS group again saw a greater drop in insulin levels), blood pressure among the ATKINS group was significantly lower than all the other groups, including nearly four times lower than the OR-NISH group.

This groundbreaking study was published in the March 6, 2007 issue of *Journal of the American Medical Association*.

Dr. Gardner admits this was a smaller study and that his research should not be misconstrued as an endorsement of the Atkins low-carb diet. However, he did say the previous rush to judgment about the low-carb nutritional approach was probably a bit premature.

"This [study] is more evidence for shifting to low-carbohydrate diets," he said.

He added that the average weight loss among the ATKINS group was only about 10 pounds each and that several of the groups had people who lost 30 pounds or more, which proved that there are multiple ways to lose weight. However, Dr. Gardner admitted there were limitations in his study that are impossible to measure, including whether the dietary changes are the key to permanent weight loss or if there are qualities about individuals that make them more prone to success.

"We need to find out what internal mechanisms are at work in people to make them successful and bottle it up somehow," he exclaimed.

He said there was a noticeable drop in performance among all groups when they were left to do their respective diet on their own following the eight weeks with a nutritionist. Dr. Gardner believes the support the dieters received was a key to their success early on regardless of the plan they were using. This is proof that having a weight loss buddy could be a beneficial ingredient for people desiring weight loss.

Foreshadowing his future research on carbohydrates as it relates to obesity, Dr. Gardner wants to study whether there is a limit on the carbohydrate intake for people to consume for weight loss.

"Is there a threshold on the continuum of carbohydrates consumed," he asked. "Is it below 40 percent [of calories], 30 percent? That's what I'd like to know."

Regarding his decision to conduct this study comparing the Atkins diet with three other higher-carb diet plans, Dr. Gardner said he feels the low-fat diet has been too heavily publicized and recommended without seeing any real beneficial results to make a dent in the health and obesity crisis we now find ourselves facing.

"People have been asking about diets for years," he stated. "We think it's time to give them some answers."

Although there have been widespread concerns about what is allegedly lacking in the Atkins diet, the researchers concluded that this particular diet is just as good a place to start for people who are committed to losing weight and living a healthy lifestyle.

"These findings [in the study] have important implications for clinical practice and health care policy," the researchers remarked. "Physicians whose patients initiate a low-carbohydrate diet can be reassured that weight loss is likely to be at least as large as for any other dietary pattern and that the lipid effects are unlikely to be of immediate concern."

Convincing the medical community of this fact is now the real challenge. How much longer will they continue to ignore monumental studies like this one while millions upon millions of people keep getting fatter and sicker than they've ever been before following the low-fat recommendations, hmmm? Interestingly, this study was underwritten with grants from the NIH, the Community Foundation of Southeastern Michigan, and Human Health Service. Will this funding trend for low-carb research from our nation's top health entities continue based on the positive response Dr. Gardner found in his study about the Atkins diet? We shall see.

Saturated fat consumption reduces inflammation, fat in the blood

In a study published in the November 29, 2007 issue of the scientific journal *Lipids*, lead researcher Dr. Jeff S. Volek, PhD, RD from the Department of Kinesiology at the University of Connecticut and his team of outstanding researchers (including Dr. Richard Feinman, Dr. Stephen Phinney, and Dr. Cassandra Forsythe, among others) tested the various components of metabolic syndrome comparing a carbohydrate-restricted diet with a low-fat diet in overweight men and women over a 12-week period. The study participants were split into one of two groups:

VLCKD—(very low-carb ketogenic diet) — 1504 calories
Fat/Protein/Carbohydrate ratio of 59/28/12

OR

LFD — (low-fat diet)— 1478 calories
Fat/Protein/Carbohydrate ratio of 24/20/56

What did Dr. Volek and his team of researchers find? Total saturated fatty acids in the blood actually decreased in the VLCKD group while the anti-inflammatory markers also "significantly decreased." Meanwhile, the LFD group, which consumed two-thirds less saturated fat than the VLCKD group, saw an increase in total saturated fat in the bloodstream despite reducing fat intake. This was totally unexpected as the conventional wisdom regarding saturated fat consumption is that it causes an increase in inflammation which leads to a worsening of metabolic syndrome conditions and overall health. But that's not what happened.

"A very low-carbohydrate diet resulted in profound alterations in fatty acid composition and reduced inflammation compared to a low-fat diet," the researchers concluded.

So what are we to make of this research in light of all we've ever been told about saturated fat? Doctors and nutritionists have long told their patients with metabolic syndrome symptoms to eat a low-fat diet and now science like this one is showing the shortsightedness of this unproven recommendation. Livin' la vida low-carb is making great strides behind-the-scenes because it is an excellent way to reduce triglycerides and other essential health markers related to inflammation.

Dr. Volek says his study shows how a controlled-carbohydrate nutritional approach is "adding to the evolving picture of improvement in general health beyond simple weight loss in keeping blood glucose and insulin under control." And he believes hyperinsulinemia is at the root cause behind obesity, diabetes, and a whole host of other preventable diseases that all improve with the use of a low-carb diet.

Interestingly, the Volek study is only a small portion of a much larger study. The full study shows even more improvements in blood lipids (cholesterol) with the stunning conclusion that "lowering total and saturated fat only had a small effect on circulating inflammatory markers whereas reducing carbohydrate led to considerably greater reductions in a number of pro-inflammatory" markers. Dr. Volek says this puts the onus of health risks back on the consumption of carbohydrates.

"These data implicate dietary carbohydrate rather than fat as a more significant nutritional factor contributing to inflammatory processes," he stated.

Meanwhile, Dr. Richard Feinman from the biochemistry department at SUNY Downstate Medical Center says this new research demonstrably shows why carb-restricted diets work so remarkably well.

"The real importance of diets that lower carbohydrate content is that they are grounded in mechanism: carbohydrates stimulate insulin secretion which biases fat metabolism towards storage rather than oxidation," Dr. Feinman explained. "The inflammation results open a new aspect of the problem. From a practical standpoint, continued demonstrations that carbohydrate restriction is more beneficial than low-fat could be good news to those wishing to forestall or manage the diseases associated with metabolic syndrome."

Most damning against the low-fat diet hypothesis is the fact that although there was three-fold higher saturated fat consumption by the VLCKD group, it was the LFD group that experienced higher saturated fat in the blood.

"This clearly shows the limitations of the idea that 'you are what you eat,'" Dr. Volek explained. "Metabolism plays a big role. You are what your body does with what you eat."

I like that — *you are what your body does with what you eat.* And that's why I'm livin' la vida low-carb because I have all the confidence in the world that my body will do amazing things for my weight and health with the low-carb foods I consume. It already has! I've already experienced the benefits of controlled blood sugar and insulin levels, reduced triglycerides, lower blood pressure, increased HDL "good" cholesterol, and so much more than I could have ever expected from a high-fat, low-carb diet. It's hard not to appreciate something like this when your life has been so radically changed for the better. Now the research is showing us why.

Dr. Feinman succinctly repeated and summarized what I've written about often regarding saturated fat consumption on the low-carb lifestyle in the following statement about this study.

"I think even if you allow for tremendous error, it says that if carbs are low, saturated fat doesn't have much effect on the plasma composition," he remarked.

And that is why I don't worry about how much saturated fat I consume as long as my carbs are reduced. Now we have solid science to back it up!

A high-fat, low-carb diet does not raise cholesterol

Research published in the medical journal *Mayo Clinic Proceedings* in 2003 found some good news about the impact of a high-fat, low-carb diet on cholesterol levels in patients with atherosclerosis. Lead researcher Dr. James Hays, a cardiologist from the Newark, DE-based Christiana Care Health Services, observed 23 obese heart disease patients over a 6-week period on a high-fat, zero-starch diet after they had previously been put on a cholesterol-lowering statin drug treatment like Lipitor or Crestor. They remained on their drug treatment during the study, but something amazing happened within the course of the research. Each of the participants was told to eat more fat and that half of their calories must come from saturated fat! Wow! They were instructed to eat this way for six weeks in a row. Can you imagine how these people reacted to this? I bet there were a lot of jaws on the floor when they were instructed to eat more saturated fat!

At the end of the six weeks, the median weight loss was 5.2 percent of their body weight and similar amounts of body fat. Even more important was what happened to cholesterol — it remained steady while total triglycerides dropped significantly. Dr. Hays said he would expect this trend to continue for up to one full year. Here we are six years later and the results of this research are being proved anecdotally over and over again by people who are deciding to start livin' la vida low-carb for themselves! If you were skeptical about low-carb before, are you starting to become a believer in it now?

Improved bowel health from a low-carb diet

Now we have another health benefit from livin' la vida low-carb: improved inflammatory bowel disease (IBD), aka Crohn's disease and ulcerative colitis. Research from New Zealand shows low-carb living greatly IMPROVES bowel health.

Lead researcher Dr. Richard Gearry, MBChB, PhD, a consultant gastroenterologist from the New Zealand-based Christchurch Hospital and a senior lecturer at Otago University's Christchurch School of Medicine, and his researchers observed 100 patients with IBD over a six- to eight-week period and noticed that a low-carb diet helped ease the pain associated with this condition in over half of them. The study participants were treated at Box Hill Hospital in Victoria, Australia and Dr. Gearry decided to feed them foods that would not cause inflammation in the abdomen and bowel. Interestingly, the foods that do cause problems with IBD sufferers have a certain macronutrient composition that is well-known to most medical professionals.

"Doctors have known for a long time that patients know what affects their condition and causes symptoms," Dr. Gearry noted. *"Dietitians and doctors and scientists looked at this more closely and identified a number of foods that can cause abdominal pain and diarrhea."*

Wanna see a few of these culprit foods that make IBD worse? Check out this list: wheat, onions, milk, ice cream, apples, honey, legumes, and other fruits. The one thing these foods have in common is they are all high-carb foods.

"Often they are sugars and carbohydrates that are not absorbed when they pass through the bowel and when they get into the colon they can ferment and produce gas and pain," Dr. Gearry explained.

So, it's no surprise why livin' la vida low-carb worked so well for these patients with IBD. It's healthy for them and keeps their symptoms at bay. Best of all, the low-carb lifestyle was so simple and pleasurable enough to the study participants that they wanted to be on it.

"Most patients found that the diet was easy to implement and that the taste was acceptable, which is very important if people are to follow this diet," Dr. Gearry added.

The findings of this study were presented at the 2008 Australian Gastroenterology Week conference in Perth. Dr. Gearry is hopeful his research on the low-carb diet for Crohn's disease is embraced worldwide as a viable treatment option for this and other bowel conditions.

A hormone explains why low-carb diets burn fat so efficiently

Two different research teams have stumbled upon the discovery of a hormone in their studies that actually works as the very mechanism behind why fat-burning is so functional on a low-carb diet. The lead researcher on the first team, led by Dr. Eleftheria Maratos-Flier who serves as an investigator in the department of endocrinology, diabetes and metabolism at Beth Israel Deaconess Medical Center as well as an associate professor of medicine at Harvard Medical School, saw something peculiar happen to mice over a

30-day period that she fed a high-fat, low-carb diet — their lipid profile remained constant and didn't go up!

Dr. Maratos-Flier says this seemingly contradictory finding has to do with a hormone called FGF21, or fibroblast growth factor 21. It is found in the liver and is responsible for producing ketones when people consume a low-carb diet. These ketone bodies are then used to provide as much as 70 percent of the energy needs of someone eating this way.

This discovery did not go unnoticed by the researchers. Unfortunately, instead of promoting the Atkins diet as a means for lowering body fat, they instead turned to the possibilities this discovery could have on future pharmaceutical opportunities.

"We think these findings would increase the desirability of a drug that (might work through this mechanism) to increase fat oxidation in the liver," Dr. Maratos-Flier said.

Why try to make a pill that will replicate what the Atkins diet has already been shown to do a beautiful job of doing? This is just more irresponsible extrapolations pulled from an excellent study showing a high-fat, low-carb diet is beneficial. Get your head out of the sand already! She does acknowledge that this switch to fat-burning mode in the mice only happened when FGF21 was found in higher concentrations — either on a low-carb diet or during starvation. Contrary to what the naysayers say, these two are not the same.

The lead researcher on the second team, Dr. Steven Kliewer who is a professor of molecular biology at the Dallas, TX-based University of Texas Southwestern Medical Center, also found FGF21 breaks down stored fat in animals consuming a high-fat, low-carb diet as well as fasting.

"[A high-fat, low-carb diet] turned on a starvation response, even when the animals were feeding," Dr. Kliewer noticed. "They switched from using carbohydrates to fat stores as an energy supply."

Dr. Kliewer said this is a natural reaction in animals to a shortage of food which causes them to move less and sleep more in order to store up energy. He was surprised that a single hormone could literally "flip the whole metabolic profile" and that it can actually serve as a balancing mechanism for consuming too many calories.

"What's really exciting is that mice with excess FGF21 — even when they are fed — look like they have fasted," Dr. Kliewer found.

Somewhere up in heaven today, Dr. Atkins has got to be smiling from ear to ear. This is exactly what he was talking about when he described his diet as giving people a "metabolic advantage." The fact that science is just now catching up to what the late great Dr. Robert C. Atkins was sharing decades ago proves he was a man long before his time (I'll discuss the legacy of this amazing man who changed my life forever in an upcoming chapter of this book).

Dr. Kliewer admitted that this fat-burning process "makes sense" when you stop and think about it.

"During fasting, the liver hormone communicates with adipose tissue to send fat to the liver," he said. "It turns on the metabolism of fat into ketone bodies — and at the same time, it sensitizes the animals to going into torpor to conserve energy."

He added that there is an "obvious possibility that FGF21 accounts for the proposed positive effects of the Atkins diet — including weight loss and an increase in [HDL] 'good' cholesterol."

While Dr. Kliewer states that FGF21 might explain why the Atkins diet works, Dr. Maratos-Flier brought up the argument that this is only true in mice right now and it is unclear of the impact on humans. I suppose she's simply unable to believe the same results could be true in humans as well. To her credit, Dr. Maratos-Flier is planning on studying FGF21 levels in human subjects next over a period of a few days, although it would be better to do longer term studies of weeks, months and years. Perhaps that study will lead to longer studies.

Both of these studies were funded by the National Institutes of Health (NIH) as well as Takeda Pharmaceuticals, the Robert A. Welch Foundation, the Betty Van Andel Foundation, the Smith Family Foundation Pinnacle Program Project Award from the American Diabetes Association, and the Howard Hughes Medical Institute. The results of both of these studies were published in the June 2007 issue of the scientific journal *Cell Metabolism*.

Describing this research as "the most exciting" study he has ever worked on, Dr. Kliewer wants to continue looking at the role of FGF21 in increasing lifespan.

"Starvation and restricted diets are linked to some fascinating physiology including longevity," he noted. "In the long term, I would like to investigate the role of FGF21 in aging, since caloric restriction has been linked to an extended life span in many species."

It certainly sounds fascinating to see a low-carb diet being observed in this manner. Who knows what the implications could be. We'll be watching!

Gene found in fruit flies may explain the efficacy of low-carb

Not a lot of people know what the medical condition known as "metabolic syndrome" is, but chances are many people are walking around right now with it and haven't got a clue that they do. The quadruple threat of obesity, insulin resistance, heart disease, and high cholesterol is literally destroying the health of millions of people who stand to benefit from making some basic changes in their diet. That's the conclusion of some research that found an impressive new treatment option for people who have metabolic syndrome and even explains the mechanism behind why the Atkins diet is so effective in combatting it.

Lead researcher Dr. Sean Oldham, assistant professor at the Burnham Institute for Medical Research, found a single gene discovered in Drosophila fruit flies that helps to regulate vital regulators such as insulin, glucose and fat metabolism in the body. A mutant form of the gene called TOR, an acronym for the "target of rapamycin" gene that is present in virtually every plant and animal in the world, was created and bred with the fruit flies so Dr. Oldham and his fellow researchers could follow the gene's pathway to see what impact it would have on them.

What they found was the mutant TOR was directly responsible for reducing the influence of that gene on the body and led to a lowering of blood glucose levels and cholesterol. Additionally, an insulin-signal mediator in the body called FOXO was also blocked to show improvements in the glucose and cholesterol levels. Interestingly, the fruit flies with the mutated TOR lived longer than the control group of fruit flies.

Before this study, the exact function of the TOR gene was unknown as it relates to insulin-regulation and metabolic syndrome. It certainly provides scientific evidence in support of the Atkins diet for controlling metabolic syndrome.

"This study provides the first direct evidence that reducing TOR function could be clinically beneficial to counter insulin resistance, metabolic syndrome and diabetes," Dr. Oldham explained. *"We believe further studies on fruit flies are invaluable to discovering more details about this pathway, and will give us indispensable insight into pathological aspects of aging and senescence."*

The study's findings appear in the August 8, 2006 issue of the scientific journal *Cell Metabolism.*

What does all of this mean for people who are livin' la vida low-carb? Well, actually, this is NOT new information for us because we already knew the Atkins low-carb approach is an excellent way to control insulin levels and blood sugar. Dr. Oldham said his study revealed "unexpected and novel levels" of insulin regulation and lends credence to the much-maligned low-carb weight loss plan over the past few years.

"This study provides the first details of how TOR may... [work in the] coordination of weight reduction effects caused by caloric restriction and, in humans, it may explain the effects of the Atkins diet," Dr. Oldham said.

He added that the lowering the TOR function could very well be the treatment option researchers have been looking for regarding metabolic syndrome and insulin resistance. They will use this information to begin working on new drugs that would reduce TOR levels in the body, Dr. Oldham added.

Why would they do this when the study just concluded this can happen naturally in the body by livin' la vida low-carb? How is taking an expensive new drug with whatever side effects it will have supposed to change the bad lifestyle habits of the people eating sugar and excessive carbohydrates? Do these people who want these drugs think they will have the luxury of eating junk food all day as long as they just take their pill? Ugh!

You don't need a drug to control your obesity or metabolic syndrome. The answer really is as simple as making a lifetime commitment to a new way of eating that has improved the weight and health of tens of millions of people worldwide. That's livin' la vida low-carb, baby!

Dr. Oldham's study was supported by a grant from the National Heart Lung and Blood Institute of the National Institutes of Health, and with support from The Fishman Fund.

High-fat, low-carb diet drops insulin levels significantly

A study out of Israel published in the September 29, 2008 issue of the scientific journal *Acta Pædiatrica* by lead researcher Moshe Phillip, MD, Director of the Institute for Endocrinology and Diabetes in the National Center for Childhood Diabetes at Schneider Children's Medical Center of Israel, shows a random side-by-side comparison of three specific dietary approaches on the weight and health markers of 55 obese youth.

They were put on one of the following diets:

HIGH-FAT, LOW-CARB
MODERATE FAT, LOW-CARB
HIGH-CARB, LOW-FAT

The study participants had their health and weight markers measured after an overnight fast at baseline, following 12 weeks on their specific diet plan, and then again after nine months. What were the results? While there was "no significant differences" between the three groups in terms of body mass index and body fat percentage changes, there was one very clear distinction between the low-carb and low-fat diet. Insulin!

Insulin levels did the whole dipsy-doodle thing when they "decreased significantly" on both of the low-carb diet groups. The high-carb low-fat diet didn't fare so well with controlling insulin. But this is not surprising. As Gary Taubes shared in his book *Good Calories, Bad Calories*, carbohydrates drive insulin which leads to obesity and disease. Is it any wonder why the low-carb diets were far superior to the high-carb, low-fat one in controlling this essential blood sugar stabilizing hormone? It may not be to you and me, but this is big news to the medical establishment apparently.

Dr. Phillip and his research team concluded that while the weight loss was similar among all of the diets and that low-carb diets "apparently have no advantage over high-carbohydrate low-fat diets" in that respect, the plummet in insulin levels in the two low-carb groups is what they describe as "noteworthy" since Type 2 diabetes, the result of consistently high levels of insulin, is becoming more and more prevalent in kids and teenagers suffering from metabolic syndrome.

"The impact of low-carbohydrate diets in obese and insulin-resistant youth warrants further investigation," the researchers concluded.

Absolutely this subject should be studied more and the findings from that research should be shouted loud and clear for people far and wide to hear.

SCD-1 gene in the liver turns carbs into stored body fat

Research on the negative impact of carbs on weight and health sanctioned by the National Institutes of Health (NIH) is adding yet another layer of scientific truth and confirmation to what most of us who are livin' la vida low-carb already know. Lead researcher James M. Ntambi, PhD, Katherine Berns Von Donk Steenbock Professor of Biochemistry and Nutritional Sciences at the University of Wisconsin-Madison, and his team of researchers have discovered a specific gene in the liver known as SCD-1, short for stearoyl-Coenzyme A desaturase 1.

It turns out this SCD-1 gene may be the culprit in why some people who eat a high-carb diet keep gaining and gaining weight while others who consume the same diet don't. Apparently, this gene actually causes dietary carbs to be turned into stored body fat rather than being broken down for energy. Conversely, mice that did not have SCD-1 in their liver were able to use the carbohydrates instead of having it turn to fat.

Dr. Ntambi even fed a starchy, sugary diet to mice without SCD-1 in their liver and the excessive carbohydrates were used up and not stored. In other words, the carbs were not a contributing factor to any weight gain in the mice without SCD-1. But normal functioning livers in the control mice with the presence of SCD-1 saw just the opposite happen — the high-carb diet they consumed quickly poured on the body fat by eating the exact same food.

In the battle against the bulge, Dr. Ntambi said his study shows that genetic liver function seems to play a more critical role than thought that may react differently in people with varying levels of the SCD-1 gene.

"It looks like the SCD gene in the liver is responsible for causing weight gain in response to a high-carbohydrate diet, because when we take away the gene's activity the animals no longer gain the weight," he said. "These findings are telling us that the liver is a key tissue in mediating weight gain induced by excess carbohydrates."

The results of this study were published in the December 5, 2007 issue of *Cell Metabolism*.

As much as the current health experts talk about how consuming a high-carb, sugary diet is perfectly fine for people to manage their weight, along comes a monkey wrench in that theory that is invariably tied to genetics. It makes you wonder just how many people are walking around with this SCD-1 factor going on in their liver.

And the eye-opening results of this study are not lost on Dr. Ntambi who believes this study should open the door for even more research into the damning role of carbohydrates in weight gain and producing excessive stored fat. He sees this as a solid first step in bringing about major changes in how obesity is treated in the future. If it can be determined that SCD-1 exists in a more concentrated form among the overweight and obese, then the golden opportunity to offer a natural, dietary solution like livin' la vida low-carb to them exists and should be actively promoted to them.

"We think that obese individuals, in general, may have higher SCD activity in both the liver and in adipose tissue," Dr. Ntambi explained. "So, they may have a higher capability of converting carbohydrate into fat."

This is some of the most amazing research in favor of low-carb as a viable option for people struggling with weight issues to come out over the past few years because it lends credibility to the idea that lowering your carbohydrates is a very good thing for a whole lot of people. It's an exciting development for people like me who found merit in this way of eating independent from what my doctor and common societal knowledge told me was right. I believe this study could be a godsend for others who struggle being overweight, too, because it could convince them to take charge of their own weight and health like I did.

Perhaps this is the kind of research that will finally get the traditionalists in the medical industry to think outside the box and realize there is something more to the idea that consuming sugar and foods that turn to sugar in the body are unhealthy and not conducive for weight management because of a genetic predisposition. Whether that has ever been clearly articulated before, it certainly has now with this study.

"This is a very good example of a diet-gene interaction," Dr. Ntambi noted.

In fact, this research is part of an ongoing look at other parts of the body where SCD-1 may exist, such as the liver, muscles, brain, pancreas and adipose tissue to see what would happen. When SCD-1 was nonexistent, it didn't matter how many carbohydrates the researchers fed the mice — they didn't gain a single pound! It makes me wonder if my wife Christine is fortunate enough to have a low amount of SCD-1 in her body since she can get away with eating a lot more carbs than I can and maintain her weight. I'm so jealous!

Interestingly, Dr. Ntambi found a peculiar and distinctive dichotomy among those mice that lacked the SCD-1 gene — they GAINED weight on a diet higher in fat versus a diet high in sugary carbs and low in fat which protected their health as well. In other words, a low-carb diet provided no weight management benefit to them which lends credence to my philosophy that people need to find the nutritional plan that works for them and follow that individualized program to properly take care of their own weight and health.

So what does all this mean? The first thing that pops in my mind is how meaningless it is to have universal health recommendations for the general population. Plus, I'm thinking out loud here, but there ought to be a test where people can determine what level of SCD-1 is in their liver. I'm not a doctor, but it doesn't seem like this would be very hard to do if you had a blood test of the liver conducted. Those who have a strong presence of the gene should be placed on a strict low-carb diet regimen and those with little to no SCD-1 (ostensibly thinner by default) would be placed on a strict high-carb, low-fat diet.

In the mice that did not have any SCD-1, glucose production was basically shut down which prevented excessive insulin to be created in the body but subsequently led to an increased risk of hypoglycemia, or low blood sugar. Additionally, glycogen stores are not able to be created because the oleic acid, which helps with the breakdown of carbs, is rendered useless since the body converts them into energy.

"It looks to us that if you don't have enough oleic acid — which the SCD enzyme makes — then the carbohydrate does not proceed through normal glucose metabolism," Dr. Ntambi concluded.

To confirm this, the researchers added oleic acid supplements to the diet of these SCD-1 lacking mice and their metabolism returned to normal function. But it looks like the more carbs consumed, the higher amount of SCD-1 is present which can produce an overflow of oleic acid which then leads to stored fat and thus obesity. So it's never a good idea to go too overboard on the carbohydrates, simple or complex, as has been previously suggested and encouraged many times before by supposedly educated health "experts." Dr. Ntambi agrees.

"Too much carbohydrate is not good," he remarked. "That's basically what we are saying."

Well, it's about time somebody in the medical research world said it and I hope this is merely the start of an exciting new trend. My desire is that this research will continue moving forward by Dr. Ntambi and other courageous researchers willing to let the data speak for itself without being dictated by any preconceived notions or low-fat dogma.

Epilepsy seizures controlled by a high-fat, low-carb diet

A Colorado-based father of three named Michael started a web site called AtkinsForSeizures.com to help educate the population about how the Atkins diet can help treat and manage epilepsy. After he started reading about the research on epilepsy conducted by The Johns Hopkins Pediatric Neurology Center which recommended the low-carb, high-fat *Ketogenic Diet* written by John Freeman, he knew he had found some hope that his little girl could finally get some lasting relief from her seizures by implementing the low-carb lifestyle. Michael and his wife Tammy had tried everything, including six different drug treatment options, but they all had failed until they put their daughter on low-carb. Today these parents proudly proclaim that their daughter doesn't take ANY drugs to manage her epilepsy and only has 15 seizures each day now rather than the 100+ she used to suffer from when she was highly medicated!

THANK YOU Michael for stepping up to the plate and being a shining beacon of light for the thousands of families who feel so hopeless and helpless about what to do about the seizures that their loved ones endure. You took what could have been a nightmare story in your family and turned it into something very positive in an effort to help others. You are a BIG HERO in my book and I am so glad I found your web site. Also be sure to check out Dr. Deborah Snyder's book *Keto Kid* about how a ketogenic high-fat, low-carb diet helped her son Bryce control his epileptic seizures as well.

Low-carb beats Mediterranean, low-fat diet for weight loss, health

A well-publicized weight loss study comparing a low-carbohydrate, Mediterranean, and low-fat diet was released and published in the July 17, 2008 issue of *New England Journal of Medicine*. All the headlines were screaming about how the Atkins diet is best and livin' la vida low-carb is champion of them all. It was in virtually every newspaper, local and national television news outlets, and all the health and weight loss blogs — A BIG STORY!

And because it put low-carb living in such a positive light as compared with the low-fat diet or the much-beloved Mediterranean diet, you would think I'd be a happy camper touting this study as the best thing to happen for low-carb in a long while. But I can't get too thrilled about yet another study that shows such insignificant weight loss on a low-carb diet after two years and doesn't really require the participants to adhere closely to anything resembling the Atkins weight loss diet. This puts me in the minority I'm sure, but I have to say this is one big reason why I was disappointed with the study.

For those of you who missed it, lead researcher Iris Shai, R.D., Ph.D. from the S. Daniel Abraham International Center for Health and Nutrition in Israel, put 322 "moderately obese subjects" on one of three specific diets for a two-year observation:

LOW-CARB — Two months of 20g daily and slowly increase to 120g maximum for the duration of the study. Calorie-restriction was not required for this group.

MEDITERRANEAN — Calorie restriction of 1500 daily for females, 1800 daily for males consuming a diet with 35 percent fat from olive oil and nuts while consuming fish and poultry in place of higher-fat cuts of meat like pork and beef.

LOW-FAT — Calorie restriction of 1500 daily for females, 1800 daily for males consuming a diet with 30 percent of calories from fat as recommended by the American Heart Association (AHA)

Before I share the results, I have a few preliminary comments to make. While 20g carbs is indeed the Induction phase of the Atkins diet, 120g is nowhere close to ANY written phase of the Atkins diet — ever! Why do they put people on a low-carb diet and then let 'em go to town eating carbs later? 50 grams of carbs a day or less would be closer to correct.

I do like the fact there were no constraints on calories with the low-carb group and they just naturally kept their calories in check eating this way. The Mediterranean diet group looked fine, but I was surprised to see the low-fat diet group to include so much fat. While the AHA may consider a 30 percent fat diet to be low (and it is relatively speaking), it doesn't come anywhere near the kind of low-fat diet that infamous low-fat guru Dr. Dean Ornish suggests obese and unhealthy people go on to lower their weight and improve their health. His plan is a 10 percent fat diet with upwards of 70-80 percent carbohydrates. That's not what they did with this study which is too bad since it supposedly shows the difference between low-fat and low-carb.

Let's take a look at the results of this less-than-spectacular study: The LOW-CARB group lost the most amount of weight with 12.1 pounds followed by the MEDITERRANEAN group who lost 10.1 pounds and bringing up the tail was the LOW-FAT group who only shed 7.3 pounds. The researchers also observed what happened to HDL and triglycerides on these various nutritional approaches and the results were not at all shocking to those of us paying attention to our health — LOW-CARB saw a greater increase in their HDL "good" cholesterol and a more significant decrease in their dangerous triglyceride levels making their ratio of HDL/total cholesterol much better than the other groups.

Additionally, the A1C levels an important marker in blood sugar health, as well as their C-reactive protein levels, a key marker looking at dangerous inflammation, both improved more with the LOW-CARB group. By the way, rather than spending upwards of $100 at your doctor's office, you can now check your personal A1c levels at home for just $9 at Wal-mart with the Reli-On A1c testing kit (Reli-OnA1c.com). Everyone should know their A1c number.

As for the actual sources of fat and protein in the LOW-CARB group, low-carb researcher Dr. Eric Westman from Duke University asked Dr. Shai to clarify what kind of foods were consumed by members of the low-carb group. The notion that the researchers pushed a "vegetarian low-carb diet" as had been reported in the media is NOT what was done.

Here was Dr. Shai's response to Dr. Westman's inquiry:

This is kind of funny that some could think of a "vegetarian low-carb" diet. Is it a new suggested strategy? Could be an interesting idea but this wasn't the case here. Our low-carb diet was based on Atkins, the participants read the book, and the recipes were more or less comparable to what you know in the states.

Beef is the main red meat. What could be different? People here [in Israel] would not mix in the same meal meat and butter, a salad is considered a very rich one and not a lettuce based, and the main dressing is olive oil. As for beverages, it's the same kind that industry makes money on everywhere.

For example, a plate could include: fish or fried/not bread coated chicken/ or red meat, broccoli and mushrooms coated with eggs, roasted eggplants, vegetable salad (peppers, cucumber, green leaves, not lettuce) with olive oil dressing. I understand that some of the low-fat people find it hard to believe that such a low-carb diet was tremendously favorable within 2 years in a well designed study, but these are the facts and the science of tomorrow, with the next long-term studies in the pipeline, may confirm or not these findings.

So, as you can see, the LOW-CARB group did indeed follow more of a conventional Atkins diet approach in terms of the specific foods they ate, not a "vegetarian low-carb diet" as was widely reported by the media and mocked by the current health "experts." Although I'm not particularly overjoyed by this study out of Israel, that doesn't mean I don't appreciate the way it helped carry on the conversation about low-carb living across mainstream America and globally. If this excites people and gets them interested in learning more about the healthy low-carb lifestyle, then that's awesome!

Metabolic syndrome improved with the use of a low-carb diet

Published in the November 2005 issue of *Nutrition & Metabolism* was a study heralded as a "classic light bulb moment" and a scientific breakthrough for people who believe in livin' la vida low-carb. Dr. Richard Feinman of SUNY Downstate and Dr. Jeff Volek from the University of Connecticut were looking at the features of metabolic syndrome and discovered carbohydrate-restricted diets improve each of those factors. Metabolic syndrome includes anything that increases the risk of diabetes, stroke and heart disease, such as obesity, high triglycerides, low HDL "good" cholesterol, high blood sugar, hypertension, and insulin resistance.

While conventional wisdom has always been to lower your fat intake to improve metabolic syndrome, what Dr. Feinman and Dr. Volek could not believe is the fact that a low-carb lifestyle change, which tens of millions of Americans have used to lose weight and get healthy, is precisely what is needed to ward off each of those risk factors associated with it and the data has been right there the entire time.

"It's been staring us in the face for years," said Dr. Feinman. "Now we've connected the dots."

Medical experts have been looking for a way to treat metabolic syndrome for many, many years and now they have their answer: It's livin' la vida low-carb.

"Make a list of the features of metabolic syndrome, then make a list of the things that carbohydrate restriction is good at fixing. They're the same list. Somehow, we never really noticed that," Dr. Volek explained.

We're glad you did, Dr. Volek. He added that controlling insulin production is the key to treating metabolic syndrome.

"We know the cause of metabolic syndrome is often linked to disruption of insulin," Dr. Volek continued. "Thus, the key to treating metabolic syndrome is to control insulin, and carbohydrates are the major stimulus for insulin."

Your body turns virtually every morsel of non-fibrous carbohydrates into sugar which can create a multitude of problems for the body which become evident in the symptoms characterized by metabolic syndrome. But the researchers didn't just stop there. Guess what kind of diet made metabolic syndrome get worse, not better?

"The most obvious factor in the obesity epidemic is the drastic increase in carbohydrate consumption in recent years and the decrease in fat consumption, so the story is consistent," Feinman remarked. "I think people have learned the value of reducing carbohydrates during the media popularization of low-carb diets, but they are still making it hard for themselves by also trying to reduce fat, when fat seems to be much less important a factor than carbohydrates."

Low-fat diets are worse than low-carb plans because they exacerbate metabolic syndrome rather than improve it. These study results challenge the premise that a low-fat, low-calorie, portion control diet is the only way to lose weight and get healthy. The government should use this new research to help them start properly educating the American people about the positive effects the low-carb lifestyle can have on their health. While livin' la vida low-carb certainly helped me lose a whole lot of weight, I think I appreciate the fact that I am so much healthier now than I have ever been before.

Medical "experts" will now be faced with a conundrum: Do they continue recommending the same old dietary information they've been telling patients for years or do they tell them they should start restricting their carbohydrate intake for health reasons?

"I think official agencies are trying to back off from recommending high-carbs and low-fat across the board, so I think there are real signs of progress," Feinman noted. "The bottom line is that if you reduce carbohydrates, you can be less concerned about your fat intake, and that often makes it much easier to stick to a beneficial new diet or lifestyle change."

But with all research that has been published on how maintaining stable blood sugar is much more important for controlling your health than restricting your fat intake, I think I'll be sticking with low-carb for a very, very, very long time. Like forever! One-fourth of all adult Americans currently have symptoms of metabolic syndrome which could be treated with low-carb.

The only question that remains now is whether the medical community will swallow their pride and recognize this way of eating as a healthy treatment option for their patients. People will lose weight and find the lasting way to keep it off and get healthy — at last! The feeling of accomplishment that comes from being free from weight and health problems is just too amazing to describe in words. You just have to do it to know what it's like!

As you can see, the health benefits of low-carb are plentiful and research will continue to confirm this way of eating as the nutritional powerhouse we know that it is. I am so encouraged to know there are some absolutely phenomenal talents coming up through the ranks of higher education who are dedicated to looking further into the subject of livin' la vida low-carb.

Working behind the scenes of this low-carb science movement are some especially gifted and intelligent individuals who are literally putting themselves and their reputations out there amongst their peers in the research community because they would dare share positive information as it relates to low-carb diets. I have the greatest respect for so many of these people, especially the young ones who will be around for the next 40, 50, or 60 years adding layer upon layer of evidence to continue proving the veracity of the low-carb lifestyle. Here is a quick list of some of the up-and-coming young trailblazers you need to know about:

Dr. Eric Westman, **Dr. Will Yancy** and **Dr. John Mavropoulos** from Duke University
Anssi Manninen from the University of Kuopio Medical School in Finland
Dr. Alex Johnstone from the Rowett Research Institute in the UK
Dr. Jeff Volek and **Dr. Cassandra Forsythe** from the University of Connecticut
Dr. Matthew R. Hayes from the University of Pennsylvania

I was very pleased to see a story in 2007 where Dr. Hayes talked about the electricity happening within the research circles behind-the-scenes regarding low-carb diets because I have long held the belief that the future of low-carb acceptance in the public arena hinges on the breadth of research coming out in support of this way of eating.

"There is this strong interest in the field in carb-restricted diets in the treatment of obesity," he said. "That [interest] comes from a number of controlled clinical trials that demonstrate overweight or obese people, maintained on low-carb diets, are successful if they adhere to the diet."

This has brought about a "hot debate" in the diet world that shows no signs of cooling off anytime soon. The next lesson takes a good hard look at how low-carb diets have made a direct impact on food companies that have traditionally promoted high-carb junk products. By refusing to acknowledge the growing low-carb trend, they've seen dramatic profit losses that threaten to permanently cripple their business' ability to make a profit.

LESSON #10
Influence of low-carb on high-carb food companies significant

"Traditional food companies (specifically multi-national food companies) should have learned that in the race to maximize profits, the ingredients in their food products were making the world's population fatter, unhealthier, and more susceptible to metabolic disorders. They could have learned to make what people want (and need) by offering foods that don't negatively affect their metabolism, waistline, blood sugar, and overall general health. They could have also learned that serving a variety of different dietary needs could go hand-in-hand with their overall corporate goals."

— **Andrew DiMino**, Founder and President of CarbSmart.com

The message is getting out there and more people now than ever before are starting to believe it. Consuming carbohydrates in the form of excessive sugar, flour, and even starchy vegetables is extremely unhealthy and should be avoided as much as possible. Regardless of your dietary philosophy, cutting out refined (white bread and sugary, high-fructose corn syrup-sweetened foods) and starchy carbs (like rice, pasta, and potatoes) is a nutritional must if you want to control your weight and improve your health dramatically. And the impact of such an epiphany happening in the minds of Americans is hitting some of the most famous American junk food brands hard.

First we'll take a look at the continued financial losses for the doughnut franchise Krispy Kreme which blames an increase in ingredient costs and fuel prices with the substantial losses they suffered totaling $5.9 million by the third quarter 2008 (compared with just $798,000 in the third quarter of 2007) following multiple bankruptcies and store closings within the Winston-Salem,

North Carolina-based franchise in 2005, 2006, and 2007. Krispy Kreme CEO Jim Morgan says it has been the bad economy causing his company's fiscal failures.

"I am certainly not satisfied with our results for the third quarter," he explained. "However, we are and have been taking the necessary steps to transform this company, and we're doing that despite the current economic conditions which are affecting consumers."

And yet I believe the real reason is that people are beginning to see doughnuts for what they really are, a nutritionally deficient junk food. And thus, customers are starting to avoid them more and more.

But none of this really concerns Krispy Kreme franchisee and CEO of the Westward Dough Operating Company named Lincoln Spoor who owns the famous doughnut units located in the Las Vegas area. He says he is not worried about the financial impact on his business of low-carb plans such as Atkins and South Beach which all encourage people following them to stay away from sugar and avoid these kinds of wasted carbs.

"There was a time when our corporate franchisor had said the Atkins diet is hurting us," Spoor recalled. "I don't subscribe to that view. I think what's happening is people are very smart about what they eat these days. They ration their calories. You do, I do."

"We are saying, 'You know what, I'm rationing my calories or I'm on a diet but you know what, I really want something great. I really want something best of class, so if I cheat, and everybody cheats, then I'm going to cheat with the best.' That's what we do. People cheat with our doughnuts. They cheat with Häagen-Dazs ice cream, they cheat with Mrs. Fields cookies, they cheat with In-N-Out burgers."

People who are not serious about their weight loss plan may cheat on their diets but not everyone cheats. Whatever reason this company thinks is why their business has suffered, one thing is certain, as people become more informed and take control of their health, junk food businesses are sure to continue to decline.

Some people can eat just one doughnut and be satisfied with that. But there are many people who are like I used to be when I weighed 410 pounds who cannot stop feeding the sugar monster once it starts. I could have easily downed 6-8 doughnuts at one time and not even have thought twice about it back before I started livin' la vida low-carb. But not anymore.

Today, just the thought of one bite of a doughnut makes me literally sick to my stomach. Do they still look good? Sure. Do they even smell good? Of course they do. But I know they cannot be a part of my healthy lifestyle change...ever again! Once I go down that path, there's no turning back. Spoor disagrees.

"If you've gone off your diet if you've cheated a little bit and you've done that, it's worth it. You're like, 'You know what? I've cheated, I loved it, and I'm glad.'"

Mr. Spoor seems to be a normal-weight man and I have no idea if he has ever suffered from being overweight in his life. But as one man who has struggled with being addicted to sugar and severely obese, I realized a long time ago that sugar can no longer be a part of my healthy lifestyle.

By the grace of God and through a unique visualization method of referring to anything made with sugar as rat poison I used back during my weight loss in 2004 and wrote about in my first book, I was able to take back control of my weight and health. I am now going on over five years without allowing the large quantities of sugar that I used to consume on a daily basis to even cross my lips. There are just too many damaging effects that sugar can cause that it's better to completely do without it as much as possible and I encourage others who go on low-carb to do the same.

Being the businessman that he is, Spoor said he is tinkering with some products to try to appeal to people who are on a diet.

"We're working on a 100 calorie doughnut and a reduced sugar doughnut. And the key, of course, is to make it taste as close to our signature product as you can get. You do that two ways: One is by using the new sweeteners that are out there today, and the second is by reducing the portion. You go into any of the stores today, in the candy rack, all those candy bars are a lot smaller today than they used to be and the calories are lower and the sugars are lower and the fat calories are lower and that's one way of doing it."

There is already a 100 calorie doughnut; it's called a doughnut hole! Even a reduced sugar doughnut will still be jam-packed with white flour carbs that turn to sugar in the body. Not good! Spoor said these new "diet" doughnuts along with a whole wheat doughnut will help him appeal to the diet-conscious consumers.

Unfortunately for Krispy Kreme, none of those doughnuts will be acceptable to people who are serious about health.

Sugar is sugar and carbohydrates are carbohydrates. Carbs drive a massive hormonal release in the body which raises blood sugar and insulin levels leading to pre-diabetes, metabolic syndrome, and obesity. This connection is clicking for so many people because the message of livin' la vida low-carb that is outlined in books like *Good Calories, Bad Calories* by Gary Taubes is having a ripple effect on our culture.

According to CalorieKing.com, an original glazed Krispy Kreme doughnut contains 22g total carbs, 10g sugar, and 200 calories. I don't know anyone that eats just one of these; especially if they are hot and fresh. Multiply that times five and you've got over 100g carbs, 50g sugar, 1000 calories, plus you're starving an hour later from the insulin response. People are not finding this acceptable anymore, and are realizing that regular doughnut consumption will destroy your health.

Next we look at the fate of Interstate Bakeries, makers of the world-famous creme-filled snack cakes Hostess Twinkies as well as Wonder Bread. The Schiller Park, Illinois-based company filed for bankruptcy in 2004 because of declining sales and, like Krispy Kreme, is struggling to become viable again as a company. They were forced to close down their Southern California bakeries due to their financial difficulties.

Despite the obvious nostalgia we all experience when we see foods like Twinkies and Wonder bread, these are different times now in 21st Century America. Obesity and diabetes are much more common today than they were just two or three decades ago when I was growing up as an American child and people are becoming wiser about what they are feeding themselves and their children.

The sudden influx of damning research on key ingredients in Twinkies and Wonder Bread like sugar, trans fats, and carbohydrates and their impact on health has acted as a tsunami of bad news for companies like Interstate Bakeries. This information has literally armed consumers with better information about how to make the best choices for their diet they and their families are eating. Customers who are parents noted the trend away from Twinkies and Wonder Bread because of the growing evidence against carbohydrate consumption despite the fact it was such an integral part of their lives growing up.

Moms today are becoming much wiser about healthy living than my mom was during the low-fat heyday when I was a kid growing up in the 1980s. The perception about sugar and white flour is much more negative than it used to be, although we still have a long way to go. Thankfully the message is seeping into our culture about reading food labels and this is showing up in the loss of revenue for companies like Interstate Bakeries.

Again, according to CalorieKing.com, a Twinkie has 27g total carbs, 19g sugar, and 150 calories in just one Twinkie. Of course, nobody just has ONE Twinkie as they come packaged in two or three at your local convenience store. Three Twinkies would be over 80g total carbs, nearly 60g sugar, and 450 calories. Although the fat content of Twinkies is less than a Krispy Kreme doughnut, the sugar in these is horrific coming from a mixture of both sugar and high fructose corn syrup.

As for the Wonder Bread, CalorieKing.com shows the total carbohydrates as 12g and 60 calories per slice. This may sound innocuous, but it's almost all white flour — a surefire way to spike your insulin levels no matter what you put between two slices.

Seeing the lack of any real media coverage of the companies that make Krispy Kreme doughnuts, Twinkies, and Wonder Bread all struggling and going through labor cuts and bankruptcies to deal with their financial woes reminds me of how stark the difference is when a low-carb company went through similar financial circumstances in 2005 — Atkins Nutritionals. The company with the namesake of the late great Dr. Robert C. Atkins was literally run through the mud by a relentless media and the current health experts they quoted in their stories who were all dead set on bringing the company to an end.

Look at these headlines that ran at the time:

"Atkins Files for Bankruptcy as Low-Carbohydrate Trend Fades"
"Thin times for Atkins diet"
"New Atkins Diet Plan: Chapter 11"

"Low on Carbs, and Funds, Atkins Files for Bankruptcy"
"Atkins bubble bursts as stars get fed up with diet"
"Doughless Atkins diet goes belly up"
"The beginning of the end for Atkins?"

Citing all kinds of experts in both business and health, story after story trumpeted the end of the "Atkins craze" as the news about the bankruptcy spread from coast to coast via radio, television and the Internet. But all of this doom and gloom was really much ado about nothing because most people who even casually follow business news realized Atkins Nutritionals, Inc. had been in financial trouble for quite a while. This news did not come as a shock to anybody in the low-carb industry despite the comical feeding frenzy that ensued across the media about this announcement.

When the Atkins diet was burning white hot in 2003 and the first part of 2004, everybody and their momma was trying to cash in on the biggest weight loss trend in the history of the United States. Carb this and carb that started popping up on food packaging everywhere you looked. Even companies that couldn't care less about low-carb products saw dollar signs and tried to capitalize on the success that the Atkins diet was having. Atkins Nutritionals, Inc. paved the way for many companies to get in on the low-carb bandwagon. Well, at least that's how they were trying to market most of what they put on store shelves — even if the vast majority of them were not low-carb at all.

Predictably, when these other companies started pumping out products like there was no tomorrow, the market became so overly saturated with low-carb products that I'm sure most consumers were left scratching their heads about what to purchase. The market forces have been in place ever since making the necessary adjustments based on the buying habits of the low-carb consumer. The line of bars and shakes distributed by Atkins Nutritionals, Inc. are certainly no exception to this.

While the Atkins bars continue to be the market leaders among healthy diet nutritional bars, some of the other products offered by Atkins Nutritionals, Inc. probably needed to be discontinued a long time before. That was the reality of the situation that was difficult to swallow when everything used to fly off the shelves like it was going out of style. Atkins Nutritionals, Inc. and other companies were so successful in the previous years before their bankruptcy and they did not purge certain products that just needed to go away. Businesses deal with these kinds of inventory problems every day of the week and the low-carb industry is not immune to it. The key is to find those products that do sell well and push them hard. So, was the Atkins Nutritionals bankruptcy the end of low-carb as we know it? Not hardly!

Although the bankruptcy announcement by Atkins Nutritionals, Inc. was truly unfortunate, it really meant nothing regarding the future of low-carb. Low-carb living continues to be the weight loss option of choice for people who are fed up with the failed low-fat, low-calorie, portion-controlled diets that are shoved down our throats by current health experts, the government, and the media. It doesn't matter what they have to say about the Atkins diet, those of us who've made low-carb eating a real lifestyle change with incredible results know better not to listen.

The good news is Atkins Nutritionals emerged from their bankruptcy quickly and strongly, scaled back their product line to the best of the best (although they are beginning to come out with some truly fabulous products again to enhance your low-carb lifestyle), and revamped the Atkins.com web site with a celebrity spokesperson in Courtney Thorne-Smith (ABC-TV's *According to Jim*) in 2009. I am confident that they are poised to continue providing the low-carb consumer with products to assist them as they lose and maintain their weight — the Atkins way, which is livin' la vida low-carb! The anti-Atkins people were desperately hoping the company would go under and just go away back in 2005.

But that didn't happen.

Atkins Nutritionals survived their bankruptcy as well as a frivolous lawsuit by a man named Jody Gorran who had his case thrown out of court after years of dragging the good Atkins name through the mud (financially supported by the animal rights group People For The Ethical Treatment Of Animals). Today, Atkins Nutritionals is stronger and thriving as a result of their restructuring and refocus on the market that made them who they are. If Krispy Kreme and Interstate Bakeries had made such a resounding comeback like this, then don't you think it would make front page news in the Business section with a headline like, "Low-Carb Diets Deceased, Doughnuts and Bread Come Back to Life?"

There's an excellent book on this subject you should check out by a man I interviewed on my podcast show in 2009 named Hank Cardello who penned *Stuffed: An Insider's Look At Who's [Really] Making America Fat*

(StuffedNation.com) to help companies balance their need for a profit with the responsibility to offer healthier options for their customers.

While I feel bad for the thousands of people who lose their jobs because of store closings, it is impossible to seriously deny that the low-carb trend did not have some kind of cause and effect impact on this happening. As more and more people begin choosing healthier eating options for themselves and their families, bread and junk food companies will need to adapt to the changing consumer needs and offer products that fit the bill.

My wife and I used to love going to our local bread outlet store and loading up on loaves of bread, sweets and rolls. We'd spend about $20-30 and get a month's worth of bread products. It was inexpensive food, but it was also chock full of mostly empty carbohydrates that we did not need. When I started livin' la vida low-carb in 2004, we had to stop going to that store and haven't been back since. There's nothing there we can buy anymore and I'm sure their bottom line has taken somewhat of a hit as a result!

As for sweet products still selling well for snack food companies, that'll change when people realize it is the sugar they are eating that is contributing to their obesity problem. If companies hope to stay in business they'd be wise to become educated in healthier types of products to offer their consumers.

And if you are seeking good quality sugar-free and low-carb food options, be sure to check out the wide selection of products available from 10-year low-carb retail veteran Andrew DiMino on CarbSmart.com. You may already be familiar with the CarbSmart name from the Breyer's ice cream label. But he's got an entire online store full of some truly remarkable low-carb products you can trust and believe in. Give them a try sometime and let me know what you think.

Coming up in the next lesson learned from livin' la vida low-carb, I am excited to share with you the latest cutting-edge research showing how low-carb living can help to prevent both cancer and neurological diseases like Alzheimer's which many are starting to describe as Type 3 diabetes of the brain. You will probably not find this information anywhere else in any other diet and health book that is currently out there and you will be armed with the latest scientific developments on these critical topics.

LESSON #11
The best way to prevent cancer and neurological disease is low-carb

"The way cancer doctors image (identify) cancer is by looking for cells that only burn glucose (sugar). Low-carb starves these same cancer cells. The brain burns glucose, but too much (DrMcCleary.com), noted pediatric neurosurgeon, author of *The Brain Trust Program (2007)* and *Bald is Beautiful: Guide for Living with Childhood Cancer (2009)*

One of the most oft-quoted books against the consumption of animal fat and protein because of its alleged cancer-producing properties is *The China Study* released in 2005 by Dr. T. Colin Campbell. The premise of the book is that since the Chinese people have lower incidences of cancer, it must be because of the lack of meat in their diet. Of course, this assumes that China has the lowest rates of ALL cancers and that's just patently false — a fact conveniently omitted from *The China Study* book that you will hear vegetarians and vegans quote from so often. Current research contradicts much of what was in Campbell's book.

But let's face it — when it comes to our health in the 21st Century, one of the worst things you could ever hear from your doctor is the dreaded "c" word. Yes, I'm referring to cancer. I'd be very surprised if ANY of you reading this right now have not at all been impacted by this horrible disease personally, either through a family member or among your circle of friends. It comes on like a roaring lion and grips hard seeking to devour and destroy everything it touches.

I've seen it personally in my own life with the former Minister of Music at my church named Steve Dyar. He was diagnosed with esophageal cancer in December 2006, went through some grueling chemotherapy treatments, before heading home to be with the Lord in 2007. Cancer is ruthless and is not a respecter of persons. It doesn't care who you are and will seek to destroy your life completely.

Thankfully, there are some things we can do as a dietary defense for defeating cancer. Never mind the fact that a high-carb diet has been shown in numerous studies to be linked to a variety of cancers that I'll talk about in this chapter, including brain cancer, pancreatic cancer, esophageal cancer, kidney cancer, breast cancer, and prostate cancer, among others. With that said, here is a superb list of specific vitamins and nutrients you should consume to put yourself in the best position to ward off cancer nutritionally. It's not guaranteed, but having a preventative plan in place is better than no plan at all.

A DIETARY DEFENSE FOR DEFEATING CANCER

Less than a hundred years ago cancer was a very rare disease indeed. In fact, it was so extraordinarily rare that patients with cancer were prominently discussed in medical textbooks and journals as anomalies. Thanks to the "many benefits" of our modern, "balanced" diets, cancers are now widespread, affecting more than 30 percent of the entire population of this planet. The skyrocketing cancer rates are, not unsurprisingly, completely in accordance with the skyrocketing intake of overly-processed, nutritionally empty carbohydrates from sugar, starch and corn syrups.

Cancer therapies have done little to improve survival rates since the "war on cancer" was declared in the 1970's. Actually, nothing that can be cured now could be cured then. So clearly the best approach to cancer is prevention. Traditional diets, containing animal and plant foods farmed by nontoxic methods, are rich in factors that protect against cancer. Many of these protective factors are found in the animal fats. Vegetarianism does not protect against cancer. In fact, vegetarians are particularly prone to cancers of the nervous system and reproductive organs.

So what are the nutrients that protect against cancer? They are:

Vitamin A: Strengthens the immune system and is essential for mineral metabolism and endocrine function. Helps detoxify. True vitamin A is found only in animal foods such as cod liver oil; fish and shellfish; and liver, butter and egg yolks from pasture-fed animals. Traditional diets contained ten times more vitamin A than the typical modern American diet.

Vitamin C: An important antioxidant that prevents damage by free radicals. Found in many fruits and vegetables but also in certain organ meats valued by primitive peoples.

Vitamin B-6: Deficiencies are associated with cancer. It contributes to the function of over 100 enzymes. Most of this vitamin is available from animal foods.

Vitamin B-12: Deficiencies are associated with cancer. Found only in animal foods.

Vitamin B-17: Protects against cancer. Found in a variety of organically-grown grains, legumes, nuts and berries.

Vitamin D: Required for mineral absorption and is strongly protective against breast and colon cancer. Found only in animal foods such as cod liver oil, lard, shellfish and butterfat, organ meats and egg yolks from grass-fed animals. Traditional diets contained ten times more vitamin D than the typical modern American diet.

Vitamin E: Works as an antioxidant at the cellular level. Found in unprocessed oils as well as in animal fats like butter and egg yolks.

Conjugated Linoleic Acid (CLA): Strongly protective against breast cancer. Found in the butterfat and meat fat of grass-fed ruminant animals.

Cholesterol: A potent antioxidant that protects against free radicals in cell membranes. Found only in animal foods.

Minerals: The body needs generous amounts of a wide variety of minerals to protect itself against cancer. Minerals like zinc, magnesium and selenium are vital components of enzymes that help the body fight carcinogens. Minerals are more easily absorbed from animal foods.

Lactic Acid and Friendly Bacteria: Contribute to the health of the digestive tract. Found in old fashioned lacto-fermented foods.

Saturated Fats: Strengthen the immune system and needed for proper use of the essential fatty acids. The lungs cannot function without saturated fats. Found mostly in animal foods.

Long-Chain Fatty Acids: Arachidonic acid (AA), eicosapentaenoic acid (EPA) and docosahexaenoic acid (DHA) help fight cancer on the cellular level. They are found mostly in animal foods such as butter, organ meats, cod liver oil and seafood.

Co-enzyme Q10: Highly protective against cancer. Found only in animal foods.

Conversely, here are some of the compounds found in processed foods that have been linked to cancer:

Trans Fatty Acids: Imitation fats in shortenings, margarines and most commercial baked goods and snack foods and strongly associated with lung and reproductive organ cancers.

Rancid fats: Industrial processing creates rancidity (free radicals) in commercial vegetable oils.

Omega-6 fatty acids: Although needed in small amounts, an excess can contribute to cancer. Dangerously high levels of omega-6 fatty acids are due to the overuse of vegetable oils in modern diets.

MSG: Associated with brain cancer. Found in almost all processed foods, even when "MSG" does not appear on the label. Flavorings, spice mixes and hydrolyzed protein contain MSG.

Aspartame: An excitotoxin in diet foods and beverages and associated with brain cancer.

Pesticides: Associated with many types of cancer. Found in most commercial vegetable oils, fruit juices, vegetables and fruits.

Hormones: Found in animals raised in confinement on soy and grains. Plant-based hormones are plentiful in soy foods.

Artificial Flavorings and Colors: Associated with various types of cancers, especially when consumed in large amounts in a diet of junk food.

Refined Carbohydrates: Sugar, high fructose corn syrup and white flour are devoid of nutrients. The body uses up nutrients from other foods to process refined carbohydrates. Tumor growth is associated with sugar, HFCS as well as starch consumption.

Special THANKS to Sally Fallon from the Weston A. Price Foundation (WestonAPrice.org) for providing the research and background for this information. Now that we know how to combat cancer by supplementing our diet, let's examine some of the major cancers that could possibly be prevented by simply switching to a healthy low-carb nutritional approach according to the latest scientific studies supporting this claim:

KIDNEY CANCER

An Italian study provided the shocking revelation that a diet rich in white flour-based bread consumption is directly linked to the most common type of kidney cancer there is called renal cell carcinoma (RCC). This research may be the most damning evidence yet against eating a high-carb diet for health and is proof yet again why livin' la vida low-carb truly is a healthier way to eat for the rest of your life.

Lead researcher Dr. Francesca Bravi, from the Milan, Italy-based Institute of Pharmacological Research "Mario Negri," and her fellow researchers conducted a large controlled study of 2301 Italians adults to determine if diet and nutrition played any significant role in the development of RCC. Dr. Bravi said this is an extremely controversial subject among dietary researchers and she wanted to see if a link existed.

"To our knowledge, no other study investigated the role of cereals on RCC," Dr. Bravi remarked about the reason for her research.

One-third (767 study participants, including 494 men and 273 women) were already diagnosed with RCC when the study began and the other two-thirds (1534 study participants, including 988 men and 546 women) were used as the control subjects in the study because they had not previously been diagnosed with the disease. In fact, there were two control subjects matched up by gender, age, and location for each RCC-diagnosed case. For everyone who participated in the study, Dr. Bravi and her team looked at their lifestyle, where they lived, who they interacted with, what kind of medical history each of them had, and other appropriate measurements at the beginning of the study.

The participants were also required to take a food frequency questionnaire consisting of 78 questions about food and beverage intake to determine what the average weekly diet was like for them over the previous two years to see if any of the foods they consumed may have played a role in the RCC. Alcohol consumption was also assessed in a separate set of questions. What they found was a "significant direct trend in risk" of developing RCC when foods like bread, pasta, rice, milk, and yogurt were consumed. Here is what the study found regarding the probability of increased risk of the onset of RCC for eating any of the following foods:

Bread — 94 percent increased risk
Pasta — 29 percent increased risk
Rice — 29 percent increased risk
Milk — 27 percent increased risk
Yogurt — 27 percent increased risk

The researchers suggest that the greater risk of RCC from these high-carb foods "may be due to the high glycemic index of these foods and their possible involvement in insulin-like growth factors." At the same time, Dr. Bravi found that many of the following low-glycemic, low-carb foods were actually protective against RCC because they decreased the risk of developing it:

Poultry — 26 percent decreased risk
Processed meats — 36 percent decreased risk
Vegetables — 35 percent decreased risk

Dr. Bravi said these foods were "inversely associated with RCC risk." In fact, she went on to say that there was "no relation" to RCC found in coffee, tea, soup, eggs, red meat, fish, cheese, fruits, potatoes, sugars and desserts.

"Decreasing risk was associated with increasing intake of poultry, processed meat, and all vegetables, both raw and cooked," Dr. Bravi noted in her study.

Vegetable consumption, which is a staple among most healthy dieters including those on low-carb, has long been found in studies to contain many vitamins, carotenoids, flavonoids and phytosterols — all of which are good for your body and help to keep you healthy.

"The results of this study provide further indications on dietary correlates of RCC, and in particular indicate that a diet rich in refined cereals and poor in vegetables may have an unfavorable role on RCC," the researchers concluded.

The study entitled "Food Groups and Renal Cell Carcinoma: A Case-Control Study from Italy" was published in the October 20, 2006 issue of *International Journal of Cancer.*

While the dieting world has been exposed to a lot of crazy diets over the years, this study confirms how bad for you diets rich in cereal and grain products really are. And let's not forget about the government-recommended USDA Food Pyramid and accompanying dietary recommendations. Are they going to back away from these suggestions for grain intake in light of this study? It's doubtful.

This is yet another reason why you must take control of your own health and never allow the government to tell you what is good for you. This study is proof positive they are simply not looking out for the best interests of you and me. As for me, I'll keep on livin' la vida low-carb proudly because I can be confident my weight will be controlled and my risk of developing renal cell carcinoma is much lower than it would be on the typical high-carb Standard American Diet (SAD). It is SAD indeed.

ESOPHAGEAL CANCER

Lead researcher Dr. Vijay S. Khiani from the Cleveland, OH-based Case Western Reserve University and his team looked at esophageal cancer rates as reported by the Surveillance, Epidemiology, and End Results (SEER) program from 1973 through 2001 as well as the average carbohydrate intake of Americans over the same time period as derived from a USDA program called the National Nutrient Data Bank. While avoiding declaring any explicit link between carbohydrates and esophageal cancer, Dr. Khiani confidently stated that eating a carb-heavy diet can and will lead to obesity which then leads to a predisposition to the development of gastroesophageal reflux disease (aka GERD). Continuing the downward spiral, GERD increases the chance of the onset of Barrett's esophagus which is the very last step before the full-blown development of lower-esophageal adenocarcinoma or cancer of the esophagus.

Using linear regression analysis from both sets of information, Dr. Khiani said there was a "significant relationship between the incidence of esophageal adenocarcinoma and per-capita consumption of carbohydrates in the American diet." He noted that in 1973, the average daily carbohydrate consumption in America was 400 grams. Nearly three decades later, the average carbs consumed each day had jumped to 500 grams. This additional 100 grams of carbohydrates consumed daily by Americans directly correlates with the six-fold jump in esophageal adenocarcinoma cases — from just 2,500 in 1973 to an average of almost 15,000 annually through the year 2001 and still rising. Dr. Khiani revealed the results of his study at the American College of Gastroenterology 2006 Annual Scientific Meeting in Las Vegas, Nevada in a presentation entitled "Ecological association of rising incidence of esophageal adenocarcinoma with dietary carbohydrate intake."

So, which high-carb foods are the biggest culprits according to the researchers? Cereal products, high fructose corn syrup, processed foods, and fast food staples such as hamburgers and French fries. Unfortunately, Dr. Khiani and his researchers stopped short of pointing fingers at the root cause of the problem or offering suggestions about what to do with the information contained in his study. Dr. Khiani asserted his study does not promote "fad diets" such as "total carbohydrate avoidance" or even the more mainstream Atkins or low-carb diets that are out there advocating 20g daily for the first two weeks followed by up to 40-60g daily carbs for the weight loss phases and 60-100g daily carbs for weight and health management.

"We don't know at this point," Dr. Khiani explained. "Further research still needs to be done to determine whether there is a direct causal relationship" between carbs and esophageal cancer.

It almost seems painful for scientific researchers to acknowledge something good about livin' la vida low-carb. Even the researcher himself is non-committal about the stunning conclusions his research makes regarding eating a high-carb diet. The final conclusion from the study confirms the truth about eating carbs for people concerned about esophageal cancer.

"This ecological study provides evidence for the hypothesis that excess carbohydrate intake in the U.S. population may partially account for the increased trend of incidence rate of adenocarcinoma of the esophagus," the researchers said. "It s possible that obesity resulting from excess carbohydrate intake may be an intermediate link."

People enjoying the healthy low-carb lifestyle have long known eating excessive carbs can make you fat and now this study along with other research that continues to pour in shows it can be detrimental to your health as well. Go on a low-carb plan ASAP! Do it not just to manage your weight if you are overweight or obese, but to ward off diseases such as diabetes, metabolic syndrome and even esophageal cancer as we have seen in this study. It's a decision you will never regret!

PANCREATIC CANCER

Pancreatic cancer currently accounts for 2 percent of all new cancer cases and 6 percent of deaths from cancer annually. The development of pancreatic cancer results from the release of high levels of insulin when glucose metabolism is disturbed. One of the most common reasons for this is the introduction of excessive sugar in the body. Researchers have only now realized for the first time that there is a connection between sugar intake and the development of pancreatic cancer.

Lead researcher Susanna C. Larsson from The Department of Environmental Medicine at the Swedish-based Karolinska Institute and her research team observed data from 77,797 men and women ages 45 to 83 from 1997 through 2005 to see what impact sugar from soft drinks (mostly high fructose corn syrup) and other sources had on their risk of developing cancer in the pancreas. This study gathered information from two large population-based studies — the Swedish Mammography Cohort and the Cohort of Swedish Men.

The study participants answered a 96-question food-frequency and lifestyle survey for the researchers to come up with the data used to analyze the correlation between sugar consumption and cancer of the pancreas. By the end of the study, the researchers found that there were a total of 131 cases of pancreatic cancer that they say can be traced directly to the "consumption of added sugar, soft drinks, and sweetened fruit soups or stewed fruit." For those in the study who consumed five or more servings of added sugar daily, there was a 90 percent (nearly DOUBLE!) increase in their risk of developing pancreatic cancer. Even more startling is the fact that it only took two servings of sugary sodas daily to bring about this higher risk.

"Consumption of sugar-sweetened soft drinks, which contain large amounts of rapidly absorbable sugars, induces a rapid and dramatic increase in both blood glucose and insulin concentrations," they wrote.

As for the coffee and tea drinkers who added sugar to their favorite beverage at least five servings per day, the risk jumped 70 percent. Keep in mind the study considered a serving of sugar as one teaspoon or lump although many people often use much more than that in their beverages. Other sources of sugar intake from fruit soups and stewed fruits with extra sugar increased the risk of pancreatic cancer by 50 percent. The American equivalent of these foods includes any canned fruit packed in heavy syrup or other frequently consumed food products with high amounts of added sugars.

"The researchers have now been able to show that the 'risk of developing pancreatic cancer is related to the amount of sugar in the diet," the report showed.

The results of this study appeared in the November 2006 issue of *American Journal of Clinical Nutrition.*

So what about this research connecting a high-carb, high-sugar diet with pancreatic cancer? We have already seen evidence that sugar leads to heart disease, obesity, addiction, and many other physical and mental ailments. Now we can add cancer to the mix. What further evidence is it going to take before we start seriously considering sugar as the real health threat that it is? This is why I described sugar as "rat poison" in an entire chapter of my first book because it can quite literally make you sick and even kill you. Anyone who thinks that sugar can be part of a healthy lifestyle should begin to question the logic of that kind of thinking. That conclusion certainly doesn't make any sense in light of the latest scientific evidence like this study.

Larsson stated that pancreatic cancer could possibly be avoided with a few minor changes in the diet.

"It is perhaps the most serious form of cancer, with very poor prognoses for its victims," Larsson explained. "Since it's difficult to treat and is often discovered too late, it's particularly important that we learn to prevent it."

Somebody tell me what the difference is between cigarettes and sugar (something naturopathic physician Dr. Scott Olson wrote about in his book *Sugarettes*)? Both are highly addictive and lead to various forms of illness, including cancer. They are easily available for purchase by the consumer and many people use them. But there's one distinction — cigarettes have been given a stigma by those who have lobbied to warn people about the dangers of smoking them. In fact, that warning is placed right there on every single pack of cigarettes sold in the United States.

What about sugar? Not that I'm advocating necessarily putting warning labels on foods that contain it, per se, but where are the public service announcements, the real-life stories of those who have been negatively impacted by consuming sugar, the outcry from the public? It's nonexistent because people have not been given the information about what sugar is doing to them. Even with studies providing damning information about sugar consumption, most people will just shrug their shoulders and go on about their lives eating a honeybun and washing it down with a Super Big Gulp full of sugary soda without thinking twice about it. This seems reckless to say the least.

The researchers said it as clearly as they possibly could that there is too much evidence pointing in the direction of a progression of illnesses, specifically those conditions present in the ever-growing population of people with metabolic syndrome, caused by eating and drinking too much sugar which then leads to the increased risk of pancreatic cancer.

"Evidence is mounting that abnormal glucose metabolism and hyperinsulinemia may be involved in the development of pancreatic cancer," they wrote. "Conditions such as diabetes mellitus, a high body mass index (BMI, in kg/m2), and physical inactivity, all hallmarks of insulin resistance, have been directly related to the risk of this malignancy."

While the incidence of pancreatic cancer is still miniscule, Lasson reminds people that it is "important to learn more about the risk factors behind the disease" to best prevent it from happening in the first place. Will the world take heed of that warning or will more people need to die before we take it seriously? Sugar is very bad news for anyone attempting to live a long and healthy life, but nobody seems to care. We go on about our lives as if there are no consequences to poor decision-making regarding our health and then we wonder what went wrong when we are afflicted with a devastating and deadly calamity like cancer.

BRAIN CANCER

Research supervisor Dr. Thomas Seyfried, professor of biology at Boston College, led this study featuring a high-fat, low-carb product called KetoCal. The nutritional label for each 100g serving of this powder drink product shows it contains 90 percent fat (72g), 15g protein, and just 3g carbohydrates. It is also heavily fortified with all the essential vitamins and minerals for a nutrient-dense diet. This product has been marketed for used with epileptic children to help control their seizures, but Dr. Seyfried and his team of researchers wanted to see if KetoCal could improve the condition of those suffering from brain cancer.

Although KetoCal was used in the study, the company did not pay for this study except to donate the products that the mice involved in the study consumed. But the results of this study were not so much about any particular product as much as it was about the remarkable findings of how health improves dramatically on a high-fat, low-carb diet. The researchers implanted into the brains of male laboratory mice two kinds of malignant tumors and then divided them into three distinctive dietary groups:

GROUP 1 — Low-fat, high-carb mouse chow
GROUP 2 — Unlimited amounts of the high-fat, low-carb KetoCal
GROUP 3 — Restricted amounts of the high fat, low-carb KetoCal

What were the results of the study? GROUP 1 and GROUP 2 did not see improvements in the brain cancer. However, GROUP 3 saw a 35-65 percent reduction in the growth of the brain tumors and extended their life survival rates longer than the control groups. Moreover, the overall health of the high-fat, low-carb GROUP 3 mice was enhanced compared with the low-fat, high-carb GROUP 1. The results of this study were published in the February 21, 2007 issue of the scientific journal *Nutrition & Metabolism*.

Describing the high-fat, low-carb diet as a "novel alternative therapy for malignant brain cancer," Dr. Seyfried believes the results his team found should lend credence to finding a more natural, just as effective, and economical way to fight this devastating condition.

"While the tumors did not vanish in the mice who received the strict KetoCal diet, they got significantly smaller and the animals lived significantly longer. And compared to radiation, chemotherapy and surgery, KetoCal is a relatively inexpensive treatment option," he said.

Since brain cancer is a leading killer among the cancers in both adults and children, researchers have been looking for less invasive ways to provide long-term management that will reduce the size of tumors by using the knowledge we already have about what feeds the cells of this cancer. What the high-fat, low-carb diet does is basically starve tumors from getting any glucose (sugar), something we have learned from other research actually feeds cancer cells.

So, despite the low-fat diet that GROUP 1 ate, it was the high-carb content that prevented their brain tumors from seeing improvements. Interestingly, although opponents of livin' la vida low-carb have made a mockery of ketosis and the ketone bodies that are produced on a low-carb diet, the truth of the matter is tumor cells cannot effectively metabolize them and, thus, cannot grow. Do you think you're gonna hear that on the 6 o'clock news anytime soon?! Yeah right!

What's most revealing about this study is the fact that it shows a positive step in the right direction with health as a result of going on a low-carb diet. We always hear the naysayers talking about how unsafe and ineffective this "dangerous fad" diet is for people to go on. But clearly the evidence from the research that is coming out is showing just the opposite is true. There will come a day sometime in the future when livin' la vida low-carb will be the preferred and quite possibly recommended dietary approach to treating obesity and disease in the United States of America. It won't happen soon, but I honestly believe that day is coming. I only hope to stick around on this Earth long enough to see it happen in my lifetime. It could happen within the next 50 years. Wait and see because I strongly believe it's coming sooner rather than later!

PROSTATE CANCER

Lead researcher Dr. Song-Yi Park, from the Cancer Epidemiology Program, Cancer Research Center of Hawaii at the Honolulu-based University of Hawaii, examined data from the Multiethnic Cohort Study which took place from 1993 — 2002 featuring 82,483 men who were 45 years old and older at the beginning of the study. Detailed records of what each of the study members ate were recorded for Dr. Park to observe. Overall, there were 4,404 instances of prostate cancer which the researchers determined were not caused by the consumption of calcium or vitamin D from the dairy products the study participants ate. Also, the total volume of dairy products was also not a factor in the development of prostate cancer. This was true across all racial and ethnic groups.

Instead, Dr. Park and his researchers noticed something rather peculiar about the kind of dairy products that were ingested by the study participants and how that impacted their risk for developing prostate cancer. It turns out that there was a 12 percent decrease in the risk of developing prostate cancer for those who drank whole milk. Conversely, there was a 16 percent increase in the risk of developing prostate cancer for those who drank 2% or skim milk. In other words, it is the fat in the milk and dairy products consumed that provide protection against prostate cancer, which flies in the face of everything we've ever heard about diet and health.

With over 500,000 new cases of prostate cancer and another 200,000 deaths annually (and the statistics have been steadily rising since the early 1990s), this research bursts the bubble on the low-fat dogma we have been forced to believe for the past thirty years! This study appeared in the October 8, 2007 issue of *American Journal of Epidemiology*.

Of course, Dr. Park's research is not going to be easily accepted by those who buy into the whole notion that a low-fat diet is protective against various forms of cancer and other health ailments. But this large-scale study is certainly going to challenge the wisdom of that hypothesis. The researchers do admit that the only potential downside to their study is the fact that it relied on self-reporting data provided by the study participants about what they ate which has the potential for inaccuracies from poor memory of the foods they consumed. But that's just a smokescreen that will be thrown up to challenge these remarkable findings.

In anotherr study, Dr. Park and his researchers used data from the Multiethnic Cohort Study to see if the specific kind of fat made a difference in the prostate cancer risk. They looked at total fat, saturated fat, monounsaturated fat, and polyunsaturated fat as well as n-3 and n-6 fatty acids. The dietary cholesterol, meat (broken down to reflect total amount of meat, red meat, processed meat, and poultry) and fish consumed, and the amount of fats from meat were all recorded for the men in the study. Of the 4,404 men who developed prostate cancer, 29 percent of them had advanced tumors. Interestingly, the researchers said the type of fat and meat consumed showed no association with overall prostate cancer risk or tumor development.

The researchers put it succinctly this way: *"We found little evidence of any relation of fat and meat intake with prostate cancer risk within any of the four racial/ethnic groups."* It can't get much plainer than that! This study was published in the September 15, 2007 issue of *International Journal of Cancer*.

When asked to elaborate on the findings of the study, Dr. Park was cautious about recommending a high-fat diet which he claims begins a chain of events that could lead to cancer.

"Although diet is likely to influence prostate cancer risk, the intake of total and saturated fat do not appear to be important contributors," he exclaimed. "However, because high intake of fat can lead to obesity as well as other cancers, the consumption of high fat foods should be limited."

While I can appreciate the veracity of these findings, I must respectfully disagree with Dr. Park regarding the relationship of fat consumption to obesity. As long as you keep your carbs reduced, a high-fat diet is not harmful for an increase in obesity and obesity-related diseases. His personal commentary regarding dietary fat notwithstanding, Dr. Park is at least shining a light on the faulty research that has long been allowed to reign as the gospel truth because it has never been challenged. The inconsistency of the data should be the impetus for even more research that should provide more answers about the role of meat and fat in a healthy diet rather than making ludicrous dietary recommendations based on old research. Dr. Park agrees.

"Our findings did not support any association between intake of fat, fatty acids, cholesterol, or various meats and prostate cancer risk," he concluded.

Another research study on low-carb diets and prostate cancer was published in the November 13, 2007 issue of *The Prostate*. It's exciting news for men who are concerned about prostate cancer. Lead researcher Dr. Stephen Freedland, a urologist from the Durham, NC-based Duke University School of Medicine, observed 75 male mice who were fed an isocaloric diet of either a zero-carb, very high-fat diet (84 percent fat), a high-carb, low—fat diet (72 percent carbs, 12 percent fat), or the traditional Western diet (40 percent fat, 44 percent carbs). Each of the mice was injected with cancerous cells after 24 hours on their new diet. The mice that ate the zero-carb diet actually lost up to 15 percent of their body weight compared with increases by the low-fat and Western diet groups. In fact, they needed more calories to try to even out the body weight of the mice. Interesting!

But even more fascinating is what happened after 51 days — the size of the tumors in the zero-carb diet group were 33 percent smaller than the Western diet group and survival was longest among the zero-carb diet group. Dr. Freedland credits a decrease in insulin production that happens when you consume fewer carbs for the stunted tumor growth in the mice. The researchers were very hopeful about the results this study could have on humans.

"If this is ultimately confirmed in human clinical trials, it has huge implications for prostate cancer therapy through something that all of us can control, our diets," Dr. Freedland exclaimed.

Yes it will be!

"We are planning to start clinical trials" starting in 2008, Dr. Freedland said at the time of his study. "The results of this study are very promising, but of course much more work needs to be done."

Beyond specific cancers like the one I've mentioned, cancers of all kinds are beginning to show signs of improving with a low-carb lifestyle change. There was a fantastic article published in the September 17, 2007 issue of *Time Magazine* that details the use of a high-fat, ketogenic low-carb diet on cancer patients to see what impact it would have on their condition. The findings of the researchers had the entire world buzzing about the health benefits of the low-carb lifestyle yet again.

In the article entitled "Can A High-Fat Diet Beat Cancer?" researchers Dr. Melanie Schmidt and Ulrike Kammerer, both from the University of Wurzburg in Germany, implemented a high-fat, low-carb ketogenic diet on the most dire of cancer patients who had run out of treatment options. Without the use of any medications, they simply required the participants to slash their carbs and eat more fat. By getting rid of virtually all the carbs in their diet, especially sugar which feeds cancer cells, the researchers replaced that energy with healthy fat sources including hempseed and linseed oils, soy-based proteins, and animal fats and proteins. It's a supercharged version of the Atkins diet and more closely resembles the original low-carb diet plan from the late great Dr. Robert C. Atkins released back in 1972 called *Dr. Atkins Diet Revolution* which you can still get a copy of on Amazon.com.

According to the *Time* story, this high-fat, low-carb treatment goes back much further than Dr. Atkins to 1924 when a German Nobel Prize winning scientist named Otto Warburg put forth what would be known as the "Warburg effect" which concluded in the words of Warburg that "the prime cause of cancer is the replacement of the respiration of oxygen in normal body cells by a fermentation of sugar."

Warburg said NEARLY A CENTURY AGO that cancer THRIVES where sugar resides. If you're interested in reading more about the incredible work of Otto Warburg and the continuing research into his findings today, then be sure to check out the most comprehensive book I've seen on this subject entitled *The Hidden Story of Cancer* by Professor Brian Peskin (thehiddenstoryofcancer.com/cancerbook).

So, the thinking goes like this: remove the sugar (and the carbohydrates that turn to sugar in the body) and replace it with fat, then the cancer cells will die. It was a BRILLIANT hypothesis that was lauded among the scientists and health advocates of his day, but somehow it has been forgotten by many in our modern culture.

Not for Dr. Schmidt and Kammerer, though. They've taken Warburg's lifetime of work and run with it. By removing sugar from the diet of cancer patients, can they stop the spread of cancer before it is too late? The whole world is watching with hopeful anticipation that this could be exactly what is needed to bring cancer under control. Modern-day scientists researching and using a high-fat, low-carb diet such as Dr. Larry McCleary, Gary Taubes, Drs. Mike and Mary Dan Eades, Dr. Eric Westman, Dr. Mary Enig, Dr. Richard Bernstein, Dr. Jeff Volek, Dr. Stephen Phinney, Sally Fallon, Dr. Barry Groves, Dr. Jay Wortman, Dr. Annika Dahlqvist, and Dr. Mary C. Vernon, among a multitude of others have all laid the basic groundwork for furthering the theory that this method of eating is the optimal nutritional approach for living as healthy as you possibly can. And the concerns that people have about a high-fat diet are unfounded as long as you combine it with a low-carb approach as these German researchers are doing with the ketogenic diet being used on cancer patients.

This experiment has been dubbed "The Wurzburg trial" and is underwritten by a German food company named Tavartis which seems to stock a line-up of high-protein, low-carb products. So begins this journey to cancer-free living for some who have lost all hope when chemotherapy and other treatments failed them. It's not a certainty, but it is another option that many are never even told about. Painful and arduous cancer treatments such as surgery, radiation, hyperthermia and autohemotherapy are so aggressive and potentially life-threatening that a more natural and quite possibly much more effective treatment like a ketogenic diet could be a welcoming prospect for those dealing with this most dreaded of modern diseases to afflict the human body.

Sadly, Schmidt said a few of the cancer patients who attempted to eat a sugar-free diet couldn't handle not being able to drink sugary sodas and eat chocolate. Have you never heard of diet soda and sugar-free, low-carb chocolate bars? You don't have to give these things up; you simply replace the sugary ones with a healthier version instead. And for a chance to live much longer than you expected, isn't it worth making a small sacrifice like giving up sugar to make that happen? This goes beyond my ability to comprehend.

By the end of the three-month study, the researchers were able to see five patients survive the high-fat, low-carb cancer treatment with incredible results!

Here's what happened to them:

- They all remained alive and the cancer did not overtake them
- Their illness remained stable or even improved
- The tumors in their body grew slower, stopped, or even shrunk

AMAZING! And these improvements didn't go without fanfare within the lab where this was happening either. Kammerer said it was nothing but "positive reactions and an increased interest" in how this high-fat, low-carb diet was doing what it was doing. She is cautiously optimistic, though, since it was not a resounding success with all the patients. But this is an excellent first step in figuring out what methodology for treating cancer should be heading into the future. Interestingly, one of the experts in the *Time* column stated that the reason more clinical studies like this haven't been conducted is because of the close ties the medical establishment has to the pharmaceutical industry which would stand to lose billions of dollars annually if an all-natural cancer treatment were promoted.

The Wurzburg trial is only the first of many low-carb cancer studies that are coming down the pipeline. There's one happening in The Netherlands right now and another one in Germany. While expectations are high, they are all being careful about proclaiming this ketogenic treatment option as the be-all, end-all for treating cancer. Just like with weight loss, a high-fat, low-carb diet isn't for everyone. It's all a matter of how the individual will respond to such a dietary regimen and at the stage of cancer they have. If a ketogenic strategy can be implemented early enough, then perhaps there is greater hope for those individuals. Rather than waiting to start livin' la vida low-carb until a last resort when nothing else has worked, why not try making it your first option for getting the cancer under control before it can spread? That certainly seems to make sense to me.

In a study published in the August 17, 2009 issue of *Proceedings of the National Academy of Sciences*, lead researcher Don Ayer out of the Huntsman Cancer Institute and a professor in the Department of Oncological Sciences at the University of Utah found that restricting the amino acid glutamine will halt a cell's ability to utilize glucose in patients who have cancerous tumors.

"Essentially, if you don't have glutamine, the cell is short-circuited due to a lack of glucose, which halts the growth of the tumor cell," Ayer said.

His next area of study will be to test theories about the interaction between a certain protein and gene can control glucose uptake by cells.

"If we can understand that, we can break the cycle of glucose utilization, which could be beneficial in the treatment of cancer," he noted.

Exciting stuff! And let's not forget all the negative health implications of eating a high-carb diet, including high blood pressure, insulin resistance, lower HDL cholesterol and high triglycerides, the onset of Alzheimer's disease, diabetes, and negligible weight loss. Why would you want to go through all of that whether you have cancer or not? How about avoiding these by going ahead and implementing a delicious and healthy low-carb lifestyle today so you'll arm yourself against whatever ailments may come your way?

Unfortunately, not all the recent scientific research on cancer has been positive for low-carb diets when headlines blared from coast to coast that the Atkins diet leads to colon cancer. Unlike all the studies I just shared with you, this one was trumpeted heavily on all the television news outlets, newspapers, and online news web sites the whole world to see. You couldn't miss this one when it came out in June 2007.

To most people passively paying attention to the news that day this story ran, you'd probably think to yourself, "Why would anybody in their right mind go on the Atkins diet?" Man, that low-carb diet must be really bad news if it can cause cancer. Who would even risk doing that diet ever again after this research proves it? I'm so glad I read that headline." You may laugh at my description of how people probably interpreted this study, but I'm telling you that's the exact conclusion and reaction that most uninformed people make upon hearing this kind of news about livin' la vida low-carb.

It's time to hear the facts about whether the Atkins low-carb diet actually leads to colon cancer. This is the information you just won't get in any of those headlines from the media. If you want to be enlightened, then let's get started!

First, let's look at the study itself. Lead researcher Harry Flint, professor in the Gut Health Programme at the UK-based Rowett Research Institute, and his fellow researchers observed a mere 19 "healthy but obese men" who had a BMI ranging from between 30-42 and placed them on intermittent diets consisting of various amounts of carbohydrates over three distinct phases of the study. Here are those three phases in the order they were conducted:

PHASE 1 — The men ate a very high-carb diet consisting of 400g carbs daily for three days in a row at the beginning of the study. This was the number of carbohydrates that is supposedly "needed to maintain their weight" (though if I ate that many carbs today I'd gain 15 pounds by tomorrow morning!)

PHASE 2 — Then, for the next month the men cut their carb intake down by 60 percent to 160g daily. This was still a fairly high-carb diet, but a little closer to what is deemed healthy by most of the government dietary recommendations.

PHASE 3 — Finally, the men had their dietary carb intake slashed again for the next four weeks to 85 percent of the PHASE 2 carb allowance and just 6 percent of the original number of carbs consumed by the study participants in PHASE 1 to 24g daily. This level of carbs most closely resembles the Induction phase of the Atkins diet of the three phases.

During this 9-week experiment, Flint and his researchers took stool samples from the study participants to measure for bacteria and the level of butyrate, a fatty acid chemical prevalent in the gut that has been found to reduce cancer in rats. What they supposedly found in this research is what precipitated all the news headlines. According to the researchers, there was a four-fold decrease in the amount of butyrate in the study participants after their four-week stint on PHASE 3, or the "Atkins" stage of the research.

Flint was shocked because this change in butyrate was "the largest ever re-ported in a human dietary trial." This was supposedly the first such study on the impact of livin' la vida low-carb on bacteria in the gut.

"The results provide strong evidence that butyrate production is largely deter-mined by the content of a particular type of carbohydrate in the diet that the bacteria in our guts can utilize," Flint explained. "But this doesn't automatically lead to the conclusion that reduced butyrate production causes colon can-cer."

Even still, Flint believes his study confirmed what previous research has al-ready found.

"Studies in cell culture have also suggested a link between butyrate and colon cancer," he said. "This study is part of a general inquiry into how to prevent obesity in humans."

The researchers acknowledge that the Atkins low-carb diet is "highly effective" for weight loss, BUT...

"In the long run, it is possible that such diets could contribute to colorectal can-cer," Flint warned. "It is a preventable disease, and there is evidence that poor diet can increase your risk."

We can only assume Flint believes low-carb fits the description of a "poor diet" since he calls it "extreme" and not good for the long-term. Sigh. The argument that low-carb is only good for weight loss in the short-term has been thrown around by misinformed people for a long time. Flint said his study is going to render even more shocking results to "give a fuller picture" when it finally ap-pears in a medical journal.

"We would like people to get the best of both worlds," he contended. "That means knowing in greater detail what goes on in the gut when on a low-carb diet."

Go ahead and go on the Atkins diet for "short-term bursts" to boost your weight loss efforts, but don't you dare do it over the long-term unless you want some rather severe health issues to deal with, Flint concluded.

"It should be possible to lose weight by taking out sugar and starch and maintaining some of the fiber that supports bacterial activity in the intestine," he stated.

Flint is convinced that "long-term deprivation of carbohydrate...causes damage to the gut" and he intends on doing more research on the butyrate/colon cancer connection in humans. Okay, so there you have it! That's the bad news that is supposed to be making low-carb very unappealing to the casual observer. And if I wasn't already really paying close attention to all the research coming out about livin' la vida low-carb, then I'm sure I would be scared half to death to even try it, too.

But let's share a few facts that were missing about Flint's study.

1. It is a small, unpublished, NON-clinical trial study.

This is a vital point. It's one thing to talk about your study, but yet another to have the results of that study got through the peer-review process to look at the veracity of the results based on other research. Perhaps Flint is working on that, but it's disingenuous for him to take this to the media talking about 19 obese guys who were fed a high-carb diet for over a month before putting them on low-carb. I wonder if the results would have been different if PHASE 3 would have been implemented first.

2. We have no idea what foods the men ate on their "Atkins-like" diet.

As we know, the phrase "Atkins diet" has simply become synonymous with a low-carb diet. This has become all-too-common with people who say they are on the Atkins diet when they have obviously never cracked open the book by the late great Dr. Robert C. Atkins. It would be good to know what kinds of carbs were consumed among the 24g that were allotted each day. At this point, it's a mystery!

3. Low-carb INCREASES fatty acids in the blood not decreases them.

This is a metabolic truth that was completely missed by the "experts" featured in the news stories about this study. The higher the fatty acids in the blood, the less need there is for having them in the colon. Livin' la vida low-carb saturates the body with healthy fatty acids.

4. Ketogenic diets (like PHASE 3) use ketones for nutrition.

Once again, we have another basic metabolic truth that was overlooked. The body can make its own carbs through a process known as gluconeogenesis. Ketone bodies are what kept our early ancestors fueled up eating a very low-carb diet.

5. Low-carb diets reduce weight, lower insulin, and increase ketones.

The proof is in the pudding (low-carb, of course!). You lose weight when you go on a low-carb diet and your insulin production is significantly reduced which is why low-carb is an excellent treatment option for diabetics. Those increased ketones energize your body and allow you to burn stored fat while remaining active.

6. It's a leap of faith to speculate based on only one measure of study.

If I wanted to duplicate this study in the same manner or even in a slightly different manner than Professor Flint did it, then I can't help but wonder if I would come up with a different result (especially if the low-carb diet came first!) It's stretching the imagination to think one unpublished study of 19 men warrants as much ink in the press as this study did but we've seen it happen before and I have no doubt it will happen again.

7. Diets that are very low in carbs actually TREAT cancer.

The more we look at cancer, there's a trend beginning to grow — remove the sugar and excess carbohydrate from the diet so the cancer can't feed off of it and you can reduce your risk of getting a variety of cancers.

8. High-carb diets may be linked to all kinds of cancers.

Using deductive reasoning, if low-carb diets starve cancer cells and keep them from spreading throughout the body, then it's safe and accurate to say that high-carb diets do the opposite — they feed cancer cells and allow them to grow at will to do their damage to the human body. If you want to have a real health headline that is both shocking and backed up by growing scientific evidence, then run with that one!

9. Foods on the Atkins diet have LOTS of butyrate in them.

This is the irony of all ironies. While Flint and his gang bemoan the lack of butyrate on this "Atkins-like" plan they fed their study participants, check out the following acceptable low-carb foods consumed on the real Atkins diet along with their very high butyrate content:

Butter: 3,230mg
Parmesan Cheese: 1510mg
Swiss Cheese: 1100mg
Cream: 1080mg
Cheddar Cheese: 1050mg
Gruyere Cheese: 1050mg
Edam Cheese: 1000mg
Gouda Cheese: 1000mg
Feta Cheese: 775mg

10. Gut bacteria reduction only happens in the absence of vegetables.

If you are consuming the recommended levels of vegetables in your diet as required on the Atkins diet, then gut bacteria should not be reduced. It's when people attempt to do "Atkins" on their own assuming they know what that means that gets them in trouble. Do yourself a favor and read the book!

Shifting gears from the subject of cancer, I'd like to take a look at how livin' la vida low-carb can help with brain health — another area of health like cancer where the research has absolutely exploded in recent years.

There's an emerging new form of diabetes of the brain that is becoming so rampant that neurologists and medical researchers are now describing it as "Type 3 diabetes." I first heard about this in 2007 when I interviewed low-carb neurosurgeon Dr. Larry McCleary about his book called *The Brain Trust Program*. According to a study published in the February 2009 issue of *Proceedings of the National Academy of Sciences*, lead researcher Dr. William L. Klein, Professor of Neurobiology & Physiology and of Neurology at the Evanston, IL-based Northwestern University, and his team concluded that insulin protects the brain from toxic proteins that lead to Alzheimer's disease which they acknowledge is indeed this "Type 3 diabetes" of the brain. They added that treating the neurologically-diseased and Alzheimer's patients with insulin and a diabetic prescription medication called Avandia can improve brain function and should be used as a routine treatment option for people suffering from these conditions.

Why would we want to be pumping insulin and diabetes drugs into people who are dealing with a terrible disease like Alzheimer's when previous research in 2006 has already shown changing to a low-carbohydrate nutritional approach gives the brain the preferred fuel source it craves — ketone bodies — to function at optimal levels and effectively reverse the impact of Alzheimer's disease? And we know from a 2005 study that the use of a hyperketogenic diet consisting of a very high-fat, very low-carb nutritional intake to effectively treat and cure conditions such as Parkinson's, Alzheimer's and Lou Gehrig's disease has also shown great results to those who have tried it.

Plus, we can thank Swedish researchers who have already demonstrated to us that high blood sugar levels and Alzheimer's disease are indelibly connected. So, wouldn't it stand to reason that controlling the blood glucose in the body would help to manage diseases of the brain like Alzheimer's?

According to the NIH-related National Institute on Aging web site (nia.nih.gov), research is already underway looking at the impact of an insulin nasal spray on memory for patients with Alzheimer's disease. Their thinking is to squirt the insulin directly into the brain through the nose to avoid the hypoglycemic response that would happen if it was injected in the traditional way into the arm. But like Type 2 diabetics who are told to keep eating sugar and carbohydrates as long as you just give yourself insulin shots, this is the WRONG approach to helping people dealing with Type 3 diabetes, aka Alzheimer's disease. Why not encourage carbohydrate-restriction to these patients? Then the need for insulin and diabetes medications like Avandia becomes irrelevant because blood sugar and insulin are controlled naturally through their diet and thus treated just as effectively if not better.

There's only one teeny tiny little problem with this solution to those who provide health care for these patients: nobody makes any money off of treating Alzheimer's sufferers with a low-carb diet. I hate to be cynical, but it's hard not to be when you see this same scenario play itself out over and over again after a phenomenal study comes out clearly identifying a problem that could be solved with livin' la vida low-carb. And yet a drug or other revenue-producing medical substances like insulin are pushed on to people as the "best" and many times the "only" treatment for dealing with a preventable disease.

Whenever you hear a researcher or doctor say that the only way you can treat a disease is through medication or surgery as your first choice, then you should immediately question it. From all I've seen in just the few short years of looking at this subject of health as an educated layperson, there are almost always natural ways to manage health conditions — especially with the proper diet. Most of your health centers around metabolic issues whether the medical world will ever acknowledge that or not. It's what makes the miniscule one or two weeks of nutrition courses offered to medical school students so inadequate for dealing with the real world cases they'll encounter with their patients day in and day out.

As harmful as we know carbohydrates can be in the body of someone who is insulin resistant or dealing with other common high blood sugar/high insulin issues like diabetes and metabolic syndrome, the first course of action that should be taken is placing those particular patients on a high-fat, low-carb diet immediately. If after 90 days of this kind of treatment there is no improvement, then possibly looking at prescription drugs and/or insulin could become a part of the conversation. But this should only be as a last resort when the diet has failed to correct the problem.

Yet from what I've seen both scientifically in the literature as well as from anecdotal stories of the changed lives of real people, the low-carb diet approach will not fail if it is given a fair chance to work. And practitioners don't need to try to encourage their patients to sneak in so-called "healthy" whole grains or low-fat foods to screw with the results. Give patients a copy of *Dr. Atkins' New Diet Revolution* to read and then encourage them to soak it all in on their way to getting better for good.

Is it really too much to ask for dietary changes to be the first consideration for a period of time before resorting to more risky pharmceutical approaches to treating preventable diseases? I don't think so. We need to end the pill-popping madness and stop encouraging the production of more and more drugs to treat every disease known to mankind! Livin' la vida low-carb might not cure every ailment — but it sure hits a lot of them.

Low-carb neurosurgeon Dr. Larry McCleary was gracious enough to provide his thoughts on this study which I think you'll find an insightful read.

This is an interesting study.

To summarize: The researchers were studying nerve cells in tissue culture. This means they were not in a brain, but had been placed in a growth medium (like what they do to grow bacteria on a Petrie dish). The cells came from the hippocampus (one of the primary memory centers in the brain).

They looked at the neurons for evidence of Alzheimer disease type of pathology (such as build up of amyloid beta pathology) in the untreated neurons. They then added insulin to some similar nerve cell cultures to see what difference it made. When this was done, they noted a marked decrease in amyloid beta pathology (which is a positive change). They did the same thing with Avandia (a Type II diabetes medication that increases the response to insulin, or enhances insulin sensitivity) — basically sprinkling it in with the nerve cells. They saw similar benefits in the nerve cells — those being less amyloid beta pathology.

The take home message from these studies is that somehow both the addition of insulin or Avandia did something beneficial for the nerve cells.

Amyloid beta does several bad things to nerve cells. By binding to specific receptors (binding sites located on the surface of the nerve cells) it causes oxidation and decreases neuroplasticity — the ability of nerve cells to make connections, or synapses, with other neurons. It can even kill nerve cells. These findings decrease memory function. Both insulin and Avandia applied directly to the neurons markedly decreased these findings.

The interpretation of these observations from a clinical perspective is as follows:

1) Enhanced insulin signaling in the brain is good for brain cell function and metabolism. Insulin signaling can be enhanced directly be applying more insulin to the nerve cells, or by making the nerve cells more sensitive to the insulin that is already present (as demonstrated by the beneficial results obtained when Avandia was added).

These findings have been applied to humans by administering insulin intra-nasally to humans with mild Alzheimer disease. The patients showed improved memory when this was done.

The importance of these observations for someone with Alzheimer disease (a disorder with no current cure) is as follows: that insulin taken intra-nasally may temporarily improve function in a condition with no cure. Avandia may be slightly helpful in this context as well.

To fully understand what happens in the brain damaged by Alzheimer disease, you need to know that insulin signaling in the brain declines. (This is another way of saying that the brain becomes insulin resistant — just what happens to the body when diabetes develops.) That leads to the formation of amyloid beta pathology and nerve cell and synaptic loss.

From a health perspective, it makes the most sense to make lifestyle choices that maximize total body insulin sensitivity. That means eating right, exercising regularly and avoiding stress — to name a few things. They represent the best way to be healthy from both a brain and body perspective. When this is done, insulin signaling in the brain improves (and injecting insulin intra-nasally is not needed.)

As we become insulin resistant, the levels of insulin rise in our bloodstream. Since insulin in the brain comes from the blood, one might think that brain insulin levels would rise in tandem with blood insulin levels. THIS IS NOT THE CASE! When insulin levels in the blood rise, insulin levels in the brain actually fall to below normal levels. This occurs partially because the brain transports much less insulin from the blood into the brain cavity. Lower brain insulin levels mean less robust insulin signaling and result in enhanced amyloid beta pathology and nerve cell loss. The best way to prevent this is by keeping blood insulin levels low and this is best done by eating reasonably — meaning avoiding excess calories and excess carbs.

While Dr. G. Pasinetti has done work showing calorie and carb restriction helps prevent AD from developing and improves function, there are some individuals in such advanced states of pathology that these interventions don't work and it is only for those individuals that intra-nasal insulin and so forth might be considered.

The best approach is to eat right and prevent the situation from developing in the first place.

So, from my perspective, the research studies done by Dr. Klein SUPPORT what you have been saying all along. That is, that eating right is healthy for the body and brain by maintaining insulin sensitivity in both. His studies merely document that by demonstrating that good insulin signaling in the brain is beneficial for brain health.

I hope this helps.

Thanks,

Dr. Larry McCleary

But as I previously noted, there has been some truly remarkable research that provides compelling evidence demonstrating several amazingly positive benefits of a very low-carb, high-fat diet in the treatment of Parkinson's, Alzheimer's, Lou Gehrig's disease, epilepsy and other brain-related diseases. Let's take a look at the studies behind a few of those now:

PARKINSON'S DISEASE

Lead researcher Dr. Theodore B. VanItallie, from the St. Luke's-Roosevelt Hospital Center in New York, believed that a "hyperketogenic" diet would serve as an excellent natural remedy for Parkinson's disease because the excess ketones in such a diet consisting almost entirely of fat would trick the body into healing itself without the use of drug therapy. If you think the Atkins diet is restrictive having a fat/protein/carbohydrate ratio of 60/25/15, then this ultra-low-carb diet used by Dr. VanItallie on his study patients may be considered insane by some people. Hold on to your hats, folks, because he had them on a 90/8/2 diet! You read that right...a ninety percent fat diet!

Five Parkinson's disease patients followed this unorthodox diet plan for just four weeks and guess what? Their balance improved, their tremors and shaking ceased, their overall mood was much happier. This study was published in 2006 in the journal *Neurology*.

The once sacred hard-nosed belief that fat can play no role in a healthy diet is clearly out the window now. Several trials and other recent studies looking at dietary treatment of medical conditions has found that people suffering from neurodegenerative disorders like Parkinson's, Alzheimer's and Lou Gehrig's disease can see unbelievable improvements in their condition just from something as simple as virtually eliminating their intake of carbs and protein.

High-fat diets are theorized to benefit people with brain tumors by keeping them from growing bigger. But this isn't a new treatment option. As I shared previously in this book, a high-fat ketogenic low-carb diet has been used for nearly 90 years to treat epilepsy patients, mostly children, to reduce the number of seizures they have. Not surprisingly, the medical community isn't so quick to embrace this "extreme" version of a low-carb diet.

This kind of puts all the negative comments about such mainstream low-carb diet plans such as the Atkins, South Beach, Protein Power, and even the Zone diets in perspective, doesn't it? If these diets are as supposedly dangerous and unhealthy because of their lack of carbohydrates at levels between 15-20 percent of caloric intake, then what are these naysayers gonna say about a diet with just 2 percent carbs?!

So why does this kind of diet help with these awful diseases? The body goes from metabolizing sugar to a much better fuel source — ketone bodies. However, many of the current health "experts" believe a ketogenic diet is unfeasible for people because they supposedly can't stick to it. And, of course, we hear from dietitians who say they are concerned about all that fat causing heart-related health issues and that eating so much fat is unhealthy and undesirable for people to stick with. So I suppose they would prefer these patients eat a 55/25/20 diet known as the Standard American Diet (SAD).

What about just putting these patients on the Atkins diet to see how they would react? Dr. VanItallie actually said the Atkins diet does not produce enough ketone bodies to adequately treat the diseases. This should be Interesting news to the media and current health experts, that Atkins doesn't make enough ketones because it allows too many carbs! This business about the Atkins diet being "no carbs" and that you have to have carbs to survive has been exposed for everyone to see now.

Enough of the propaganda about livin' la vida low-carb, it's time to take a serious look at some of these therapeutic aspects of this amazing dietary approach. Excessive ketone levels are perfectly harmless and even beneficial in a lot of ways. Lab studies have found ketone bodies preserve organs during blood loss and create neurological changes in mice regarding Parkinson's, Alzheimer's, and Lou Gehrig's disease. Studies are still ongoing and it will be exciting to see the results as they continue proving yet again how the healthy low-carb lifestyle has been given a premature bad rap. Scientific research is once again leading the revival of low-carb living and will continue to do so in the years to come.

Regarding brain tumors, it seems the cells in these tumors are starved of blood sugar on a ketogenic diet and can't use ketone bodies for energy. What that means is the growth of these tumors stops and the ketone bodies actually provide nourishment for the healthy cells in the brain. How cool is that? Next up for Dr. VanItallie is yet another new Parkinson's disease study that takes the best elements of the 90 percent fat diet and mixes it with a modified version of the Atkins diet. The same five Parkinson's disease patients who participated in the previous study have been asked again to participate in the new study.

ALZHEIMER'S DISEASE

In March 2009, I conducted one of the most incredible podcast interviews to date with Dr. Mary Newport (CoconutKetones.com) who I first found out about after reading a *St. Petersburg Times* story about how feeding her husband coconut oil had greatly improved his Alzheimer's disease. It was such an extraordinary story of health triumph that I just had to book her for an interview to tell this remarkable chain of events to my listeners. She shared with me and my listeners about the glucose connection to Alzheimer's disease, how ketone bodies are the preferred fuel for brain function, and why medium chain triglycerides (MTCs) found in coconut oil were a miracle for her husband's condition.

This was one of the most stunning personal testimonies of how a high-fat, low-carb ketogenic diet can dramatically improve health I've ever heard in my life. You can't help but be a believer in high-fat, low-carb diets after listening to Dr. Newport gush about her husband Steve overcoming his tremors, regaining cognitive function, and ultimately defeating his Alzheimer's. Look up Episode 240 of "The Livin' La Vida Low-Carb Show with Jimmy Moore" (TheLivinLowCarbShow.com/ShowNotes) to listen to this extraordinary interview. The latest research is backing up what Dr. Newport has found happening with her husband.

Lead researcher Giulio Maria Pasinetti, M.D., Ph.D., who serves as director of the Neuroinflammation Research Center and as professor of Psychiatry, Geriatrics and Adult Development as well as in the Fishberg Department of Neuroscience at the Mount Sinai School of Medicine, used experimental mice to observe the beta-amyloid peptides in their brain to see if they could be reduced. Dr. Pasinetti wanted to see if simple dietary changes could bring about improvements in neurological conditions such as Alzheimer's. What he found was that a calorie-restricted, low-carb diet did exactly that while the mice that were fed a high-calorie, heavy-saturated fat diet showed increased levels of beta-amyloid peptides. This study appeared in the July 2006 issue of *Journal of Biological Chemistry*.

Based on his research, Dr. Pasinetti believes simple changes in the kind of foods eaten can improve the function of the brain, especially in patients who are diagnosed with the memory-altering Alzheimer's disease.

"Both clinical and epidemiological evidence suggests that modification of life-style factors such as nutrition may prove crucial to Alzheimer's disease management," Dr. Pasinetti remarked. "This research, however, is the first to show a connection between nutrition and Alzheimer's disease neuropathy by defining mechanistic pathways in the brain and scrutinizing biochemical functions."

Sweet! While the Atkins/low-carb approach has been generally considered primarily as a weight loss mechanism, researchers are proving it has a lot more benefits as a way to manage various health conditions, including diabetes, cholesterol, bone health, and now Alzheimer's, just to name a few. But this isn't the only study conducted on the low-carb approach to treating Alzheimer's.

Researchers from the Stockholm, Sweden-based Karolinska Institute presented their 9-year study of over 1,100 people at the 10th International Conference on Alzheimer's Disease and Related Disorders in July 2006. What they found during their research is that people with high blood sugar levels are at a higher risk of developing Alzheimer's disease. Previous studies have already shown a link between Type 2 diabetes and Alzheimer's, but this research revealed that even pre-diabetics who have not developed full-blown diabetes yet are in danger of getting the brain-altering Alzheimer's disease.

The Alzheimer's Association has already predicted the number of cases of Alzheimer's disease is expected to quadruple by the year 2050 as the progression of this disease correlates directly with the diabetes epidemic that is now underway. Now we are seeing the unintended consequences of our inability to consider all the treatment options for diabetes. With the most recent research pointing to the low-carb approach as the best way to help diabetics control their blood sugar levels without the use of medications, why wouldn't we want to use this miraculous way of eating to slow down the rates of Alzheimer's disease as well? The evidence is clear to anyone who is paying attention and can still comprehend what is going on here. Diseases of the brain such as Alzheimer's are very likely caused by the excessive amounts of sugar we are putting in our mouths which is then leading to the twin health epidemics of obesity and diabetes that brings us back to a higher risk for developing these awful diseases.

Can't we just stop this madness by recommending the low-carb lifestyle as a healthy, permanent way to not only maintain your weight, but also to prevent all of these diseases from inflicting us with unnecessary medical conditions? If low-carb has been shown to work so well in the treatment of all of these conditions, then why wouldn't our doctors want to prescribe it as a natural cure? It just doesn't make sense to me at all.

As I mentioned earlier in this chapter, Dr. Larry McCleary is leading the way promoting a carbohydrate-restricted diet for those people dealing with a variety of brain health issues. I was privileged to interview him about this subject at my blog in September 2007 and I'd like to share portions of that interview with you discussing what he wrote about in his book *The Brain Trust Program: A Scientifically Based Three-Part Plan to Improve Memory, Elevate Mood, Enhance Attention, Alleviate Migraine and Menopausal Symptoms, and Boost Mental Energy.*

1. Today we have a bona fide expert in the field of brain function and the surprising metabolic connection. He is Dr. Larry McCleary, a brain surgeon currently serving as the Director of Research for the Advanced Metabolic Research Group as well as the former acting Chief of Pediatric Neurosurgery and former Director of the Neuroscience Research Program at the famous Children's Hospital in Denver, Colorado. A world-renowned speaker who has been published extensively in some of the most prestigious medical journals dedicated to brain health, Dr. McCleary is THE go-to man for all things related to the brain.

It's an honor to have you with us today, Dr. McCleary, and we look forward to gleaning from your knowledge and experience in this interview. What first got you interested in brain health and is it everything you expected it to be? What has been most surprising to you about this particular field of medicine that you never would have expected going into it?

Hi Jimmy. It's great to be with you today.

As a pediatric neurosurgeon I took care of thousands of very sick brains. They were suffering from blood clots, infections, birth problems, tumors and traumatic insults. I was always searching for things that could help these sick brains recover and stay healthy.

Early in my career, I had the pleasure of working with a neuroscientist who was investigating the therapeutic potential for certain nutrients to improve brain function. Hollywood types were always stopping by to hear about the latest brain health tips from Dr. Harry Demopoulis. I had the opportunity of experiencing the dramatic impact of some of these brain-healthy compounds first hand.

So when I moved to Denver Children's Hospital I continued the research. Working hand-in-hand with the Neuro-Rehab Division at the hospital, we provided the children under our care with a mix of essential fats, medium chain triglycerides, amino acids and other nutrients. We were convinced that these sped up brain recovery and enhanced mental function. The take-home message for me was if they could help the sickest of brains they could certainly help our brains as we aged.

2. Brain health entails more than most people even realize as you so brilliantly share in your book entitled *The Brain Trust Program*. It is an outstanding resource that I was privileged to review and in it you share a three-part method for actually improving brain function through the use of diet, supplementation, and brain exercises. How does your novel new approach differ from the most common ways to correct brain abnormalities and conditions?

Jimmy, I think we have all heard that the brain burns glucose, or sugar. So if that's the case, then giving it lots of sugar must make it work better. Although that might seem logical, the science doesn't back it up. Just the opposite, there is a groundswell of medical evidence that documents how too much sugar can make the brain shrink, wither, atrophy and just plain work badly.

If you want to age your brain just eat the typical diet most Americans consume. That will lead to memory, attention and mood difficulties and will hasten the path to Alzheimer's. The Brain Trust Program builds upon this concept and provides the science behind the recommendations.

3. Many eyebrows will certainly be raised when people find out what a "brain-healthy diet" actually looks like. Foods like fish, berries, green leafy vegetables, eggs, avocados, nuts, seeds, and coffee — conspicuously all low-sugar and low-carb, by the way — are highly recommended by you for maximized brain function. It falls right in line with the latest research for neurological diseases.

Essentially, you are stating that the health of the brain is directly tied to blood sugar levels in the body — something that medical literature confirms. I'm sure some of your colleagues will no doubt scoff at your contention that a simple nutritional approach is what is needed to preserve this most vital of our organs.

What led you to go down this path for treating your patients? Have you seen similar or better improvements in brain health compared with prescription drugs and other treatment options?

As you well know, prescription drugs usually act on a single metabolic, or cellular, pathway. By increasing or decreasing a specific function, drugs might be able to treat something like an under-active thyroid. However, all of the diseases associated with aging such as heart disease, arthritis, thinning of bones, memory loss and stroke are hardly changed by drug therapy. The key question is why.

As we have seen, drugs act on a single highly specialized pathway. The diseases that cause most concern today involve disruption to multiple cellular pathways. That is why the pharmaceutical industry has failed us. We need a solution that improves MANY cellular functions. This is the very act of eating well. It is also closely tied to our DNA and evolutionary history. Simply stated, that is why nutrition is so important and so beneficial.

4. There's a lot of controversy right now being discussed over the role of artificial sweeteners in a healthy diet. In terms of their impact on the brain, what do you think about the most popular sugar substitutes being used these days, including Nutrasweet (aspartame), Sweet 'N Low (saccharin), and Splenda (sucralose)? What about the claim that these substances are merely excitotoxins that fool the brain into thinking they are sugar and, thus, the body responds in the same manner as sugar?

How about the plant-based stevia which is set to be approved as a sweetener by the FDA soon? Is it safer? Or is it just better to eat pure cane sugar, honey, and other natural sources of sugar in moderation as some studies have suggested for good brain health rather than risking any adverse side effects from these alternatives?

Most of the artificial sweeteners share a dark chemical side with the drugs that are prescribed like water in this country. Both share the fact that they are chemicals to which the body has never been exposed. For this reason they may be patented. When this occurs only one manufacturer may produce them and the profit margin is high. That is what is driving both industries.

Since the body has never seen them before, they may cause problems in certain people. This has been documented abundantly in the drug and artificial sweetener arena. For these reasons I would stick to fruits (which contain natural sweeteners) and spices (which are akin to stevia). I think we all must realize that sweetness is an acquired taste and just as we have been conditioned by the food manufacturing industry to crave sweets, we can de-condition ourselves be choosing natural foods. In time we will lose the urge to eat foods containing such additives.

5. Nutritional supplementation has become a multi-billion dollar industry these days with people taking every vitamin they can get their hands on in an effort to improve their health and ward off disease. Drugstore shelves are full of everything from A to Z, but who knows what to take? And are there better quality supplements people need which are not easily found in stores?

What are the absolutely essential supplements that everyone should be taking to give their brain the best potential for maximum function? Are there any supplements or gimmick "brain health" products out there that should be avoided like the plague?

I think this is a very important question. We are a society looking for a "quick fix" or magic bullet. I think we all know that those don't exist. That is why proper nutrition is so important and remains the cornerstone of a healthy lifestyle. Once a good diet is in hand, there are a few nutritional supplements that can aid the aging brain. I discuss these in the Brain Trust Program. Basically they reinforce the effects of a healthy diet but add nutrients that are specific for the insults associated with aging.

There are a number of products that make egregious brain health claims. That alone should be a tipoff. Be careful to choose manufacturers who use quality ingredients, avoid sources that incorporate heavy metals and make sure they deliver what the label says.

6. A large part of your book includes some simple, but effective exercises for the brain. Why is this oft-neglected part of brain health so

important and what are the benefits to setting aside time each day to do this? Can't people just read or do a crossword puzzle and work their brains enough? What happens to those people who fail to exercise their brain beyond their regular, day-to-day activities?

The brain goes through "phases" if you will as it develops. When we are children, we soak up information like sponges. Learning is effortless. Difficult things like picking up language skills come easily. As we age the brain "solidifies" and becomes less flexible. This is not bad because by this time we know what we need to do to function in society to be successful.

The down side is that we can get "fixed in our ways" and lose the ability to look at things in novel ways. That is why a mentally challenging outlook on life is vital. It keeps the cobwebs away and stimulates ALL the important areas of our brain. That is what keeps us mentally young.

For this reason we need to continually be stimulating our brains in novel ways. This means reading books, solving problems, social interactions, doing puzzles, and even exercising. Aerobic activities, weight training and balance and coordination drills such as ping-pong, jump rope and trampoline activity activate different brain regions and keep us mentally young.

7. Diabetes has become the health crisis of our time with millions of new cases popping up every year while its twin epidemic obesity continues to get worse and worse. We all know about Type 1 and Type 2 diabetes, but what about this new version some researchers are calling "Type 3 diabetes" which is the new way of referring to Alzheimer's Disease because of the impact sugar has on this condition? What has been your experience with treating brain diseases like these through innovative dietary improvements compared with the recommended Standard American Diet?

Type 3 diabetes as you have referred to, was a phrase coined by researchers at Brown University. It suggests that the brain is unable to effectively use glucose as a fuel, much the same as the body of a diabetic can no longer use glucose as a fuel. The ability to deliver a low, stable and continuous supply of glucose to the brain is what makes it most happy.

The dramatic spikes, surges, or continuous excessive supply delivered by today's diet is toxic for the brain. It is now well-known that insulin resistance, glucose intolerance, or the worst form of sugar problem — diabetes, ages the brain and doubles the risk for all types of memory problems and even Alzheimer's disease. As you have suggested, the types of fats and carbohydrates in our diets are key in accomplishing this goal.

We need to include more of the brain-friendly omega 3 fats and veggies and fruits (especially berries), and less of the refined carbohydrates such as cakes, cookies, and breads and trans fats in items like margarine.

8. Many of my readers who deal with less severe brain conditions like migraine headaches, menopause, hot flashes, dimming of the senses, brain fog, and memory loss will be pleased to learn that you actually recommend a specific "cocktail" for each of these in your book. Fascinating! Each of these contains all-natural and healthy ingredients that will supercharge your brain and make it better and stronger than ever.

Give us an example of your most prescribed "cocktail" for a common brain ailment. How quickly can people expect to find relief for their condition using these treatment options and will they need to keep up these regimens for the rest of their lives?

Many common conditions of the brain are directly related to its inability to produce the energy it needs to get through the day. Our brains are being asked to do more today than ever before. They consume energy 10 times faster than the rest of the body. Our dietary and lifestyle choices impair the brain's ability to meet these energy needs which depend upon glucose.

The suggestions I make in The Brain Trust Program depend on an alternative energy source the body developed millions of years ago for times when the brain couldn't depend upon glucose. This alternative fuel is ketone bodies which are merely partially burned fats. They are burned differently than sugars and the brain loves them.

They have been shown to help a multitude of brain afflictions from memory loss to migraine headaches to hot flashes. They are generated in the body from a nutritional supplement called pure MCT (medium chain triglyceride) oil that is available from high end vitamin stores or on the internet. When consumed the results and response can be surprising and may be measured in days! Another easy way to produce ketone bodies is simply by restricting carbohydrate intake.

9. You are a big believer in the body's use of the ketone bodies that form in a carb-restricted state for optimal brain health. What has your research on ketones shown you to make you so confident that they are an excellent replacement for glucose as fuel for the brain? What is your professional response to those who oppose a low-carb nutritional approach as an unhealthy, dangerous, fad diet that is potentially harmful and deadly over the long-term?

Fad diets come and go. The diet we cut our evolutionary teeth on is essentially a low-carb diet that generates high levels of ketone bodies. You need look no further than the brains of children with intractable seizures to see how miraculous ketones are for brain health and function. They work where all drugs fail by increasing the energy available for the nerve cells and keeping them from becoming over-excited which is after all what causes seizures to develop in the first place.

10. THANK YOU for sharing a few moments of your time with us, Dr. McCleary. You truly are one of the leading voices in the health debate over the veracity of low-carb diets for health and the information you have provided about brain health and function in your new book and in this interview today is absolutely incredible. What is the ultimate take-home message that you hope people will remember (no pun intended!) about *The Brain Trust Program*?

We all age and our brains age — but at different rates. As this occurs, there is a period when the brain cells weaken, but before they die. This is when we have symptoms, but also when we can make a difference. If we change our diets, lifestyles and level of brain stimulation we can "nurse" a sick brain cell back to health. But the sooner you start, the better the outcome! So don't wait...jump start your brain now before it is too late!

While the jury may still be out on the positive role of a low-carb diet on such debilitating health conditions like cancer and neurological diseases, you certainly can't argue with the results seen in the studies so far...and the many more that are sure to come in the near future! The next lesson turns our attention to those radical vegans and vegetarians who would like nothing more than to see the entire world eat the same way they do. And the most zealous activists supporting a veggie-only diet can (at times) display some of the most bizarre and awkward behavior you've ever seen in your life. I've seen it for myself over the past five years and will share some of my most outrageous personal encounters I've had with them. Prepare to be entertained!

LESSON #12
Whatever you do, don't rile up the vegetarians and vegans

"I spent a whole month as a vegan one day. Seriously, after all the debates involving intestine-length, canine teeth and gut pH, one fact remains that usually quiets most vegans: there has never, in the history of man, been a society, race, or nation that has survived, let alone thrived, without consuming animal products."

— **Mark Sisson**, author of *The Primal Blueprint: Reprogram Your Genes for Effortless Weight Loss, Vibrant Health, and Boundless Energy* and uber-popular low-carb blogger at MarksDailyApple.com

Upsetting vegans is something that just sort of happens naturally when you have a popular low-carb blog talking about the health benefits of meat-eating like mine does. While I have enjoyed writing about the virtues of eating a low-carb diet for several years now, some of the most radical and outspoken people in the world of health and nutrition are the anti-meat, rabbit food-eating members of this small sect of the population. This is not to say that everyone who is vegetarian or vegan acts this way, perhaps only the ones who comment on my blog. I've got a few examples of this I want to share with you in this chapter of my book.

Okay, somebody tell me something. Why in the world would two very attractive women write a book about weight loss when neither one of them have spent a day in their life struggling with their weight? Well, that's exactly what Los Angeles, California natives Kim Barnouin and Rory Freedman did with their in-your-face attempt to explain to us why women who are overweight got that way. You've probably heard of their book *Skinny Bitch* by now and at least they described themselves accurately! If that extremely profane and totally unnecessary title doesn't grab your attention right away, then perhaps the world's longest subtitle might:

A No-Nonsense, Tough-Love Guide for Savvy Girls Who Want to Stop Eating Crap and Start Looking Fabulous

It's obvious from the start that this isn't gonna be the same old kind of diet book we have all become accustomed to in the past. That in and of itself is not necessarily a bad thing, but it does appear these two ladies have a rather large axe to grind. And you quickly figure that out as soon as you start reading this book with all of its *&#@% *#$#* slamma-jamma graphic idiolect. In an obscenity-laden wasteland of literary refuse, Barnouin and Freedman, one a former model who has studied nutrition and the other a former Ford Model who had been involved in the field of diet and nutrition for more than a decade, quickly let you know what they think about a wide variety of health-related topics. Some are ones that I would agree strongly with them about ("Soda is liquid Satan") and others I obviously disagree just as strongly with them on ("You are a total moron if you think the Atkins Diet will make you thin").

Well, ladies, as much as I agree with you about sugary sodas, I guess you're gonna have to call me a "moron" because that's exactly what the Atkins diet did for me! I was transformed from a 410-pound ticking time bomb on the verge of a certain fatal heart attack down to an athletic and healthy man ready to live a long and healthy life. Now I'm "Livin' La Vida Low-Carb" and I'll never be the same again!

But for Barnouin and Freedman, none of that matters to them because they seem to be members of the radical minority in this country who choose to eat a vegan-only diet. What that means is no meat, no eggs, no dairy, no coffee, not even diet soda because they oppose artificial sweeteners, too — nothing that even touches or comes close to meat! Their recipe for healthy living includes whole grains, fruits, and vegetables and now they're trying to convince women that they too should turn to the vegan lifestyle to become what they've always wanted to be — skinny, happy, and ready to take on life.

If the language and attitude presented in this book are even a smidgen of what Barnouin and Freedman are like in real life, nobody's gonna want to be around them. Could it be that meatless diet of theirs is actually making them cranky and irritable because they're constantly hungry all the time?! Freedman admits that she started down the vegetarian road when she received some literature from PETA (People Eating Tasty Animals!). She was so moved and convinced herself that people were getting sick because of eating meat that she decided to write this book so she could help others "make intelligent and educated decisions about food."

According to the sample menu, you get to eat fresh apple juice with oatmeal, nuts, and fruit for breakfast, grilled soy cheese with a tomato slice and small salad for lunch, and fake vegan ground beef, vegan mashed potatoes, with corn and spinach for supper. This kind of fake food does not sound very appealing to me.

That book along with another pro-vegan book I referred to previously called *The China Study* has been heavily promoted by vegans over the past few years and many of them have let me know how much they don't appreciate the things I say about their cherished diet like I did with *Skinny Bitch*. A woman from the UK named Mary was not a happy camper with what I had to say about vegans despite the fact that the authors of that book had described a person who eats the Atkins diet to get thin as a "total moron."

"Well, it seems that Jimmy Moore has an axe to grind. He wants to sell his own diet book!"

I have no axe to grind and I'm not the angry one. In fact, my readers know me as a pretty happy-go-lucky kinda guy, ya know? Sure I wrote a book in 2005 about my low-carb weight loss experience because many people asked me to so it could encourage them to start on their own weight loss journey. And now I've got another book in 2009 to show people that low-carb is much more about improving health than anything. I have no vendetta against people who want to be vegans if that's the lifestyle change they so desire.

"I think the Atkins diet can make you thin, but it is not famous for making you healthy (Dr. Atkins himself suffered from hypertension, and died of something suspiciously resembling a heart attack — though his widow refused to allow an autopsy so we can't be a hundred percent sure. He had suffered a heart attack before)."

It's well-documented why the Atkins diet is a very healthy way to eat, lose weight, and live a better life. I've detailed it all in this book. Additionally, the "Dr. Atkins died of a heart attack" campaign has been shot down by the truth that Dr. Atkins died of unfortunate injuries he endured during a tragic slip and fall accident on ice in New York in 2003. Let the man rest in peace.

"And the Atkins diet is not guaranteed to make you popular, even if it does make you thin. (So much is forbidden on Atkins that it is the calorie restriction that makes you lose weight. You would be a couple of kilograms lighter too, if it weren't for the constipation.) All that B.O., flatulence and eczema can wreak havoc on your social life."

I assume the forbidden foods she mentions are bread, potatoes, pasta, rice, etc. But since when is being popular more important than being smart and healthy? It's quite easy to eat in social situations when you know which foods are actually good for you and which ones to pass up. Constipation, BO, flatulence and eczema are not typical problems on a low-carb diet.

"I am a vegan by the way, and eat puddings, drink coffee, have snacks. (Obviously the author of the above rant is worried that veganism is an attractive diet, and wants to make it look incredibly restricted. He wants to see my fridge!) I eat lots of fruit of course, but also pancakes occasionally, homemade muffins, rich deep chocolate mousses...If anyone wants recipes check out our website and visit the forum."

There are plenty of treats on a low-carb diet and these snacks she mentions are not even remotely attractive to someone in control of their blood sugar.

"And I do have an axe to grind, and don't mind who knows it. I want people to eat the best food they can, not dress up decomposing flesh in a mushroom sauce, and call it dinner. Would you really eat it if you thought about what it was?"

I do think about it and what I think is that it's called survival and making good use of the resources God provided us. I don't believe eating meat is wrong especially when the animals who give their lives for us have had a good life which is why I recommend eating grass-fed, free-range organic meats and animal products.

"Oh and I don't make any money out of this. So at least my opinion is unbought."

My opinion is not bought, otherwise I would have drifted to the low-fat side by now, because there is much more money to be made over there! Low-carb is not the popular choice at the moment and if I was in this for the money I'd be a poor business man indeed.

It really doesn't matter to me how you lose weight if you need to, but that you actually follow through on your commitment to change. That is the central message of everything I write about. I cannot overemphasize this enough: I really don't care which method you choose to lose weight, just do it! That, to me, is the bottom line.

While I admittedly lean towards a low-carb lifestyle personally for me because it has made my life better, I do not oppose anyone doing whatever they think will work for them to put their health back in order. I just don't need anyone telling me what I have to do to be healthy ever again. Put the information out there and let people decide for themselves. I have been threatened for slander on my blog by one vegan named Simon:

"I think it is fair that Mr. Moore retract his statements about the vegan diet...implying that vegans don't drink coffee, soda, etc. or he will be defending himself in court for slander! If he knew anything about the vegan diet he would know it is such a variable diet rich in taste, texture and nutrients and the best diet for the environment in general. Please use quality articles with substance as people might soon lose interest in your articles."

I felt no need to retract anything since I was simply repeating what was said in a published book by Kim Barnouin and Rory Freedman, and that is not slander. Legal threats don't bother me because I haven't done anything to warrant such action. It's fine if you disagree with my opinion, that's the beauty of living in the United States of American where people can have an open debate of ideas without the risk of being silenced.

While I will never agree that veganism is healthy I will gladly defend the right of vegans to express their opinions and hope they would afford me the same courtesy. It's time to stop this bickering about this "my way is better than yours" mentality and simply state your case for why people should choose low-carb, or low-fat, or the vegan lifestyle. In the end, I trust people to make the best choice for them!

A vegan who regularly reads my blog wrote me the following e-mail wanting to know why I choose to engage a debate about veganism when I don't agree with them. Here's what he wrote:

"Wouldn't your time be better spent arguing for a low-carb lifestyle instead of arguing against a vegan lifestyle? I am, in fact, a vegan, but this e-mail isn't meant to persuade you to adopt my lifestyle. All I ask is that if you feel free to criticize other dietary choices, perhaps you could be more prepared to have your own choices criticized. And finally, if your blog is really devoted to promoting a low-carb lifestyle and not to criticizing other lifestyles, perhaps it's time to call a truce and get back on topic."

I do welcome and appreciate feedback of all types and certainly can understand the concerns of someone like this. While I certainly make no bones about supporting the low-carb lifestyle, I have also tried to provide information for my readers about other nutritional lifestyle choices to help them make the best decision about what eating method can work for them. I've blogged about the low-fat diet, low-calorie diet, Slim-Fast, LA Weight Loss, "The Biggest Loser" diet, cookie diets, coffee diets, and much more.

Obviously, none of these have anything to do with the low-carb lifestyle, but I talk about them anyway because they interest me from the perspective of a low-carber who has seen success on this particular way of eating. Again, I am not required to stick with just talking about low-carb at my blog, although I do attempt to incorporate my experiences doing low-carb with whatever I am blogging about.

Pretty much anything and everything that is related to health and weight loss is fair game for the theme of my web site. Regular readers already know that and also know that if the feedback I receive from a specific blog post generates enough interest that warrants a second, third, or fourth article, then that is my prerogative to continue on with it. Who says that everything I want to write about a certain topic will be covered in just one post?

As to the specific concerns, I think it would be prudent to go back and read my review of *Skinny Bitch* to see how this all started. It was two vegans who wrote a book exclaiming, "You are a total moron if you think the Atkins Diet will make you thin." Was that not meant to provoke supporters of the low-carb lifestyle in some way?

At the very least they should expect rebuttal and a book review response by the people they are offending with their statements. Someone could do the same thing at their own "Livin' La Vida Vegan" blog if they wanted to share their diet worldview, too. I welcome this kind of response to something I have written about because it tells me that I am precisely "on topic."

I really had no intention of writing so many columns on vegans, but the words and actions of certain ones made it impossible for me to ignore. Here's another response I received from a vegan.

Mr. Moore,

Has Mrs. Atkins informed you of what killed Dr. Atkins? HEART DISEASE!!! Please don't allow her to convince you it was from some genetic defect, either! I've been a vegetarian for 26 years...I'm 53. I don't look much older than you do.

Not only are you ignorant and ill informed, but skating on thin ice with a low-carb/eat-meat-til-you-drop diet. Until you have actually lived as a vegan you have nothing but your blindingly myopic opinions to guide you.

As a former meat eating Southerner from Texas raised in ranching and hunting country...I've been on both ends of the spectrum. Knocking something because you have no intentions of giving up your cruel, selfish and environmentally destructive ways because you are guilt ridden about your treatment of the innocent (and believe me that IS the case — otherwise you would try veganism before publicly denouncing it) will only hurt you and people gullible enough to follow such lame advice.

Do the world a favor — educate yourself first by becoming vegan, then learn something called "balance" in reviewing both sides of the issue. Who knows, if you succeed you may just be credible. Until then, YOU appear to be the lunatic and extremist.

Most of the general population knows that Dr. Atkins died because of nothing more than a tragic slip and fall accident on ice. I do not have an "eat-meat-til-you-drop diet" but rather a low-carb diet which saved my life. So why wouldn't I continue this diet for the rest of my life?

My decision to eat meat does not make me cruel, selfish or environmentally destructive. I always recommend people eat grass-fed organic meats whenever possible. My only guilt is that I didn't start livin la vida low-carb sooner. And the challenge to become vegan by trying it for myself is fine. However I do not feel that I should have to become vegan to understand its principles as there are many books on the subject. I'm well-educated on veganism as well as other diets.

There was another vegan woman who responded to me after reading my review of *Skinny Bitch* to express her opinions about what I had to say.

Hello Jimmy,

I actually just wanted to comment on your review of this Skinny Bitch book. Yes, I have read the book and I actually found it very informative. If you get offended easily, which YOU do, I would not recommend it, but loosen up a little! Seriously!

There is absolutely no starving of oneself in this book, I don't know where that came from. The sweets and snacks you are desperately seeking are easy to find, they are just not based on the artificial, chlorinated chemical sweeteners that you all live on. You can have cake, ice cream, cookies, "cheese", muffins, crackers, chips, popcorn...anything you want actually, just as long as it's not laden in butter and whipped saturated fat, or lard, etc. Natural sugars are OK. They won't make you fat!

You sound SO uneducated and ignorant, that I feel really bad for you and your poor heart. Congratulations on your weight loss! I just feel bad that you had to willingly put your body into a state of ketosis to do it. Your body may be smaller, but your internal organs probably hate you.

Can you actually conceive of the amount of stress you have put on your kidneys, liver, heart, brain, skin, spleen, and I really get nauseated thinking about how disgusting your colon is. RANK!!! Anyways, I hope you don't get too offended, but I just think that you should know how others perceive you.

A vegan diet is actually the most flavorful diet I have had. Decomposing dead flesh is not the most appetizing thing I could think of to eat. Your taste buds are probably way too desensitized to appreciate whole grains, veggies, legumes, and fruit (I just had a banana for a snack). It was so good!

Yes, I am vegan and I apologize for my rudeness, I was just offended by your review. If the members of this blog read the book, I guarantee that you would lose at least 80% of them, the rest of the 20% are just looking for an excuse to eat crap. How sad!

I personally have known about 10 people (close to me) that have used the Atkins program and they did start to lose weight, but they felt tired, smelly, constipated, acne breakouts, grumpy and just plain bad (according to them, because I would never try that diet). Convince me that the Atkins diet is healthy — please I would love to hear your side.

Anyways, that is all! Good luck with everything and keep smiling!!!!!!!

P.S. You shouldn't hate healthy, skinny people! It just makes you look silly. I have chosen to educate myself, just like them, and never let myself get obese. I have never starved myself, nor would I ever consider it. Stop being such a Hater!

This is proof yet again that there are all kinds that live in this world of ours. But you've got to admire her passionate desire to spread her vegan enthusiasm to the whole world. Good for her! But I don't appreciate when she and other vegans use their criticism of the Atkins diet to artificially prop up their vegan lifestyle. If you support your way of eating, then support it! Don't bring another nutritional approach down to try to make yours look better.

I have already written one book about my weight loss experience which tells you why none of those other "diets" ever worked for me and how the Atkins diet changed my life forever. And I'm indeed proud of you for choosing to eat a vegan diet if that is something that works for you. You have chosen it to control your weight and health while making it your permanent lifestyle choice. If you've read any of my writings at all, then you would know I harp on that point early and often. It really doesn't matter which plan you choose to help you lose weight and get healthy, but you need to do something.

After I shared my response to this e-mail from the vegan, she wrote me back again with some semblance of an apology.

Hey Jimmy,

I feel the need to apologize for my rude comment about your review. That is definitely your right to eat whatever makes you happy and satisfied. I really don't care what you eat and I don't know why I chose to even comment. Just the heat of the moment, I guess. A person's diet is such a personal topic, isn't it? I'm sure your colon is just fine and I'm sure you feel healthier than you did so good for you! Have a wonderful, long, healthy life!

P.S. I don't take anything back and do not regret saying them, but I am apologizing if I offended you. You are still a human being and deserve respect.

I am certainly NOT offended by a few negative comments about me or my low-carb lifestyle decision. However, I WILL stand up for the things that I know are true — including the fact that the Atkins/low-carb way of eating is based on sound nutritional science and will continue to help people lose weight, keep it off, get healthy and stay healthy for the rest of their lives. I LOOK healthy because I AM healthy! Here's to livin' la vida low-carb for many more years and decades to come!

As so often is the case when people come on my blog with opinions that challenge the low-carb nutritional approach, my readers are very enthusiastic to ask some genuine questions to get to the heart of the matter. Here's what one of them wrote about the negative comments about livin' la vida low-carb shared by the vegan reader's comments:

Are you telling me here that butter, fat, and lard aren't natural? Do you honestly believe that "natural" sugars will somehow behave differently in your body than artificial ones? Have you ever bothered to open a book that explains a little about human metabolism or even heard of a hormone called insulin or glucagon? I suggest you do some reading before you try to give anyone else health advice.

I'm always pleased when my readers offer suggestions. Let's help further educate the public by explaining what the low-carb lifestyle is all about. Be nice, but don't be afraid to share what you think. And it's really funny how the ripple effect of just one blog post can continue to make waves long after it was written. Vegans continued to come out of the woodwork to attack me and low-carb in even more e-mails, comments on my blog, and even on other blogs.

A vegan blogger named Beth Kujawski wrote on her "Finding My Voice" blog (BethKujawski.blogspot.com) about discovering my book review in a Google search while looking for a web site about the *Skinny Bitch* book. Kujawski derided my hometown of Spartanburg, South Carolina by opining that it is "where barbeque is a way of life" (what the heck is that all about?!) She says that she tried low-carb herself and lost weight on it but then somehow knew that what she was eating couldn't be good for her.

Does anyone honestly believe that they can eat steak dipped in butter for the rest of their life and be healthy? Apparently, some people do.

No wonder there are people wanting to run away from the "low-carb" label in favor of something less abrasive with such distortions as this. If people think this is the Atkins diet, then it is obvious they've never read any credible resource detailing the plan (check out registered nurse Jackie Eberstein's web page at ControlCarb.com/CCN-Lifestyle.htm to see for yourself what the controlled-carbohydrate lifestyle is all about).

Kujawski goes on to point out that "the Atkins craze has abated" because "we're not hearing about it every day on the news."

We're not seeing Atkins-approved products sprout up in every section of the grocery store anymore. Gee. Why is that? Maybe it's because people started to think that: 1) Eating nothing but protein is really frickin' expensive, 2) Maybe it wasn't the end-all, be-all path to wellness, and 3) They didn't want to live in a world without a potato.

While the media has hurled insult after insult against the low-carb lifestyle for several years now, that hardly means people aren't doing it anymore. There are still tens of millions of people in the United States alone (including a lot more Hollywood actors and even professional athletes than you realize) following this way of eating and it is making them healthier, lighter and better than ever! The proof is in the results we've seen for ourselves.

To supposedly make her point, Kujawski said she had a friend who was a "full-fledged Atkins prophet."

She would write e-mails, at length, about how great she felt - how clear-headed - and I watched as the weight dropped off. She wore smaller and smaller jeans. She tucked in her shirts. She faithfully ate her Atkins bars and meat. Atta girl.

But...

A couple months ago, I ran into her, and she was heavier than she was when she first started the Atkins diet. Uh oh.

There is no reason to say "uh-oh" here. The friend was going along great, livin' la vida low-carb and obviously hit a major bump in the road in her quest to get healthy and stay healthy. If she had stayed on her diet, she would still be healthy and thin.

Kujawski blogged about me again, calling me stupid, a meat-eating minion and a coward. It's hard to take someone seriously when they resort to name calling.

When I took all this controversy with the vegans to my podcast "The Livin' La Vida Low-Carb Show with Jimmy Moore" (TheLivinLowCarbShow.com/ ShowNotes) in Episode 32, the pro-vegans banded together and threatened the Executive Producer of my podcast Kevin Kennedy-Spaien to "sever" his relationship with me because of my comments. They flooded him with mes-sages pressuring a backlash if my podcast show was not pulled immediately.

Whatever happened to freedom of speech? I have just as much a right to speak out against veganism and in support of low-carb as they do to tell me how supposedly cruel I'm being to animals by choosing to eat them. If you don't want to eat animals, then don't.

You'll be pleased to know that my podcast producer did not back down to the pressure and actually came out stating he would "fully support" me and my right to express my opinions about livin' la vida low-carb just as boldly and proudly as I have been doing since October 2006 at the podcast.

"While we at Disc of Light (DiscOfLight.com) do not necessarily agree with every point of view espoused by our contributors — in fact, that would be im-possible since we cover opposing voices on several topics regularly — I do hold one belief very firmly. It is a great American value, too often forgotten by people of all creeds and causes in these highly charged times. It goes some-

thing like this: 'Although I may disagree with what you say, I will defend unto the death your right to say it.'"

As an olive branch to those vegans who felt their message had not been adequately portrayed, Kennedy-Spaien said he would love to have any vegans or vegetarians who "want to share your articulate and empirical thoughts on why any given dietary system is best" to submit their audio feed for a rebuttal podcast.

"I would say to those who object to Mr. Moore's views, we are willing to grant you the same respect we grant Jimmy...We encourage you to make your feelings known to the world and we will give you the soap box to do so. And we will continue to do so for Jimmy Moore as well."

Not one person took Kevin up on that offer.

However, one of my fellow contributing writers at DietDetective.com named Allena Rose Tapia promotes herself as a "moderate vegetarian," so I had high hopes that some rationality would come out of her. Unfortunately, that didn't seem to be the case.

She conducted a mock interview with a carnivore where she asked her husband to answer some questions about what it's like being a meat-eater. I thought I would try to answer her questions myself here in my book, if not on her blog.

Question: What's the one thing that keeps you from being vegetarian?

Answer: You need animal fat in your diet to be healthy, so a veggie-only diet would leave you nutritionally deficient.

Question: What about the fact that a lot of these tastes can be replicated by meat substitutes?

Answer: If you mean tofu, then no thanks! There are a lot of unanswered questions about soy that still linger out there and these concerns are being substantiated by the research. Give me a T-bone steak instead!

Question: I notice you have children. Do you worry about the environment you're leaving them?

Answer: I'm more worried about a world where a truly healthy diet of fats and proteins is shunned and they'll be forced to eat bean sprouts and tofu for sustenance. We've become too backwards nutritionally these days and it's getting worse.

Question: Why aren't you worried about it?

Answer: Because quite frankly civilization has lasted for many years longer than the past hundred or so on a high-fat, low-carb diet consisting of meat, a little bit of vegetation, and a few berries. The whole low-fat, vegetarian fad has only been around the past few decades and has not stood up to the test of time. It'll pass soon enough when people realize they can manage their weight and health on a diet with 60-70% fat — even saturated fat!

Question: You're familiar with some of the methods by which meat animals are killed and tortured. How do you get past that when you bite into a burger?

Answer: I care about the humane treatment of animals, but I don't care that they are slaughtered to become food for me and my family. And this is why I always recommend grass-fed organic meats whenever possible. It's the way I believe God intended.

Question: How much do you worry about your health in connection to what you eat?

Answer: It's the reason why I went on a high-fat, low-carb diet in January 2004 and have continued to eat that way ever since. My health has never been better than it is right now thanks to eating this way despite the fact that it goes against everything I've ever heard to be true about a healthy lifestyle. But I challenge anyone to tell me that I'm worse off today than I was at 410 pounds.

Question: Would you be willing to reduce your meat-eating days to 3 per week, plus one fish day?

Answer: Why would I want to do that? Meat not only tastes good, but it is good for you too!

Recently I have heard some reports in the media that eating "green" is eco-friendly and prevents global warming, and I'm not joking. An op-ed article by

PCRM member (Physicians Committee for Responsible Medicine) Dr. Patrice Green entitled "Save the Planet with a Vegetarian Diet" spoke about this.

"Temperatures are rising around the world, ice caps are melting, and storms are becoming more severe. Even the Chesapeake Bay and its surrounding island communities are at risk. Death tolls from the increasing heat are also rising, according to a new study from the Harvard School of Public Health's department of environmental health."

Attempting to use a hot political topic as the springboard for her promotion of the vegetarian lifestyle, Dr. Green exclaimed that "global warming can be slowed...by getting 'greener.'" But she's not talking about ditching your SUV for an electric car or purchasing those expensive new mercury-based "energy-efficient" light bulbs. No! She means your diet.

"Most people are neglecting one of the most important steps toward stopping global warming: adopting a vegetarian diet."

Why the PCRM thinks becoming a vegetarian is the answer to global warming is beyond me.

"Studies have shown that people who follow a plant-based diet are slimmer and have less risk of chronic, diet-related diseases than people on high-fat, meat-based diets. In fact, America could begin to reverse its diabetes and obesity epidemics by turning to a high-fiber, low-fat vegetarian diet consisting primarily of vegetables and fruits, whole grains, and beans, lentils and peas."

No, livin' la vida low-carb has been the one shown in study after study which I have highlighted in this book to reverse diabetes, lower body weight best, and raise your HDL "good" cholesterol while significantly lowering triglycerides among other health markers even better than that highly-touted low-fat vegetarian diet of yours. The evidence speaks for itself. Concluding that changing to a "green" diet "might be able to save ourselves — and the planet," Dr. Green I believe is simply playing on the emotions of those who subscribe to the validity of global warming.

In a letter addressed to Blue Cross Blue Shield of Vermont in late 2008, PETA claimed that since meat-eating is so unhealthy the health insurance premiums of meat-eaters in that state should be increased. Additionally, they surmise that since vegetarians and vegans allegedly live healthier, they should be rewarded with decreased health insurance premiums.

"Given the latest news about the effects of E. coli on meat-eaters — and the mountain of evidence linking meat consumption to some of our nation's deadliest diseases — this change will benefit Blue Cross Blue Shield's bottom line while also helping to ensure that your policyholders don't flat line," the PETA representative wrote in a letter to the president of Blue Cross Blue Shield of Vermont.

It's a well-known fact that there is no danger of E. coli if you stick to grass-fed beef and the alleged "mountain of evidence" against meat they keep talking about does not exist.

My contention is that those of us who consume a healthy meat-based high-fat, low-carb diet are benefiting our weight and health much more so than the vast majority of Americans who are consuming excessive amounts of processed, sugary, refined, garbage carb-laden foods that are the real culprit in obesity and disease.

Rather than admit there are multiple ways to live a healthy lifestyle besides being a vegetarian, PETA instead insisted that Blue Cross Blue Shield take action against meat-eaters to punish them.

"By giving your policy holders a financial incentive to go vegetarian — and penalizing those whose meat-based diets fuel our nation's worst health problems — Blue Cross Blue Shield could save millions of dollars in the long run," the PETA representative asserted in the letter.

Wouldn't a better plan be that you eat your diet that makes you healthy and I'll eat my diet that makes me healthy and neither one of us criticizes the choice of the other.

Thankfully, Blue Cross Blue Shield of Vermont responded by saying:

"Under Vermont law, we would not be allowed to vary rates based on the dietary and nutritional habits of various members," a representative noted. *"We have no information one way or the other if vegetarians are more healthy."*

Coming up next, we'll share about a true hero and legend in the world of livin' la vida low-carb who was an amazing man way ahead of his time when he started the low-carb revolution in earnest in the early 1970s. It's time to honor the lifetime of work of the late, great Dr. Robert C. Atkins.

LESSON #13
Dr. Robert C. Atkins was a great man
far ahead of his time

"After witnessing the benefits of Dr Atkins' low-carb lifestyle and complementary medicine ideas over almost 30 years of clinical practice, it is no surprise that accumulating research is validating his approach. There is no doubt that this will continue. Dr. Atkins deserves to be remembered and respected for his pioneering work and courage in the face of decades of brutal criticism."

— **Jacqueline A. Eberstein**, R.N., nurse at the Atkins Center For Complementary Medicine working with Dr. Atkins for three decades, co-author of *Atkins Diabetes Revolution* and founder of Controlled Carbohydrate Nutrition, LLC (ControlCarb.com)

Popular online retail giant Amazon.com celebrated their 10th anniversary in 2005 and decided to compile a list of the bestselling authors over the years to be included in their "Hall of Fame." At the top of the list was J.K. Rowling, author of the wildly popular Harry Potter book series. Rowling is definitely the queen of her domain and can write just about whatever she wants and have it sell a bazillion copies. These Potter fans are loyal as evidenced by the fact that Amazon sold more than 2 million copies of *Harry Potter and the Half-Blood Prince* before it ever released. AMAZING!

Several other famous authors, including Dr. Seuss at #5, John Grisham at #6, and Stephen King at #7 are very well-known fiction writers and have made their mark in publishing history. The Christian fiction *Left Behind* series authors Tim Lahaye and Jerry Jenkins landed at #9 and daytime television talk show and advice guru Phil McGraw came in at #11. But guess who slipped in under the radar as the bestselling health author in Amazon.com's decade of existence? It's none of than the patriarch of livin' la vida low-carb himself, Dr. Robert C. Atkins. I'm not at all surprised, but look at how they described Dr. Atkins in their little blurb about who he is:

"Creator of the famous 'Atkins Diet,' which shuns carbohydrates in favor of meat-laden protein."

Even when he's being recognized for achieving great publishing success, these people still get it dead wrong about what Dr. Atkins promoted in his books. Maybe somebody should have actually read one of those tens of millions of books that sold because they would know Dr. Atkins never promoted anything that "shuns carbohydrates in favor of meat-laden protein." That is the editorial comment of the person who reported on this list and is so far from the truth it is simply ludicrous. People who HAVE read the book know it is a high-fat, moderate-protein, low-carb nutritional approach that is backed up by solid science and a litany of anecdotal evidence in people like me who have succeeded following it.

The comment made about the #24 author on the list, South Beach Diet creator Arthur Agatston, is also incorrect:

"Created the 'South Beach Diet,' which unlike the Atkins program says carbs can be good."

The Atkins diet advocates eating carbs as well, but in a much more controlled manner than is typical of most diet plans out there.

Regardless of how people view Dr. Atkins and his books, his impact on society and history cannot be diminished. My life was personally changed dramatically for the better as a result of reading *Dr. Atkins New Diet Revolution* in December 2003 when my in-laws bought it for me as a Christmas present. I will never have to live with the burden of obesity and the health-related problems that go along with it ever again because this man had the vision to create a weight loss and weight maintenance program that really works.

I say kudos to Amazon.com for honoring a true giant in the realm of health and nutrition.

Not everyone gives Dr. Atkins his proper historical due, though. Even after his untimely death in 2003, the enemies of the Atkins diet have been out in full force to rewrite history about Dr. Atkins' stellar career where he helped millions of people lose weight, control their diabetes, and improve their health. One of the most outspoken Atkins antagonists who shares his disdain for the Atkins low-carb way of eating on a regular basis is Dr. Joel Fuhrman, author of a vegetarian book called *Eat to Live*, who also has a blog called Disease Proof (DiseaseProof.com).

In a post published in 2006 entitled "Examining Dr. Atkins' Death," Dr. Fuhrman said the whitewashing by certain people about how and why Dr. Atkins died is "distorting the facts" about what really happened to him.

"Before Dr. Atkins was hospitalized near the end of his life, he weighed about 200 pounds. Atkins' medical record showed he had atherosclerosis, coronary artery disease, had suffered from a previous heart attack, and had high blood pressure. However, many would have you believe he was merely a healthy guy who died after slipping on a patch of ice."

Can you still believe this is such a heated subject of controversy about something that happened many years ago? Dr. Atkins has passed on to meet his Creator and cannot stand up to defend his good name. Since he is no longer around to defend his good name, I will be more than happy to stand up for him! I wish they would just let the man rest in peace.

Let's address this issue of Dr. Atkins and his health at the time of his death by reviewing what Dr. Atkins' widow Veronica Atkins had to say about it in the days following this tragedy.

"I am sure that any one of you would be offended and perhaps even horrified to have complete strangers intrude into your personal family matters, especially with regard to something as intimate as your medical records or those of your loved one," Mrs. Veronica Atkins said in a statement just days after her husband died after suffering complications from a slip and fall accident in New York City.

Mrs. Atkins explained in that statement about her late husband's weakened heart that it was due to an infection, not his diet. Several medical professionals and cardiologists confirmed that the diet promoted and engaged in by Dr. Atkins was NOT the source of his condition. PERIOD! End of story! Why must this question keep coming up when it's already been settled? Could it be that anti-Atkins advocates are desperately grasping at straws to scare people away from beginning a healthy low-carb lifestyle change? Makes you wonder.

"I look forward to the day when Dr. Atkins' soul can rest in peace and I can grieve uninterrupted," Mrs. Atkins wrote at the end of her statement.

Please keep in mind when reading negative commentary about Dr. Atkins, consider the source of the information.

"The only point to be made here is these guys advocating a high meat diet are unfortunately hurting themselves too, not just their followers, but it is a shame that people have to suffer and even die needlessly from the advice of these high-meat advocates."

For Dr Fuhrman to make the giant leap that the death of Dr. Atkins proves his diet is no longer viable for people to follow for weight loss and health is like saying the passing of Michael Jackson means pop music has run its course and people should only listen to country music now. This is, of course, preposterous.

Where would I be today without the Atkins diet? High blood pressure, high cholesterol, breathing problems, Type 2 diabetes, probably weighing over 500 pounds, no sex life, no social life, sitting in front of a television moping about my health, feeling depressed that I haven't been able to find a way to lose weight, suicidal, or even six feet under along with my brother Kevin who died a premature death at the age of 41 due to morbid obesity (who I'll talk about in the final chapter of this book). All of that was avoided because I went on the Atkins diet!

Livin' la vida low-carb worked for me and I'll never be the same again because of it. Neglecting to point out the countless positive success stories of the Atkins Nutritional Approach like mine that exist in the world today is both short-sighted and narrow-minded. Dr. Robert C Atkins has changed so many lives for the better including a good many people who are reading this book right now.

When people regularly rail against low-carb so often I'm driven to carry on the torch of advocacy for livin' la vida low-carb that had been for the most part absent since the untimely death of Dr. Atkins In 2003. It was as if all the defenders of this way of eating fell off the face of the planet or suddenly decided to clam up. I for one felt that somebody needed to stand up on behalf of Dr. Atkins to defend his life's work even though I never had the privilege of meeting him prior to beginning on his plan. He left behind an incredible legacy that will continue to positively impact the lives of tens millions of people around the world for decades and generations to come. My only regret is that I was never privileged enough to shake his hand and thank him personally for helping me lose 180 pounds in 2004. I am a permanently changed man today because of the Atkins diet and nobody can ever take that away from me.

But although I can never have that fateful meeting with my nutritional hero, I got to experience the next best thing — a personal meeting in January 2006 and then a blog interview with none other than Mrs. Veronica Atkins in May 2007. As the faithful wife and loving companion to Dr. Atkins through all the ups and downs of his unprecedented medical career, nobody knew the human being she affectionately referred to as "Bobby" better than Veronica.

I've been able to meet and interview a lot of interesting people at my blog and podcast show over the past few years, but none more thrilling than this one with Mrs. Atkins. Eloquent, articulate, and ever-faithful to the mission of her late husband, you will be encouraged anew to start livin' la vida low-carb after hearing what this engaging and elegant woman had to say.

1. Words cannot adequately express how privileged and honored I am today to have with us here at the "Livin' La Vida Low-Carb" blog the one and only Mrs. Veronica Atkins. As most of my readers already know, Mrs. Atkins is the widow of Dr. Atkins who came up with the most widely-discussed diet program in the history of the world. Did Dr. Atkins have any idea this low-carb diet he stumbled upon decades ago would create such a ruckus? More importantly, did he ever really expect the Atkins diet to be fully embraced by the health and medical community?

Thanks Jimmy. It's my privilege and pleasure to be here with you and to share a little bit with you and your readers about my late husband, Dr. Atkins. Your Livin' La Vida Low-Carb blog has been an invaluable resource for health professionals and the public alike to remain informed and current on all things low-carb. Your passion equals that of Dr. Atkins — and that's saying something!

The short answer to both your questions is a resounding "Yes." Bobby certainly didn't want to create a ruckus — he hated controversy — but he had no choice. He was ridiculed and alienated by his peers for pointing out that carbohydrate restriction is the single best strategy for treating excessive levels of insulin which leads to diabetes, obesity, hypertension, heart disease and even cancer. So, of course, he felt compelled to speak out.

Certainly, he fully believed that the controlled-carb lifestyle would eventually be accepted as a healthy lifestyle choice. How could he not when he saw the evidence in his clinical practice every day where he could reverse Type 2 diabetes and prevent it in those who were at risk of developing it. My husband firmly believed that had mainstream medicine adopted his teachings, the public health crisis that we see today, where obesity and diabetes have reached epidemic proportions, could have been averted.

2. As much as he and his healthy nutritional approach have been irresponsibly chided and scorned by the so-called health experts and the media over the past few years, nobody in this world really knew Bobby Atkins the human being as well as you — his faithful companion. What are the qualities you best remember him for and is there anything about the real Dr. Atkins that you wish people would never forget?

Well, I was in constant awe of Bobby...his intellect, his honesty, his courage, his boundless energy, his curiosity and thirst for knowledge and his commitment to his patients and their rights.

One of my fondest memories is of him leaving our apartment every morning at 6:30am for the short walk to his clinic...and the worn black canvas bag (that I tried, unsuccessfully, to replace with a briefcase on his birthday!) that he carried with him wherever he went — stuffed to the gills at all times with his writings, notes and medical journals. For all his brilliance, there was a childlike quality that he never lost...and every day was an adventure for him.

I wish people knew how hard he fought to change things. Even though he knew that by speaking out he would be attacked and vilified by his detractors, he never wavered in his convictions. In his monthly newsletter, writings, radio show and media appearances over the years he spoke out about many of the issues that only now are making headlines: the dangers of trans fats, the over-prescribing of hormones, antibiotics, statin drugs, and the consumption of denatured foods such as white flour, sugar and high fructose corn syrup — which make up the majority of products that line our supermarket shelves — and their role in the obesity epidemic; he brought to light scientific evidence that heart disease is not caused by cholesterol when it was widely accepted that it was the #1 cause.

He called to task some formidable opponents — the food companies, the pharmaceutical giants, the FDA, the ADA, and the AMA — and exposed their deceptive and in many cases dangerous practices. And he was instrumental in changing policy that led to the passing of patients' rights bills.

I'd also like people to know that he was a brilliant clinician and diagnostician and not just a "diet doc," a label that stuck due to the phenomenal success of his Atkins Diet Revolution books. In his clinical practice, he treated a myriad of illnesses and succeeded in weaning patients off of their medications using diet and correcting nutritional deficiencies — something that gave him enormous satisfaction. He used the low-carb approach as the basis for all of his treatments.

Another interesting and little known fact about my husband is that at one point he wanted to pursue a career in comedy — in fact in his early years, it was a toss-up as to whether he would pursue a medical career or a career in stand-up comedy. He had a wonderful wry wit and I think he could have been a successful comedian. However, I have no doubt and neither did he that he was put on this earth to make a difference.

3. How did it make you feel when the downright malicious lies from anti-Atkins, anti-meat groups like the Physicians Committee For Responsible Medicine (PCRM) came out about your husband's untimely death following a slip and fall on ice in New York City were plastered all over the news boldly and erroneously reporting that Dr. Atkins had died of a heart attack and was obese? If you could respond directly to those who make such allegations, what would you say to them?

As you can imagine, it hurt me to the core. I'd ask this group to try and see reason, put aside their agenda and tell the truth. Unfortunately the more I hear about this group, the more I'm convinced that they are fanatics — unwilling and uninterested in seeking the truth.

They certainly showed their true colors when they illegally obtained copies of Dr. Atkins' medical records following his death and then leaked false information to the press claiming he was obese. When my husband was admitted to the hospital following his accident, he weighed 195 pounds — a healthy weight for a 6' 2" tall man. The extra weight he gained during his hospital stay was due to an accumulation of body fluids related to his treatment and linked to organ failure. However, this group chose to distort the facts to suit their agenda, which is very disturbing indeed.

Dr. Atkins had suffered from a heart condition called cardiomyopathy — which is a disease of the heart muscle caused in his case by a viral infection and was totally unrelated to his diet. He spoke openly about his condition and did a lot of research, publishing his findings to help others with this condition.

4. Carrying on the amazing work of your husband today, you head up The Robert C. Atkins Foundation where quite literally millions upon millions of dollars are being invested in those research facilities who are willing to test the Atkins low-carb diet in the battle against obesity and the twin epidemic of obesity and diabetes. How does the Atkins Foundation go about determining who gets these generous endowments and when can we expect to see the fruits of those dollars produce scientific proof of what most of us who are livin' la vida low-carb already know?

Well, many types of studies are being funded by the foundation, not just low-carb diet studies. The foundation accepts proposals from any serious non-profit organization wishing to pursue questions still needing answers in nutrition, metabolism, childhood obesity/diabetes, cancer, Alzheimer's disease, cardiovascular disease to name only a few, along with numerous advocacy and community projects.

The selection process is based on how well the study is designed, the importance of the questions being asked, the amount of funding being requested, and, very important, how we see the findings being put into practice. My goal is to impact childhood obesity and diabetes in my lifetime along with contributing to the science that shows the benefits of low-carbohydrate food choices on many other diseases.

5. Speaking of diabetes, you are thoroughly convinced that it CAN be cured and eradicated through the use of the Atkins diet and a 2006 study from Dr. Eric Westman out of Duke University has already shown that is exactly what happens when diabetics are placed on such a plan.

If such clear evidence is on the table that a low-carbohydrate plan can bring A1C levels down to "normal" while vastly lowering triglycerides, raising HDL "good" cholesterol, and normalizing blood sugars sometimes without the use of any prescription drugs or insulin, then why does the American Diabetes Association (ADA) continue to overlook the Atkins diet as a viable option for taking on this preventable disease? What is it going to take to convince diabetics to stop eating the ADA-recommended high-carb, low-fat diet and turn to low-carb as the lifestyle change they need to finally bring their condition under control?

As they say, the proof is in the pudding. And Dr. Atkins proved over and over again in his 40 years of clinical practice that the controlled-carbohydrate program is without question the correct one for the prevention and treatment of obesity and Type II diabetes. However, whenever he tried to bring his findings to the attention of the medical establishment, they were shot down for lack of supporting research studies.

Nevermind the fact that the low-fat proponents who dismissed his findings had no research to back up their theories. We now have an overwhelming amount of research which supports carbohydrate restriction as the number one therapy in the prevention and treatment of Type II diabetes. Yet they still choose to look the other way.

These organizations, the AMA and ADA, obviously have their heads in the sand when they continue to ignore the mounting scientific evidence on the impact of a controlled-carb diet on obesity and Type 2 diabetes. There is also the concern that many experts are influenced by strong lobbying groups such as the food industry and pharmaceutical giants.

Bobby would often tell me of patients who were able to get off their medications and better control their blood sugars within days of starting his program. But the tide is turning, especially on a grassroots level, as more and more people try low-carb and do well. I certainly believe that the "powers-that-be" will have to come to their collective senses and be forced to address the immeasurable damage done by the low-fat dogma.

6. I know it breaks your heart to see childhood obesity and obesity-related diseases afflicting children at record levels over the past decade. But you came across a small glimmer of hope last year when a class of 5th grade kids from a Florida elementary school did something quite

extraordinary — they refused to sell sugary candy as a fundraising avenue for their field trip to Washington, D.C. because they said it was too unhealthy. WOW, now that's a shocker in this day and age! When you heard about the bold stand against sugar of these courageous students, what did you do to help them out and have you come across any other examples of similar actions taken by students elsewhere?

As heartbreaking as it is to see the devastating effects of childhood obesity, it is equally heartening to see the ability of children to change things. When I heard about the children in Florida not having enough funds to take their field trip because they chose not to sell sugary snacks, I met with the children and of course funded the trip.

This was not my first experience with the ability of children to create change. Surely, the greatest example of the power of youth to create change is an extraordinary Canadian group called Free the Children. It was started in 1995 by two brothers, Craig and Marc Kielberger, both barely in their teens. It has since grown into an international movement of children helping children that has improved the lives of over a million children in 40 countries.

They've built over 400 schools to date, provided much needed clean water and medical supplies and set up supporting community women's groups. In 1998, they started Leaders Today, a leadership institute that empowers and inspires over 250,000 youth every year around the world to become actively involved in volunteerism to help those in need and to make the world a better place.

The Robert C. & Veronica Atkins Foundation joined with Free the Children to create a program called Life in Action, which has already been implemented in 120 Canadian schools. It's about educating children in the basics of nutrition, the importance of good wholesome, nutritious food and the avoidance of nutrient-deficient foods and sugary snacks. It also encourages regular physical activity in creative ways.

I've visited some of these schools and spent time with the children and it's just incredible to see the enthusiasm with which they have embraced this, and their eagerness to pass on their knowledge to family and friends. We are working on bringing this program into U.S. schools as well.

7. I had the privilege of meeting you for the first time in January 2006 in Brooklyn, New York at the Nutritional & Metabolic Aspects

Of Carbohydrate Restriction conference and was able to personally thank you on behalf of your wonderful husband for the Atkins diet. In January 2004, I weighed 410 pounds and my health was on the verge of collapse had I not done something about it as soon as possible.

Today, I am 190 pounds lighter and no longer taking the three prescription medications for high cholesterol, high blood pressure, and breathing I was on at the time. With literally tens or even hundreds of thousands of other Jimmy Moores out there living healthy for perhaps the first time in their entire lives because of the Atkins diet, why isn't the Atkins low-carb nutritional approach being recommended alongside the high-carb, low-fat diet by government and health organizations? What can those of us who have been so dramatically changed for the better by the Atkins diet do to convince these people in positions of power over health policy in America that low-carb should be given equal treatment?

Well, I don't believe there's anyone out there who could say you've not done your share — and certainly what we need more than anything are more Jimmy Moores! Your own story of dramatic weight loss and return to health following the low-carb approach is something that Dr. Atkins would have relished.

Unfortunately, it takes time to turn the tide of popular thinking. The slick marketing tools employed by the food companies ensures that the low-fat dogma remains ingrained in people's consciousness, and of course that takes time to reverse.

However, we are seeing some very positive policy changes take place, such as the removal of unhealthy snacks from school vending machines and healthier school cafeteria lunches being served. We have Mayor Bloomberg, Arnold Schwarzenegger and former President Bill Clinton, among others, all of whom appear to be committed to following through on children's health issues in various ways.

While we are making strides, the low-fat mentality however is still quite pervasive. For example, I would love to see a return to the day when schools will again start serving full-fat nutritious milk to children instead of the tasteless, blue-tinted low-fat substance that passes for milk and is so popular with school authorities. I doubt children are overweight because of drinking whole milk!

I am fully committed to doing everything I can to educate people with the facts and to further Dr. Atkins legacy. And to that end, my new web site (VeronicaAtkinsFoundation.org) launched just recently. My site will feature many low-carb recipes — including favorites of mine and Bobby's — all tasty, nutritious and easy to prepare. It also has a section on family nutrition.

I'm very excited to be working with Jackie Eberstein, who was one of Dr. Atkins closest colleagues, to provide a source of accurate and up-to-date information for the public and professionals alike on the low-carb approach, research and complementary medicine. Jackie Eberstein's web site just recently launched as well. Jackie is the consummate expert on all things Atkins.

8. That recent JAMA study out of Stanford University in March 2007 showing the Atkins diet was the best among four popular diets for weight loss and improved health after one year certainly gave a huge shot in the arm to the life's work of your husband as interest in the low-carb approach has been rekindled. Do you see anything else coming up on the horizon in the next year or so from the realm of research, a new book, or even from the entertainment industry that could help continue the rebirth of the Atkins diet?

Yes, that study was a wonderful validation of Dr. Atkins' work and I feel certain it will spur many more. Certainly, it lends credence to all of the studies funded to date by the Atkins Foundation which showed similar results.

Many of the initial studies funded by the Foundation have been completed and the results published. For a listing of articles already available, readers can look on the Atkins Foundation's web site. Several of our investigators will be publishing their findings in the coming year. There is a large two-year NIH study comparing the Atkins diet with a low-fat diet and the results of that should be available this coming year as well.

Gary Taubes, the journalist who wrote the eye-opening article in the New York Times magazine section is coming out with a wonderful new book (Good Calories, Bad Calories) clarifying much of the history and dogma about our current guidelines and recommendations.

Also, an independent filmmaker named CJ Hunt is finishing a documentary called The Perfect Human Diet which chronicles the evolution of our dietary habits which should be a fascinating account of our eating habits and how they have changed.

9. Despite the constant negativity that is hurled against the Atkins diet, the fact is it has left an indelible impression on our society about how people perceive carbohydrates, especially nutritionally bankrupt ones such as sugar, high fructose corn syrup, white flour, potatoes, rice, pasta, processed foods, and fast food. In the perfect world, though, what would Veronica Atkins like to see happen with all the invaluable information that was provided by Dr. Atkins in his books? Do you think future society will one day look back at all the needless criticism about the Atkins low-carb diet and shake their heads in disappointment?

Well, Dr. Atkins upset a lot of apple carts in his time! The bread, pasta, fast food and soft drinks industries lost millions because of him. He challenged the proclamations of the FDA, the AMA, ADA, and others — and in so doing incurred their wrath. However, his commitment paid off and I read recently that more than 44% of people in the U.S. are eating less carbs.

I'm so optimistic about all that is happening at the moment in the area of health — the emerging science on the safety and health benefits of the Atkins approach and the recognition that in the midst of an obesity epidemic, low-fat is not the answer. The World Wide Web of course will continue to have an enormous impact on people's ability to access and exchange information. We now have so many wonderful low-carb web sites and blogs, like your Livin' La Vida Low-Carb blog, which provide a forum for intelligent discussion and the dissemination of accurate and truthful information.

10. THANK YOU, Mrs. Atkins, for taking just a few moments of your time to spend with me and my readers today about the wonderful world of livin' la vida low-carb. You are an amazing and gracious ambassador for the low-carb lifestyle and we in the low-carb community want you to know how much we love and appreciate what you are doing to help continue the fantastic legacy of that incredible man you called husband, Dr. Robert C. Atkins. Do you have any final words of encouragement or advice to share with my readers who are already following or even thinking about going on the Atkins diet?

For anyone thinking about starting the low-carb approach, the most important advice I would give them is to read two of Dr. Atkins' most important books.

First, start with Dr. Atkins New Diet Revolution and when you're close to your goal weight, then read Atkins for Life. While I realize that in today's world of instantaneous access to information, taking the time to read a book might be considered passé, these are no ordinary books and you will find yourself referring to them again and again.

There's a wealth of knowledge contained within those pages plus they're written in Dr. Atkins inimitable style so it's never boring. And, please remember — it's a lifestyle, not a diet.

Thank you so much Jimmy for all that you've done and continue to do for the health and well-being of humanity and for being such an ardent supporter of my husband and his work.

What an incredible experience that was to interview Mrs. Veronica Atkins and I'm honored she spent time sharing some amazing memories about the man who was so instrumental in changing my life and the lives of many of my readers forever. God bless you, Mrs. Atkins, for keeping the spirit of the late great Dr. Robert "Bobby" C. Atkins alive and well. Thank you for continuing to carry on his work now and into the future through the Dr. Robert C. and Veronica Atkins Foundation (AtkinsFoundation.org).

One of the hallmarks that someone's life has made a lasting impact on the world is when their contributions to society are still being talked about many years after that person is gone. That's precisely what has happened to Dr. Atkins over the years. Ever since he was prematurely taken from us on April 17, 2003 after a tragic slip and fall accident on some ice in New York City which resulted in a massive head injury that he was unable to recover from at the age of 72, people have continued to be enthusiastic followers of his controlled-carbohydrate nutritional approach. Although I had not yet chosen to begin livin' la vida low-carb at the time of his death in 2003, I have since grown to love and appreciate all that this incredible man has done for me even after his untimely demise. My life will forever be changed for the better because of the lessons I learned from the Atkins diet.

It's no secret that Dr. Atkins suffered from a heart condition called cardiomyopathy stemming from a viral infection and most reasonable people realize it had nothing at all to do with his healthy low-carb diet. In fact, if you go back through statements he made throughout his 30+ years in the diet industry, then you will hear him speak quite candidly about this personal condition he suffered from and the many hours of research he undertook to study it to help others dealing with it as well. You probably won't hear this information anywhere else.

Nevertheless, the never-ending drumbeat of personal vilification of Dr. Atkins goes on to this very day and I'll sometimes hear from people inquiring about the circumstances surrounding his death and whether it had anything to do with his diet. I'm always happy to respond to these questions because it's an opportunity to share the truth. Here's an example of what one man wrote to me:

Hello,

I really enjoy your blog! Congratulations on the fine success you continue to enjoy.

My questions for you: Is there any truth to the stories circulating a few years ago that Dr. Atkins had arteriosclerosis and other circulatory conditions? I know the family addressed his post-coma weight gain, but can't find where they addressed these reports. Any info? If this is already answered on your blog I overlooked it, I'm sorry. Thanks for your time.

I explained to him that there are some pretty radical low-fat loving, anti-meat individuals and groups out there who will continue to rail against this way of eating because it threatens them and their low-fat way of life. It's great that they have chosen to be a vegetarian or a vegan or whatever, but that way of eating doesn't work for all of us as you well know.

He then responded with a follow-up e-mail:

Hey Jimmy,

Can you tell me, if you know, what the nature of the infection Dr. Atkins had that led to these conditions? Did his family or Atkins Nutritionals, Inc. representatives ever say?

Unless that issue is buried once and for all, there will be no end to the ammunition his enemies will have to claim that the diet could lead to long-term damage to the cardiovascular system, even if it takes 30 years to do it.

And I'll confess, it's given me a bit of cautious doubt myself, despite the benefits I've seen so far in my own weight and energy (the next blood test is several weeks away yet). I'm one of those "examine all sides first, then decide" people! Thanks again.

Man, if I had a dollar for everyone that asks me this question. Here was my reply back to him:

Yes, Dr. Atkins had issues that were present in his own health LONG before he even started his research on low-carb diets. Veronica Atkins issued a statement explaining this to the world. To me, it's as simple as this — looking at Dr. Atkins and his health is not going to prove or disprove what livin' la vida low-carb has done for me. The fact is it IS working for me and I've never been healthier in my entire life. It sounds like the same thing has happened for you, too. CONGRATULATIONS!

Ultimately, the decision about continuing on with this way of eating is yours. But ask yourself one question — How else am I going to eat healthy if I don't eat low-carb? That's just a little something to think about, my friend. THANKS again for writing.

The bottom line that I try to tell people is don't let anyone try to talk you out of your low-carb lifestyle with lies and innuendo when you know it is what's right for you. This is YOUR life and health, so anyone who disparages your decision to eat a healthy low-carb diet can just go suck on an egg (which is very low-carb, by the way!). You could tell it was like a light bulb went off in my reader's head when he wrote his final e-mail back to me:

Thank you! I never saw that statement from Veronica Atkins before and it is entirely satisfactory to me. Thanks for pointing me to it!!! As for the occasional anti-meat fanatics you get dropping by, just remember, "You will never reason a man out of something he wasn't reasoned into in the first place." I personally wouldn't waste time on them. They won't dispute Atkins on any medical, scientific or otherwise objective basis because they can't. But in their minds they don't really NEED to, either.

As you know, they view eating anything with a face as morally wrong. That (in their minds) ends all need for rational, mature discussion. No success you have will make one bit of difference to them, except to make them angrier; you are still WRONG and EVIL for eating meat, period. Hence the losers who threaten you with the heart attack bogeyman. That you tolerate them as well as you do is impressive...I have no patience for such fools. Continued success to you!

Ah, another satisfied low-carb convert...welcome to the fray, my friend! You see, even though it has been years since Dr. Robert C. Atkins has departed from us, we're still talking about him. And they'll still be talking about him in 2010, 2015, 2020, and beyond! His legacy will live on for a very long time because you and I both know he was right all along. Since Dr. Atkins had his fair share of them over the years and still does to this very day, it should come as no surprise to learn that when you put yourself out there on the Internet like I do there will be people who will judge you for what you are doing. We'll talk about these bundles of joy in my next lesson. You're gonna love it!

LESSON #14
If you put yourself out there on the Internet, people will judge you

"Keyboard warriors, shrouded in their cloaks of anonymity and odd pseudonyms, have nothing better to do but heckle those of us who only wish to help others. They're what we call 'haters'. There was a time when their words would keep me up at night. Some were racists. Others called me a 'quack' and a 'snake-oil salesman'. In fact, I deleted two fairly successful YouTube channels because I simply couldn't cope with the daily criticism. But what I've come to understand is that nowhere can you find a successful person without a band of haters behind them. They're part of the recipe for success. I love them as much as they hate me."

— **Sean Croxton**, fitness and nutrition expert at UndergroundWellness.com and popular health video blogger at YouTube.com/UndergroundWellness

When you put yourself out there as a regular and consistent daily blogger and build up a sizeable audience of readers like I have, then it should not be surprising to learn that your readership contains quite an eclectic group of people. Sure, most of my readers have a common bond around the subject of livin' la vida low-carb, but that doesn't mean we all think and believe the same way. And thank God, too! Wouldn't life be pretty drab and dreary if all of us were exactly the same? UGH! I think I'd lose my mind if it weren't for the variety that life tends to throw my way from time to time. Of course, that drives my wife Christine nuts because she loves the stability of predictability. But give me the ebb and flow of life any day of the week!

With that said, sometimes the changing tide can get a little more intense than I would prefer it, though. For example, in 2006 a major company in the United

States (you would recognize the name if I told you who it was and you've probably consumed their products many times) had a representative contact me at 11:00pm on a Friday night (yep, when the phone rings that late, it can't be good!) requesting that I remove a blog post I had previously written or they will contemplate forcing me to do so with legal action. You heard me right — they threatened to sue me! Okay, whatever, it's no big deal to me...I'll just remove the post. Sheeeez! And so I took the time to take it completely off all the web sites I write for and gladly so. Again, it's no skin off my back one way or the other.

It is not and has never been my intention to cause any harm to a business or individual with the columns I write about at my blog. I only seek to stir up debate about issues that merit further discussion by taking a firm stance on what I believe is important. Know what you believe and why you believe it is my motto. That scares some people and apparently some businesses, too. It's kind of funny that this particular company seemed to think my column about them was some sort of viable threat. Sure, I reach thousands of readers daily, but this is one of the most widely recognized brand names in the entire world with tens of millions of customers worldwide sending their legal eagles after me over a flimsy little blog post. What were they thinking?

Do I really wield that much influence that this multi-billion dollar company would come after an innocent individual for simply expressing an opinion about them that they happen to disagree with? I wonder what they would do if I took their threat to a major news outlet like the *New York Times* or NBC News? Talk about your David vs. Goliath story! I guess I should be flattered that I have a blog that even some of the biggest names in corporate America takes notice of and feels threatened by what I write. If I felt they were doing something that goes against what I believe, then I wouldn't hesitate sharing it with you and refusing to back down. That wasn't the case in this instance, so I pulled the post.

Freedom of speech and press is a precious constitutional right in the United States of America and I don't believe any company is beyond reproach from criticism. That's why I'll keep writing the way that I do and sharing my concerns when issues arise. Even still, this incident was nearly enough to make my wife Christine have a heart attack! Was it a full moon or what?! Oi!

Despite the distress that incident brought on my family, just a few days later I got the following pithy response from one of my readers about what he thinks of me personally:

god are you an idiot

Aside from the fact that God should be spelled with a capital "G" since He is the creator of the universe and everyone already knows I'm an idiot (just ask Christine, she calls me that all the time!), what's your point? Some people just have way too much time on their hands these days.

Here was my cordial response back to him:

Why, THANK YOU! I appreciate your very kind compliments and hope you continue finding what you are looking for at my blog. Take care, my friend!

Not content with leaving good enough alone, I received a quick follow-up e-mail from this person with even more personal attacks against me.

Well I did discover something amazing when I read your blog. You could find someone to marry you. That is more amazing than the amount of lard you lost.

I wonder who peed in his Corn Flakes to have him go off on me in such a personal nature like that. But, you gotta love it because at least he's sharing what's in his heart of hearts. All I can say to all the naysayers and haters of what I do at my blog is take your angst elsewhere. The mission of "Livin' La Vida Low-Carb" is all about providing an encouraging, uplifting, and positive safe haven for people desiring weight loss and better health. It beats all I've ever seen to think anyone in this world would be opposed to such a noble and sincere endeavor, but indeed there are those who would like nothing more than to see me crash and burn. As long as there are hurting people looking for hope and inspiration to help them get through another day, then I'll keep on keeping on doing my best to edify and raise up their spirits any way that I can.

Being overweight or obese is hard enough emotionally that you merely want to connect with someone who understands what you are going through. When I weighed 410 pounds prior to 2004, I would have LOVED a blog like "Livin' La Vida Low-Carb" to learn about healthy low-carb living, get the latest cutting-edge information, read inspiring stories of weight loss success, find recipes and resources to help me on my lifestyle, and have open access to someone who has already been through the journey I am taking. Hopefully, my blog is all of that for the millions who have been touched by it already. I stand ready to help anyone anytime they have a question or comment about their low-carb lifestyle and I always respond as quickly as possible to every inquiry. I can be reached via e-mail at livinlowcarbman@charter.net.

This just goes to show you that people who read blogs can most certainly come in all sorts of shapes and sizes. Everyone is welcome to visit, interact, and learn (from the largest company's right down to that guy who lives out in the boonies with a dial-up connection!). It's what blogging is all about...even if the crazies tend to come out the woodwork from time to time! Check out this one I got from a man that speaks for itself:

Look around your mid-section, you could live off that fat for 6 months. I am highly skeptical that your body needs all that fat. I'm pretty sure your gall blad-der will need removal within a few years. Though that's only if you survive the colon cancer from the 15 pounds of fetid low quality hormone laden mad cow meat adhering to your colon. Do you notice how bad your BO is and how bad the toilet smells after you go. If you don't just ask your wife. Chimp poo is nothing like that!

PS - And what is with your so-called brother being in hospice and singing karaoke? I've yet to meet a hospice patient released for a little karaoke R&R. I think somebody is looking for pity points. But if you weren't a drama llama you would not over medicate with fatty foods (formerly sugary foods in your younger years).

Does something like this even deserve to be dignified with a valid response from me? I think not (although I thought you'd get a good laugh out of it like I did!). Even still, it never ceases to amaze me how some people can be so vicious in their opposition to someone who they've never met before that they would resort to childish name-calling and mindless ridicule just to make their point.

Case in point: Check out these comments about me, my blog and my book that were posted at the page for my first book at Amazon.com. Written by someone calling themselves "SaveYourMoneyQueen" and hailing from the state of Hawaii, here is what she wrote in her "review" of my book entitled "Snore me to death...":

Jimmy Moore has the most obnoxious, self-serving blog. It is full of hype designed to promote this book. I strongly recommend that you spend a few minutes reading his longwinded blogs, and you'll soon realize what this re-gurgitated book is all about: himself. It truly is a nice story, but not required reading. Save your money and take a pass on this "inspiring" business man.

Don't you just love people like this? What do you want to bet this person never even bought my book? I would put heavy odds on it. And perhaps this person is affiliated with the sugar, potato, or pharmaceutical industry and is merely trying to smear my name and my story because they disagree with the truths I write about them at my blog and in my books (I'm not very supportive of any of those industries as you might expect). Additionally, this person could be a strong supporter of the failed low-fat/low-calorie/portion-controlled diets that plague our society and keep us fat as a nation. Putting down a low-carb suc-cess story should make 'em feel better, right?

It really doesn't matter why she wrote what she did and I certainly don't mind a dissenting voice. But I do have to chuckle that someone like this would get so up-tight about what I write about at a blog regarding the subject of livin' la vida low-carb that she would stoop to this level of immature behavior to voice her opinion. I'm glad to see such vibrant passion in the opinions expressed by this person who doesn't even know who I am from the average Joe on the street because it is exactly that kind of enthusiasm that is needed to do something about obesity.

Could it be that this person is overweight or obese and has taken offense to something I have written? I don't back down from telling the truth as I see it on virtually any issue, so that is a plausible explanation for this outburst of hatred against me. But my regular readers will attest to the fact that I also sprinkle in a fair amount of encouragement and real-life examples from my own experience and others who have been successful in their low-carb weight loss journey to truly inspire people who struggle with their weight and health as we once did.

As to the charge that my blog is "self-serving," "longwinded," and "full of hype," I have not forced anyone to read my blog ever. The incredible amount of traf-fic I see at my blog month after month comes from people who are earnestly seeking more information about the low-carb lifestyle and have found a place of refuge in "Livin' La Vida Low-Carb." I started it in April 2005 with the pur-pose of informing people about low-carb living, sharing my experiences on a low-carb nutritional program, promoting items of interest about low-carb, chal-lenging the negative stereotypes about low-carb in the media, and being a virtual friend to anyone desiring weight loss and greatly improving their health through livin' la vida low-carb. That's it. No sinister plan here. That has been my intention and will continue to be my goal for many years to come.

There is nothing wrong with me informing my readers about my life and what is happening with it. In fact, I still get e-mails from people all the time asking about how they can buy my books, where they can meet me, and when I will be coming to their area. I am humbled by the attention my triple-digit low-carb weight loss success story has received and simply want to show others that they can do it, too! That's the overriding message of everything I do at my blog and in my books.

Am I immune to criticism? Absolutely not. I've gotten my fair share of it in other forums I have written for. I don't mind it at all because I enjoy stirring people to think about the issues I bring up and not just mindlessly absorb everything they read. I appreciate honesty and don't mind thoughtful negative comments when they are focused on the issues. Criticism isn't restricted to just Amazon. com or my blog, though. Sometimes, other blogs get in on the action.

One such blog called Diet Lowdown, which describes itself as being dedicated to giving a critical eye to all things related to dieting, decided to throw down the gauntlet with a post he called "Livin La Vida Low-Carb Or Livin La Vida Loco." Describing me as a "junk food addict," the author who calls himself The Diet Meister said in his post that I might be losing weight, but I'm not being very "healthy" with the way I am eating. The Diet Meister was "shocked" and said I was doing a great "disservice" to Dr. Robert Atkins by describing my diet as the Atkins diet (actually, I call it livin' la vida low-carb). Finally, he believed I should change the name of my first book to "Livin' and Dyin' La Vida Low-Carb." OUCH! Tell me how you really feel.

Some of these issues about my personal way of eating have been discussed at great length previously, but I decided to post the following comment back to the Diet Meister at his blog:

Hey Diet Meister,

THANKS for mentioning my "Livin' La Vida Low-Carb" blog and for sharing your genuine concerns about the way of eating I used to lose my 180 pounds and keep it off. You make some valid points and I would just like to clarify them for you. The "sample" of what I eat in a day I assume came from a post where

I sent the "Today Show" an average meal for me. It was not meant to be an indication of what I eat EVERY SINGLE DAY because I don't eat the same things all the time. I even mentioned that it my post.

While you believe my diet is filled with what you would call "junk food," which I assume you are referring to the low-carb snacks and diet sodas in that category, I have seen these as lifesavers for me as I have been livin' la vida low-carb. I got some similar criticism after I posted that blog and decided to pen other posts to help people understand my philosophy about why I eat the way that I eat.

I admit in that post that my eating habits are not as strict as some people who have lost weight with low-carb. This is an ever-evolving process for me. I don't claim to have all the perfect answers to everything about doing low-carb. I'm simply sharing what I have done to lose and maintain my weight through the low-carb lifestyle.

With that said, my goal in 2004 was to lose weight, but my goal in 2005 was to successfully keep it off for the entire year. The way I see it, as long as my weight and health are not adversely affected, I have no problem consuming foods that help me get there. Will I keep doing that for years to come? Maybe, maybe not. You have to remember I was a 410 gorilla just a few years back. My blog just gives me an opportunity to tell others about how livin' la vida low-carb has changed me and is still changing me.

By the way, I eat lots of vegetables, including cauliflower, green beans, salad greens, and more as part of my healthy low-carb lifestyle on a regular basis. I mix it up so this way of eating doesn't get boring as so many people claim that it is. I can appreciate your concern about my eating habits and thank you for allowing me to clarify them just a bit here at your blog. I did indeed write a book and released it in October 2005. I think you will be pleasantly surprised by what you read and will gain a better understanding of where I came from before my miraculous weight loss.

Don't give up on me yet! I'm that flower that is just waiting to bloom. Don't rush me into sprouting before it's my time to do it. I'll get there in due time. THANKS AGAIN and take care!

Once I responded kindly and thoroughly to his concerns, The Diet Meister wrote me back and told me he appreciated what I had written. One of the pitfalls of blogging that I've noticed since I started doing this is the fact that there are brand new readers who find out about you for the very first time each and every day. Quite literally, tens of thousands of new readers stumble upon and read my blog every single week and I am extremely grateful for that.

But what inevitably happens is someone will read a single column that I have written without knowing who this Jimmy Moore character is within the context of the thousands of blog posts I have written since April 2005. Many of these critics wonder how I came up with my opinions and sometimes misunderstand what I have written. It happens all the time and I've really come to expect it. Generally I attempt to reply back to the person who e-mailed me providing links to other blog posts I have previously written for context as well as clearly explaining where I am coming from. Do I HAVE to do this? Of course not. Yet in the spirit of sharing ideas and attempting to educate people on my perspective, I cheerfully do it.

I received one such e-mail from an apparent brand new reader since he said he "spotted" a recent blog post I had written at the time about a McDonald's restaurant closing down because of competition from the neighborhood farmers' market. I individually responded to each of his criticisms about my column that he presented:

"I don't know you but I am having difficulty understanding why you seem to have so much hostility toward McDonald's."

I enjoy reading comments from people who come across my blog for the very first time. Welcome to the debate of ideas about diet, health, nutrition, weight loss, and, of course, low-carb. Please feel free to navigate around my blog and read everything that has come before the post you cited. Regarding your assertion that I have "hostility toward McDonald's," nothing could be further from the truth. My regular readers will tell you that I am all for letting a business do what it has to do to turn a profit. That's the American way and NOBODY should force a business to do anything that would stand in the way of their economic success.

I believe in the power of a democratic society without the use of strong-arm tactics like unnecessary government-forced rules and regulations. For example, I was opposed to the ban of trans fats in New York City. Does this mean I approve of the use of trans fats in the food served at places like McDonald's? Not hardly. Instead, I am a strong proponent of personal responsibility for weight and health problems rather than blaming it on a disease or making it the fault of fast food companies.

"I read that you lost a lot of weight. Congratulations on that accomplishment but the rancor in your article gives me the impression you blame McDonald's for being overweight."

THANK YOU for your compliments about my low-carb weight loss success which I chronicled in my first book in 2005. However, where was the "rancor" in my article? If you have read any of my previous blog posts, then you will quickly discover that I generally write in a very direct manner fueled by the personal experiences I have encountered as part of my miraculous low-carb weight loss experience. My intense passion should not be mistaken for opposition. I make no apologies for my writing style and can't be held responsible for your misinterpretation of what I wrote. With that said, I can without a shadow of a doubt tell you that I don't blame McDonald's for my obesity or anybody else's. Again, it goes back to my philosophy that the individual has the power to bring about change.

When there was a move for McDonald's and other restaurants to cut back on their portion sizes and calories in their menu items, I stood up for them against such a ridiculous notion. Additionally, when they voluntarily decided to put the nutritional information on the packaging of their products, I applauded their efforts. I'm not anti-McDonald's from a business standpoint and believe they could be a good company for people living a healthy lifestyle. All it would take is for them to provide better and healthier choices for their prospective customer base.

"The last time I visited McDonald's there were salads, fruit, low-fat yogurt, grilled chicken, orange juice and milk. So, what is your real problem with the brand?"

Do you think those foods make McDonald's a "healthy" place to eat? Okay, I'll might give you the plain salads (which contain sugar in them by the way!) and grilled chicken (although, even that is suspect!), but clearly the rest of their so-called "healthy" menu is loaded with too much sugar and carbohydrates to be deemed good for you. And fruit? Oh, do you mean those little apple slices that come with a container of caramel dipping sauce that is just loaded with high fructose corn syrup? Low-fat yogurt? You've got to be kidding, right? OJ? Milk? Have you looked at the carb counts of these lately? It's not a pretty picture. I provided McDonald's with a few examples of some excellent low-carb menu offerings in a letter I sent to them and blogged about, so we'll see if they take me up on my suggestions.

"I can't believe I am actually writing to you about this but in your glee over the closure, you overlook the 27 employees that are being 'displaced.' You seem elated about this and I can't understand why. I suspect these employees are 'local town folk' too as are the truck drivers, repair people and other vendors that support any restaurant."

I'm really glad you did write to me because you allow me the opportunity to address your concerns directly. Again, I wouldn't say I have "glee" over this McDonald's closing down, but rather it's not surprising considering the economic dynamics of the area. As for the employees who worked at that store, the article I quoted very clearly said they would be offered positions at another McDonald's location if they wanted it. Don't be so smug and crass to think I'm "elated" over anyone losing their job. I've been through that myself in the past and wouldn't wish it on anyone. But you move on with your life. You find something else to do to make a living and support your family. That's the way it works in a free economy, especially in the high-turnover restaurant industry.

Statistically speaking, many of the people employed at the McDonald's that shut down would have moved on in the next six months or so anyway and they can do so much better for themselves than Mickey D's. This very well may give them the impetus to get out there and find an even better job with higher pay and benefits.

Yes, it's sad when a job is lost, but it's not the end of the world. Perhaps these ex-McDonald's employees could look into working at an even better job now. If they put forth enough initiative and energy into their new job as they did selling Big Macs and French fries, then I have no doubt they will be successful. But they shouldn't expect a job to come running to them.

"You could also check this out with experts but I suspect the chances of getting a food borne illness is probably greater buying food at a local farmers market from some unknown source (not all of the items are organic as many believe) than from a national chain since the chains require their suppliers to meet certain national standards for food safety."

Oh yeah, that's worked out real well, hasn't it? Try telling that to Taco Bell or Olive Garden who got hit hard from a public relations standpoint when people got sick from food they consumed at these restaurants. There's not one shred of evidence to back your claim that food sold at a farmers' market will make you sick.

"I do not expect you to reply but I hope I have given you some points to consider."

Well, that's where you are wrong, my friend. You not only got a reply from me (I personally answer every e-mail that comes my way), but I even devoted an entire blog post to your e-mail and have now included you in one of my books. I always appreciate feedback and the attempt to share thoughts and opinions about what I blog about. Hopefully this can serve as a springboard for looking closer at the issues and create the kind of synergy that is needed to help further the education of the public about issues concerning health.

On the Internet, though, it seems everyone is a critic and that's what makes the blogging universe so much fun in my opinion. You get an unfiltered, uncensored, and sometimes irreverent and immediate response from virtually every angle you can possibly think of. And the opinions that are expressed in this format include some that would never ever be uttered in "real" life from these people. That is especially true of those who leave anonymous comments.

Over the years I have received plenty of complaints that my blog is too much this and not enough that. While I appreciate hearing feedback from a representative segment of the thousands who visit daily, the fact of the matter is I blog about what's on my mind from my perspective. I'm certainly not saying that my opinion is 100% accurate every single time I start typing and anyone who believes they are infallible should watch out for that lightning bolt coming down from the sky!

When I started writing about livin' la vida low-carb, it was with a purpose in mind and here it is: tell others about how the low-carb lifestyle can change their life through weight loss, experiencing amazing health improvements, and having a commitment to living this way for the rest of their long and healthy life. There are all sorts of web sites and blogs just like mine for the low-calorie lifestyle, the low-fat lifestyle, the vegan lifestyle, and so forth. So why not have one for the healthy low-carb way of life, too?

Unfortunately, some people mistakenly believe that I'm not allowed to be an advocate for low-carb at my blog. Why? Because a low-carb diet isn't necessarily for everyone — something I readily admit is true. In fact, I tell people all the time to find the proven plan that works for them that they'll enjoy, follow that plan exactly as prescribed by the author of that plan, and then keep doing it for the rest of their lives. If that's low-carb, low-fat, low-calorie, vegan, vegetarian, meat only, whatever, then do it! Yes, there's no doubt I'm enthusiastic about low-carb living and why shouldn't I be? It has changed my life forever. And despite some minor weight gain issues from time to time, this way of eating has afforded me some of the best health markers of my entire life. Livin' la vida low-carb is why this is happening and I want the whole world to know what it has done for me. Again, this is what my blog and books are all about.

However, after blogging about a study that came out trashing low-carb diets (it happens more often than not!) to counter all those headlines that made people believe they should eat a high-carb breakfast to lose weight, I got the most peculiar comment in response to what I shared. It was an "anonymous" comment and the person who penned it follows a low-calorie diet. While I appreciate that there are readers who come at the nutrition subject from a different perspective than me, it's a bit disingenuous on their part to expect me to change to their preferred way of eating.

Just try asking someone like low-fat diet guru Dr. Dean Ornish to talk positively about the low-carb Atkins diet and he'd laugh in your face because this dietary philosophy doesn't jive with what he personally believes is the most nutritionally sound advice for people desiring weight loss and better health. He has a right to his opinions about healthy living and people can choose to embrace or reject what he has to say. The information age we live in affords us the luxury of educating ourselves about what is true and what is not.

That's what made this comment I received from that nameless low-calorie loving reader so odd. Here's what he wrote:

While I generally agree that some of the articles you post are a bit bogus, I find that you are ever increasingly hostile towards anything non low-carbohydrate. I know you are a very strong advocate for the low-carbohydrate lifestyle, it has changed your life and you make a living from it. However, not everyone has the willpower or the drive to make such a lifestyle change.

A calorie restricted diet is not evil; it won't hunt you down and kill you. A lot of doctors and health professionals choose for their patients to restrict their calories because they can eat the foods they love. If you take a person who has never been on a low-carbohydrate diet and suddenly expect them to eat nothing but induction food for two weeks or longer, a high percent of them will fail. Even if they can later add in fruits and nuts and the like, it may be too much of a severe restriction. It may very well be that your health will vastly improve, but it does happen on a restricted calorie diet also.

I respect the work you do, and I respect your opinions, but I do not agree that you should be bashing everyone else in the process. If you had lost your weight on a restricted calorie diet, improved your health, and maintained your weight, would you not promote that and disagree with everyone else?

Jimmy, I have nothing but the utmost respect for you and your lifestyle, honestly. I do not want to cause arguments or hard feelings. I just think that a carbohydrate restrictive diet is not a magic cure nor is a calorie restrictive diet. Some will have success on one and not the other, neither is for everyone. I would just like to see a little less hostility towards other people's choices and beliefs. I respect yours, please respect mine.

Here was my response:

THANK YOU for openly expressing your concerns, anonymous. Anyone who has read my blog for any length of time knows I have often hit hard on studies against low-carb because they are simply continuing to push the message that low-carb is unhealthy while propping up a low-fat diet as the preferred way. This is not something new and you can see examples of where I've come down on the low-fat/low-calorie lie many times in the past in my blog archives. What you will see is how my general writing style has not changed very much as it relates to challenging the low-fat diet wisdom. If anything, I've toned it down somewhat from my earlier columns.

With that said, most people who read my writings know that I am all in favor of people finding the proven plan that works for them to lose weight, following that plan exactly as the author prescribes, and then keep doing that plan for the rest of their lives. If that's a low-fat and/or low-calorie diet, then who am I to stand in their way and tell them NOT to do it? There are certainly a dime a dozen support sites out there for those particular ways of eating that people can visit.

But when someone comes to the "Livin' La Vida Low-Carb" blog, I want them to be encouraged, educated, and inspired about the healthy low-carb lifestyle. This way of eating worked remarkably well for me to help shed the pounds and greatly improve my health, so I can't help but share the positive experiences and research about it. It's precisely why I started my blog to begin with.

With all the constant negativity out there about livin' la vida low-carb as exemplified in study after study, we need more people to get fired up and responding to these kinds of things. There are no checks and balances on these people who espouse low-calorie, low-fat diets. They just write assuming ahead of time that low-carb is bunk. But I know better than that because of what has happened to me and to many more people. Trust me, if you need to hear from more low-carb success stories, I'm sure they are all too happy to fill up my e-mail box with their testimonies of change.

I'm curious, though. What articles have I posted that you think are "a bit bogus?" Everything I write about is researched and accurate to the best of my knowledge. If you think I've made something up (ergo, the use of the term "bogus"), then I'm all ears. Don't throw something out there like that without providing examples. And don't misunderstand my passion for wanting to get the word out about healthy low-carb living and think that means I am "hostile." Enthusiastic, maybe, but there is no hostility in my blood. I care about people enough to tell them the truth about what is healthy.

While you believe someone can only accomplish success on low-carb if they have some miraculous willpower or drive, the reality is it takes neither of those to be successful. All you need is a steadfast resolve to make better choices for the sake of your weight and health. When people start caring enough about themselves to reduce their carbohydrate intake to control blood sugar and insulin, eat some protein at each meal for satiety, and consume plenty of fat to burn as fuel and to keep their diet delicious and healthy, then we will see some pretty major changes happening with obesity and disease in America.

As it currently stands, the low-fat, low-calorie, portion-controlled diet has been given decades to rule the nutritional roost. And what has it gotten us? More obesity, more diabetes, more sickness, and more death. We're taking more prescription drugs now than ever before and nobody is disgusted by this. This isn't me "bashing" anyone; it's just presenting the truth. Isn't it true obesity rates have gotten much worse since the great low-fat, low-calorie movement began being promoted in this country in the early 1970s? And diabetes, especially Type 2, has exploded into a literal crisis of health over that same time period, hasn't it? Who is gonna argue that we are healthier as a nation today than we were 30 years ago? Anyone?!

By the way, I did lose a whole lot of weight on a low-fat diet in 1999 and I was miserable on it. Hungry all the time, weak with barely any energy, dizzy and nauseous, and downright miserable! Although I lost 170 pounds in nine months eating that way, I gained it all back within four months when I couldn't take it anymore. With livin' la vida low-carb, that impulse to rebel against how I eat has never even remotely crossed my mind. I am more satisfied now with how I eat than I even was when I was eating whatever I desired. Now I desire those low-carb foods that my body was always meant to eat.

There are no hard feelings from me. Life is too short to be upset at anyone, let alone someone who was brave enough to share their thoughts and concerns with me (albeit anonymously). I can appreciate your perspective and am grateful you respect mine. Nobody is saying livin' la vida low-carb is a "magic cure," but it sure is dramatically changing the weight and health of a whole lot more people than we are being told about.

If low-calorie diets are working for you, then GO FOR IT! Keep working your plan and it will keep working for you. Get involved at a low-calorie supporting web site, forum, or blog and get all the inspiration you need for your chosen dietary approach. But this is "Livin' La Vida Low-Carb" and I will keep on talking about the healthy low-carb life. It's the purpose I have in my life right now and, God willing, nothing will ever keep me from fulfilling that purpose.

THANK YOU again for sharing your thoughts with me and my readers.

Just like this person who posted anonymous comments at my blog, I have always contended that people are much more assertive, aggressive, and in-your-face on the Internet than they ever would be if they were standing right in front of you. Sure, there are a few exceptions to this, but for the most part it's true. And when you can post something anonymously without any way to trace where it came from, you can multiply that willingness to say anything by at least one-hundredfold! People have their opinions and certainly don't mind sharing them regardless of the consequences.

I learned a long time ago that you had better put on a thick layer of skin if you decide to start blogging for the whole world to see, especially when it comes to sharing your own personal diet and weight loss story. Everyone has their own theories about what works and I think it's great that the World Wide Web affords us the chance to hear all of these voices and decide for ourselves what is true and what is not.

But there is some sense of responsibility for decency and class when it comes to leaving a comment, especially when it is critical. There's nothing more cowardly in my opinion than to do what I like to call a "drive-by comment" — you come into a blog, post a flaming comment anonymously, and then run away. What good does that do? Where's the debate of ideas? Just put your name and e-mail address on there at the end so that if people have questions about what you wrote about, then they can reach you. How difficult would that be? Well, I suppose they don't want to be contacted and that should make you suspicious of their remarks.

Anyone willing to give a strong opinion should never be afraid to catch some heat back from the people who disagree. It's how public discourse should be handled and yet so many people like the following anonymous reader just don't get that. I've blogged quite extensively about having "loose skin" after my 180-pound weight loss and a nameless, faceless commenter decided to leave his feedback — "drive-by comment"-styled — to one of my blog posts.

Here's what he wrote:

Everyone is being very supportive of your weight loss, but dude you are still very very overweight and borderline obese. You lost a lot of weight, but 220 pounds is not a lean weight unless you're a bodybuilder or athlete. Jesus, you've still got a good 70 pounds of pure fat to lose in order to be considered "normal."

It's seriously not "loose" skin; it's just heaps of fat that you haven't lost yet because you basically starved your body with an improper diet while not doing enough exercise.

I guarantee your body would look worlds better had you hit the weight room and treadmill six days a week and not subscribed to a fad diet that goes against nature itself. Face the facts: You lost weight too quickly while NOT exercising enough. That is not loose skin; that is fat that is backed up by emaciated muscle mass.

Don't believe me if you want, but I know what I'm saying. Your got about 60% if the way to your goal and then you stopped, thinking 220 pounds was your ideal body weight, and you neglected your body composition of muscle:fat ratio. You have no muscle and tons of fat, that's why your body looks so bad. Sure, surgery can fix this, but dedication and a gym membership will fix it as well. And before you go on saying "Well, I do work out, I do have a gym membership, etc.", have you considered you just aren't working hard enough?

Again, congrats on the weight loss, but you need to stop making excuses and face your own issue: get more dedicated to exercise and ditch the unhealthy fad diet. The human body needs carbs to fuel all of our organs, which includes the skin (the largest organ) and brain.

Nice, huh? So, tell me how you REALLY feel. Ahhhhhhh, what do you say to something like that? While there was some truth in what was expressed, there was a whole lotta crap too. This is indicative of the kind of abject hatred people have not just for those of us who wisely have chosen to follow a low-carb nutritional approach, but also anyone who is on a journey to better health and weight loss. Let's take a look at each part of this comment to separate the good from the bad from the ugly:

Everyone is being very supportive of your weight loss, but dude you are still very very overweight and borderline obese. You lost a lot of weight, but 220 pounds is not a lean weight unless you're a bodybuilder or athlete. Jesus, you've still got a good 70 pounds of pure fat to lose in order to be considered "normal."

By what standards am I "very overweight and borderline obese?" I presume you are referring to body mass index (BMI), but that's not the entire story. Yes, I'm still a big guy, but everyone who meets me says I am much taller and large structured than they expected. I'm a big guy who used to be a REALLY enormous guy. I'd love to lose more weight and am working on getting there the best I can. According to you, I need to weigh 150 pounds as a 6'3" man — ummmm, call me crazy, but that's just nuts!

It's seriously not "loose" skin; it's just heaps of fat that you haven't lost yet because you basically starved your body with an improper diet while not doing enough exercise.

I'm the first to admit some of it is indeed body fat, but I could not disagree more that I've "starved" my body with some kind of "improper diet." Have you read the latest studies on a high-fat, low-carbohydrate diet? It's stunning and I highly recommend you read books like *Good Calories Bad Calories* by Gary Taubes to get the whole story before you show how ignorant you are describing this way of eating that way. And how do you know I'm not exercising enough? I did DAILY cardiovascular exercise the entire time I was losing 180 pounds in 2004. How much MORE could I possibly do?

I guarantee your body would look worlds better had you hit the weight room and treadmill six days a week and not subscribed to a fad diet that goes against nature itself. Face the facts: You lost weight too quickly while NOT exercising enough. That is not loose skin; that is fat that is backed up by emaciated muscle mass.

I'm the first to admit I regret that I didn't "hit the weight room" sooner as I noted in the final chapter of my first book. But I did upwards of 45-60 minutes (and sometimes more!) of treadmill or elliptical training every single day of the week during my weight loss. I was afraid of gaining weight then, but I have since added weight lifting to my exercise plan with great success. What's so "fad" about eating a diet like our early hunter-gatherer ancestors did with healthy whole foods like beef, eggs, fish, nuts, and anything else they could forage for nourishment? To me, eating tofu and bean sprouts and saying you love it "goes against nature itself." How did I lose too quickly and how can you possibly know that I wasn't exercising enough? To paraphrase the former Democratic U.S. Senator from my home state of South Carolina Fritz Hollings, there's a whole lotta assumin' going on out there.

Don't believe me if you want, but I know what I'm saying. Your (sic) got about 60% if (sic) the way to your goal and then you stopped, thinking 220 pounds was your ideal body weight, and you neglected your body composition of muscle: fat ratio. You have no muscle and tons of fat, that's why your body looks so bad. Sure, surgery can fix this, but dedication and a gym membership will fix it as well. And before you go on saying "Well, I do work out, I do have a gym membership, etc.", have you considered you just aren't working hard enough?

I will agree that I could have lost more weight than I did and I'm still on that journey to get my body weight down rather than up. But I won't sacrifice my health to get there. Right now, I am as healthy as an ox despite your assertion to the contrary. Sure, my body composition could use some more muscle, but I'm working on that, too. In 2008, I grew more muscle mass than I EVER have in my entire life. I'm proud of this and know it will continue henceforth. I'm not just a member of a gym, but I have had a personal trainer guide me when I started lifting about proper form and technique. If I was a lazy slob who didn't stay committed to my workouts and exercise routine, then I could see you stating I wasn't "working hard enough." But quite frankly you don't have a clue what you are talking about.

Again, congrats on the weight loss, but you need to stop making excuses and face your own issue: get more dedicated to exercise and ditch the unhealthy fad diet. The human body needs carbs to fuel all of our organs, which includes the skin (the largest organ) and brain.

I've never made any excuses for the way I look. My pursuit has always been to become better and better as the years go by. Nobody is gonna argue with the fact that I look better and am healthier now than I did at 410 pounds. And I challenge anyone to tell me I'm not exercising enough for what my body needs to get stronger, more conditioned, and to burn calories. Could I do a little more exercise than I do now? Sure, but the scientific evidence behind cardiovascular exercise especially is shaky at best. My focus is on the resistance training, but I get in several hours of cardio a week in the form of basketball, volleyball, and other recreational competitive sports events that are a regular part of my life. As for the "body needs carbs" I simply point you to Google the term gluconeogenesis and read the upcoming chapter on this very subject. 'Nuff said!

Even a non-low-carber who lost a significant amount of weight on a low-calorie diet saw this comment from the anonymous anti-loose-skin, anti-low-carb, anti-Jimmy-Moore person and decided to give her a piece of her mind about what she thought about these comments. You're gonna LOVE this:

Alright this just peeves me off. I can't believe how people can come down on someone's success. Jimmy came ages from where he was and achieved something most people only dream about. No matter what diet you use to achieve weight loss, you can end up with loose skin. It's just a matter of fact. I get tired of hearing people spout off about how working out harder at the gym can "take care" of the extra skin.

I've lost 175 pounds by calorie counting and exercise (no I did not follow the low-carb diet) and I am plagued with loose skin. I am 24 years old and NO I *am not still overweight. If I lost any more weight, people would assume I was anorexic. I am 5'5" tall and currently weigh 120 pounds. Slabs of skin are on my stomach, arms, legs, thighs...heck, even my breasts could use some serious help. Was it because I didn't "try" hard enough, or that I did something wrong? Um...no, it's not! So stop bagging on people. I just get mad that other people can be such a**holes. Sorry Jimmy. Congrats on all your weight loss. You're amazing.*

This is why I don't ever have to respond to negative blog comments like these that come my way. There are plenty of people like this sweet lady willing to tell 'em off for me. Something tells me she'd probably tell that anonymous commenter a thing or two to his face if she had the chance. As for the anonymous commenter, I welcome criticism anytime. But how about coming out from behind your computer screen and sharing with us your name and contact information so an open discussion can ensue? Plus, if you have what you believe are the answers to obesity, then why not share them in a blog? I'd be happy to post about it at my blog so that others can see what you have to say. This isn't a competition about seeing whose diet or fitness routine is better. We're all on the same side trying to help people start to care about their health. These kind of needless "drive-by comment" attacks are totally unnecessary. Show yourself and be proud of what you have to say.

People are constantly scouring the Internet looking for ways to get skinny and healthy through that perfect nutrition and fitness plan. Some will fall for the first thing they find and think it's the best plan for them while others will spend hours researching and Googling everything they can get their hands on about their chosen program. I think it is a great thing when people get excited about losing weight and turning their health around. But I only wish they'd keep that excitement for more than a few days, weeks, or months down the road — they'd be much better off if they did. I consider it a true privilege to have the opportunity to share my low-carb success story with others and encourage them as they take this journey to better health for themselves. When I blog about the new low-carb research, recipes, news items and more, I feel I am providing people a great service that they can apply to their own lives. And it's free!

But not everyone thinks my writings are worth reading.

I received a comment under my "Before & After Pics" tab in 2008 from a man named David who challenged my right to share about the low-carb lifestyle because of what I look like in a photo of me I posted in December 2008. According to David, I have a lot more work to do on my own obesity problem before I dare share anything about the low-carb life on my blog.

Here's what he wrote in his comment:

Jimmy -

Sorry to disappoint you but I just looked at the most recent pictures of you (late 2008) and you are overweight, if not obese (medical definition here, not an opinion). Could you please tell us your current weight and height, so readers can put your nutritional advice in perspective? For the same reason that people should ignore financial advice from bankrupt individuals, people should ignore nutritional advice from overweight individuals - they have limited credibility. People should only take nutritional advice from very fit and lean individuals.

I suppose David meant for this to be constructive criticism and I can appreciate it from that perspective. Sure, it sounds mean, but I don't think he intended for it to be that way. Nevertheless, I was happy to respond to David's concerns and answer some of his questions about the work I'm doing helping others who struggle with their weight and health. Here was my response:

THANKS for your concern, David. But I post all of my daily menus and weight updates at my menus blog (LowCarbMenu.blogspot.com). I blogged quite openly and extensively about a 35-pound weight gain that happened in 2008 following my decision to start lifting weights in December 2007. The creatine I was taking along with several stressful situations in my life (a failed in-vitro fertilization cycle where my wife and I were trying to get pregnant and were told we couldn't have biological children of our own, the declining health and death of my 41-year old brother, etc.) have also made it difficult to get the weight off.

I was able to get my weight back down to 235 pounds on my 6'3" body frame through a variety of methods — just 5 pounds higher than the weight I was at the end of my original weight loss in 2004. If someone chooses not to read my blog because they deem me too fat and irrelevant when it comes to health and weight loss, then that's their prerogative. I'm not making anybody read what I write and it's a free country.

But as long as I have a platform, I'm gonna share the truth about livin' la vida low-carb because that never changes regardless of who the messenger is. Am I a perfectly fit and trim individual? No. But I used to weigh 410 pounds five years ago and I've kept off the vast majority of those pounds ever since. Do you know many people who lose significant triple-digit amounts of weight who are able to keep it off over the long-term? It's very rare. One final thought for you: what does my weight have to do with promoting the positive and healthy benefits of low-carb living so that others can benefit?

—Jimmy

The adage that you don't have a right to share your thoughts on nutrition and health simply because someone deems you overweight or obese is absurd. If I was giving people advice and telling them what to do to become the next Arnold Schwarzenegger, then I could see David's point. But that's not what I do. I encourage people to find the plan that works for them, follow that plan exactly, and then keep doing it for the rest of their lives. That is the recipe for success I have seen over the past five years of living the low-carb life and it holds true no matter how much I weigh at any given moment.

Blogging isn't about perfection or nobody would be doing it. How many people do you know who have a blog about whatever subject they care about the most and consider them the perfect representation of that topic? You could argue maybe one or two of them, but certainly not the overwhelming majority. And, again, I never pretend to be the perfect low-carb dieter. I'm simply one man who lost a boatload of weight in 2004 and has kept it off for the most part ever since. I have a critical message that so many people need to hear and nothing will deter me from sharing that with as many people as I can possibly reach until the day I die. There will always be critics of what I do, but I have better things to concern myself with than worrying about what people like this have to say about me personally.

People are dying needlessly because they haven't heard the truth about how damaging carbohydrates are to their health. Even if I was a 750-pound invalid living in the middle of nowhere USA and I was sharing about how insulin drives fat storage and carbs drive insulin levels, that truth would not be any less relevant than if I had a 6% body fat, muscular 200-pound body. Truth is truth no matter who is saying it.

Would I like to be closer to that muscleman someday? Of course! But I'm just living my life one day at a time consuming my healthy low-carb lifestyle, working out at the gym, staying active, and living a healthier life than I ever thought would have been possible just five years ago. That's why I will continue to do what I do, writing about livin' la vida low-carb, and not feeling one bit ashamed of doing so. This was what my life was meant to be and my mission is to never stop telling people about the life-changing impact of low-carb!

David, I'm sorry that a 6'3" tall man weighing 235 pounds doesn't meet your lofty standards for being able to write about diet, health, fitness, and nutrition. But I've been living this way long-term, interviewed hundreds of the best and the brightest health experts on my podcast show, and committed myself daily to continue the learning process for myself and my readers that I am confident I have something valuable that is worth paying attention to. The thousands of readers who have read my blog each and every day for years are a testament to this fact. While I appreciate your comments, I think I'll get back to work now doing what I always do — educating, encouraging, and inspiring others to make better choices for the sake of their own weight and health. That's what makes what I do so significant to my readers.

As David's comments about me clearly demonstrate, when you put yourself out there front and center as a pretty major low-carb weight loss success story, the reaction that people give you about your progress is as varied as there are people in the world. Most people applaud your accomplishments and stand in awe of your continued success. Others doubt you can keep the weight off and stay healthy over the long-term.

But sometimes you receive a "different" kind of response. It was actually very well thought out and documented by a reader on Amazon.com who read a thread I started there in August 2006 called "What Are Your Criticisms of the Low-Carb Lifestyle?" The Amazon username for the person who questioned me about my weight loss progress is 2bluesky2 and I was quite impressed by the background he did at my blog prior to writing his comments at Amazon. I do believe he was being very sincere in asking these questions in his post and I'm more than happy to address them.

Wanna see what he wrote? Here it is:

Jimmy, I want to ask you about your own weight odyssey, which you discuss frequently on your blog. In looking over your blog, I found frequent references you made to your weight. You also frequently say that your goal weight is 199 lbs. Here is a table compiled from your blog showing your weight over several years:

1999. Lost 170 lbs on low-fat diet, regained it in 4-6 months
01-01-2004. 410 lbs. Started Atkins diet
01-01-2005. 230 lbs. Lost 180 lbs in 2004 on Atkins diet.
11-27-2005. 225
08-14-2006. 240
11-21-2006. 215
12-12-2006. 215-217
12-31-2006. 220
01-31-2007. 229
02-08-2007. 220
06-05-2007. 248
06-08-2007. 235
06-12-2007. 229
06-25-2007. 223
06-26-2007. 222
07-02-2007. 219
07-05-2007. 219
07-06-2007. 218
07-19-2007. 216
07-20-2007. 212
10-04-2007. 220-225
10-09-2007. 223

The table shows your amazing 180 pound weight loss during 2004 for which you can justifiably be proud.

But the table also shows that from November 2005 to August 2006, you gained 15 pounds going from 225 to 240. By November of 2006, you had lost 25 pounds and weighed 215. But by June 2007, you regained 33 pounds and were up to 248. By late July 2007, you had lost another 36 pounds, but since then you regained another 10 pounds or so. I didn't find any listings of your weight after October 9, 2007. On your September 17, 2007 podcast, you mentioned that your weight had topped out at 253, but you didn't' mention whether that occurred in 2006 or 2007.

Achieving major weight loss, as you did in 2004, is a major accomplishment. Thereafter, consistently maintaining weight loss presents different challenges. Your 2004 weight loss is truly remarkable. But you're up and down pattern since November of 2005 seems dubious. In the past 2 years you have gained 15 pounds; then lost it and more; then regained 33 pounds; then lost it and more; then regained another 10 pounds or so. Now you are about where you were in November 2005 when you started you're up and down pattern. During all of that time, you still never reached your goal weight of 199. As you know, at 6 foot 3 inches your current BMI is in the "overweight" category (and will be until you reach your goal weight of 199). As you have recently pointed out, BMI might not fairly categorize people like yourself who have a significant sagging-skin problem after major weight loss. Still, the 199 target was your own choice, and you haven't achieved it yet.

Your huge weight loss in 2004 was an inspiring accomplishment. But most people are not facing the challenge you were looking at on January 1, 2004. I think most people face the challenge you faced in November of 2005: maintain current weight, but also hopefully lose another 20 or more pounds. Your 4-year record is awesome. But your last 2 years are erratic. Those who have a major weight problem like you had in 2004 should consider doing what you did. It accomplished a lot for you. But should your recent track record inspire those who have a much smaller weight problem? Your program just doesn't seem to be working as well for you as you deal with long-term maintenance and losing those last few pounds.

I am not a health professional or expert, but I think an effective weight management program should do three things for a person in your situation. First, within a reasonable amount of time it must get you out of the obese weight range and within, say, 10% or so of your target weight. Low-carb did that for you. Second, within a reasonable amount of time thereafter, it should get you to your target weight. Ignoring your unwanted volatility, you have been basically stuck at around 220 for the past two years. Maybe you should just redefine your target as 220, maybe not. I don't know. That's for you to decide. But if 199 is a realistic target, then low-carb is not getting you there anymore. Third, once target weight is reached, the program should enable you to maintain a stable weight with low fluctuations of, say, 2% or so over some extended period (ideally: permanently). Even if you redefine your target weight as 220, low-carb has not enabled you to achieve a stable weight over the past 2 years. You fluctuate too much. Your weight increases of 15 pounds in 2006 and 33 pounds in 2007 are alarming. Those recent gains may seem trivial in view of your major weight loss in 2004, but you are in a different league now. You are not a fat guy anymore. Your 2006 and 2007 fluctuations are very inappropriate for your present size and weight.

My quick-view evaluation:
Major weight loss? Yes!
Achieve goal weight? Not really, unless you fudge the goal.
Maintain stable weight? Nope, no way. Needs improvement.

So where does all this discussion lead? Well, you have to decide that. I think that your program needs some tinkering, and maybe some strategic rethinking. If I were to make a single simple suggestion to you it would be this: start posting your actual and goal weight on your website on a regular basis. Your readers and fans will alert you if/when you need a kick in the behind. That may be all the motivation you need to keep "weight creep" from getting out of control again. I think you will agree that your fluctuations over the past 2 years are not in your best interest. They also do not reflect well on your advocacy of a low-carb program for long-term maintenance.

In this forum you have asked for comments on low-carb. I have had my say. You may not like hearing it all, but I think my observations and comments are within the scope of what you asked for. What do you say? I look forward to your always interesting comments!

See, I told you this guy put a lot of time and thought into that post. And I can appreciate all of the comments that were shared. It's gratifying to know that when you blog there are real people who are watching you to see how you are doing. This Amazon comment is a gentle reminder of that reality and I am grateful for it. Accountability in my weight loss is one of the reasons I started blogging to begin with.

Let me begin my response by saying I do not consider this criticism by 2bluesky2 to be malicious or purposefully negative in any way. He raises questions that I'm sure others have thought about but never vocalized. From the outside looking in, he seems to make some points that ring true. But since he doesn't have the advantage of knowing what I am thinking (and that would be a good thing for him!), the reality is he doesn't have the full picture in mind.

It is true I have often talked about my weight fluctuations at my blog and gladly so. I think it is beneficial for people to realize that once you hit your weight loss goal, the journey isn't over. In fact, it really just begins. After losing 180 pounds in 2004 to get down to 230 pounds, my goal in 2005 was don't gain it back! The longest I had ever kept weight off after losing over 100 pounds was about two months before I started gaining weight. I was bound and determined not to let that happen this time.

Of course, unlike my 170-pound low-fat weight loss experience in 1999 that he mentioned, I was not miserable and tired of my low-carb lifestyle even after eating that way for a full year. Yes, the diet had become such a routine for me that I didn't think of ever going off of it again. That's a lesson that will serve anyone well who expects to keep their weight off long-term. And today I'm still happily livin' la vida low-carb.

But from the graphic that was shared about my weight ups and downs over those previous three years, the "success" of my efforts seemed pretty dismal or "erratic" as he put it. In fact, he missed the date when I mentioned my high weight of 253 pounds from early 2007 which precipitated me to try that infamous diet plan we all love to despise now that will remain unnamed until I share about it in a couple more chapters. What should be most interesting about those numbers is the fact that when my weight went up even slightly, I did what I needed to do to bring it back down again. In the past and with many other people who lose weight, when they see the "weight creep" begin to happen they just throw their hands up in the air and concede defeat. Predictably, all the weight comes pouring back on them and then some. But that isn't what happened with Jimmy Moore.

And there's a good reason for this. Am I somehow immune to the inevitable weight gain that can overtake even the person with the strongest willpower? Heck no! I'm like most people who have battled obesity their entire lives and dealt with the same temptations, frustrations, and aggravations that come with weight control. It isn't easy and anyone who tells you it is can't possibly understand.

But I do have a steadfast resolve to make smarter choices now than I ever have before. That said, let me address the premise of 2bluesky2's comments. When I began this journey at 410 pounds in 2004, I never would have thought in a million years that I could get my weight down to 230 and keep it close to there for the next five years. My track record for weight management in the past was dismal at best, so the hope of keeping weight off didn't look very good.

By the end of 2004, I was at my goal weight at the time of 230 pounds on my 6'3" body frame. It felt good being at a "normal" size and I wanted to stay there. Unlike my low-fat weight loss experience, low-carb made me feel good while I enjoyed the way I ate. That was the major switch that made this "diet" work for me this time. So I kept eating this way to maintain.

Regardless of what my weight has done over the past few years, I would say that keeping it close to the original weight loss goal is doing a pretty good job of keeping the weight off, wouldn't you? Yes, my weight has fluctuated, but that is a normal part of maintaining. Granted, you shouldn't have major fluctuations all at one time, but they can add up. Five pounds up, three down, then eight up, two down, then four up, and two down is quickly a 10-pound weight gain! This happens when you allow extra carbs in your diet for those who are carbohydrate sensitive like me. Taking your eye off the ball can cause your weight to slowly rise.

The continued journey to maintain my 180-pound weight loss success from 2004 requires that I stay challenged. It is what drove me to lose the weight in the first place and it is what drives me now. If I have a goal to pursue, regardless of how long it takes me to get there, then I am always in pursuit. But once that is removed, there is little incentive to keep that fire burning within.

For me, the low-carb lifestyle is more about eating healthy and getting my overall health under control as much as it is about my weight. When I allow foods into my body that aren't as healthy sometimes, my health and weight can suffer. It's all about finding what my body can tolerate and realizing my limits. That's a learning process you never stop doing. I know I'm eating healthy right now — healthier than I ever thought possible! The Atkins diet was indeed a godsend for me and I'll never regret one moment of my decision to begin eating this way. For the first time in my life, I feel like I am in control of my weight and health. And I am despite the minor ups and downs of my personal low-carb journey.

The difference now between my 10-15 pound weight swings and before is I know what I need to do to get my weight managed. Previously, I'd lose 100 pounds, but then gain back 125. I'm not playing that game anymore because there's too much heartache and pain involved. Instead, livin' la vida low-carb helps keep me on the straight and narrow for now and in the future. It's the best thing I have ever done for my health.

Regardless of the concerns by 2bluesky2, I think anyone who reads my writings can be inspired in their own weight loss efforts to begin this lifestyle because my track record speaks for itself — 180 pounds lost in one year and maintained for five years and counting. I challenge anyone to tell me that accomplishment is unworthy of admiration because I've worked my butt off to make it happen.

I don't believe everyone who leaves criticism for me at my blog or in my e-mail box necessarily hates me, but there are a lot of people who do. In fact, entire threads at forums have been created with the sole purpose of talking about me and my menu choices on my healthy low-carb lifestyle. I find it intriguing that people are interested in what an average guy from South Carolina eats on a daily basis.

To be honest, I've only been to these kinds of forums a few times to see what all the fuss was about when my readers would bring it to my attention. Honestly, though, I didn't really see anything productive or encouraging there from people who would choose to ridicule and scorn someone else they don't even know. The man who started one particular forum that nitpicks at my low-carb menus used to be a friend of mine who I brought on to serve as a moderator at my own low-carb forum (LivinLowCarbDiscussion.com) in 2008. He did an outstanding job in that role and everything was going along fabulously.

But when I asked him and others to tone down the references to zero-carb diets there since my forum was about low-carb and I even encouraged my friend to start his own forum to talk about that subject, he and his followers apparently thought I booted them off of my forum and now they hold resentment against me for that. I welcomed them to continue talking about healthy low-carb lifestyle at my forum as long as they didn't reference zero-carb.

Unfortunately, this didn't sit too well with many of the members there who now frequent the new zero-carb forum and thus they have rationalized their right to openly ridicule of me as they have been doing in a prominent thread at the forum since November 2008. From the sanctimonious chiding of every action I take in my life to the open display of disgust they have for me as a person, it's quite a telling story in the information age we live in that people would get so worked up over a diet and health blogger of all things. Is my life really this interesting?

I learned a long time ago when I first started blogging that you can't put much stock in the negative comments that are made about you by people on the Internet. Like I have said, people will write things on forums and in comments at blogs that they'd never say to your face. My wife Christine gets very upset when people make disparaging remarks about me, but I explain to her that she shouldn't take it so personally — because I don't. I realize we all have different ways to communicate online and some are a lot blunter than others. That's not being mean, that's just a difference in style.

I don't know if these people are just jealous of what I am able to do for a living or whether they think they are somehow more deserving of success than I am, but the holier-than-thou attitude they embrace apparently gives them the sense that they are the moral authorities and final arbiters over diet and health in the world. I've never understood people like this who desire to be "nannies" over every minutia of someone else's life. But they're not worth worrying about.

At the end of the day, my purpose in blogging and sharing about the healthy low-carb lifestyle cannot and will not be distracted by those who hold ill will towards me for whatever their reasons. The work I do at my blog and podcast show each week is much too important to so many people for me to get upset and discouraged by some annoying gnats flying around my head. I'll keep doing what I know is right and sharing with people why healthy low-carb living is probably one of the most important changes they could ever make in their lives! We'll leave the negative naysayers to their own destructive devices. There's already enough negativity in the world, so why not buck the trend and start being encouragers instead? Wouldn't that be nice?

But despite all the negative criticism that has been hurled my way over the past few years, I've also received a much larger percentage of praise from those who have been positively impacted by the work I am doing. Coming up in the next lesson, we'll learn how if you put yourself out there on the Internet, people will love you, too. And that's what makes it all worthwhile.

LESSON #15
If you put yourself out there on the Internet, people will love you

"No one will love you until you love yourself. When I started to take care of my body by eating well and exercising, I became so comfortable with myself that it didn't matter as much if the Internet loved me too. Of course, if you want to leave a comment on my blog telling me how much you love my site, I won't stop you!"

— **Jennette Fulda**, author of *Half-Assed: A Weight-Loss Memoir* and popular diet blogger at PastaQueen.com

In the midst of all the constant negativity that exists out there in the blogosphere, I'll occasionally find a singular ray of sunshine that is actually quite typical of the kind of e-mails I regularly receive from so many of my wonderful readers. The following e-mail made me smile from ear to ear when I received it because this is what blogging is truly all about to me.

Your web site is fantastic! Thank you so much for providing all this really valuable information! You're inspiring. It's really nice to see that other people have interest in this. I know it takes lots of time and money to provide this information — you're doing a good thing for health in our country and our world, thank you! Your site is very organized and your writing style is easy to read, concise, informative and engaging. Keep it up and thanks for sharing your stories, your life, your research!

That's the kind of e-mail that just absolutely makes my day and validates all the many thousands of hours I have invested into the work I do. Some people have asked me why I spend so much time writing articles, researching studies about low-carb, challenging lies about the Atkins diet in the media and from the so-called health "experts," sharing my 180-pound low-carb weight loss story, and generally educating and encouraging people about the low-carb lifestyle. There's one major reason: overweight and unhealthy people.

There are millions upon millions of people who feel like there is nobody out there who understands their plight. They have tried every weight loss product and diet known to mankind and nothing seems to work for them. Many of them are on the verge of reaching a point of no return where they just stop caring about what they look like, how they feel, and even whether they want to continue living in a world that so viciously discriminates and judges them based almost exclusively on their appearance.

Here is an e-mail I received from a man in that exact situation who said my blog motivated him to lose weight:

Hello Jimmy,

I just recently came across your site and I am inspired to no end to lose my weight now. I have been trying so hard to find the motivation to lose my weight but I was afraid that if I did I would look like a big wrinkled-up prune. I thought that my skin would have been so loose that I would be so ugly and gross.

I really appreciate your site and I will be looking in every day to stay inspired. At one time I was over 500 lbs and at the current time I am not sure how much I weigh. It is very hard to find a place to weigh myself and the places that I can is very embarrassing to go and do. This includes using scales at a scrap yard where they weigh scrap metal. I don't know how or why I got this big and I wish I had someone that could have intervened before I got to where I am now.

I was wondering what the time frame was for you losing such an impressive amount of weight is? I am now following a low-carb diet and I am walking daily for 45 minutes to an hour each time. I also started weight lifting again which used to be one of my favorite activities before I gave up on myself and my life and gained all this weight.

Well I don't want to bore you with my details and I really appreciate your site and I look forward to your future posts on the blog.

Thank you very much!

Here was my response to him:

THANK YOU SO MUCH for writing today. WOW! Reading your story makes what I do so worth it, man. My heart literally aches for people just like you because I know what it feels like to be in your shoes. You hang in there, my friend, because you WILL make it. Don't give up, don't ever give up. I'm here for you anytime.

I lost my 180 pounds in one year. It was my New Year's resolution in 2004 and the weight just melted off of my 410 pound frame. It was a lot of hard work, but livin' la vida low-carb kept my tummy satisfied as it shrunk down to where it is today at 230 pounds.

You're not alone with the embarrassment of not being able to weigh yourself on a conventional scale anymore. I had to do the same thing you did just to find out how much I weighed at the beginning of my low-carb program. I know I was bigger, but 410 was the largest recorded weight I had ever been. It's not fun, is it?

Keep up the low-carb plan and don't stop walking and lifting weights, buddy. It sounds like you've got your mind set to do this for real this time for the final time. Make livin' la vida low-carb your permanent change of lifestyle and you will see miraculous things happen for you. I will pray for God to strengthen you during this struggle and to empower you to press on when it gets tough.

THANKS for writing and check in at my blog with your comments or questions anytime. Take care, my friend.

For all of those people who wonder why I spend so much time and effort at this blog, THIS is why I do what I do. When I was writing my first book about my 180-pound low-carb weight loss experience, I was imagining what it would be like for someone with a similar weight problem that I had picking up a copy of my book and realizing that same weight loss success is definitely within his or her ability to do just like I did. While I have heard from so many people who have bought my first book and told me how it motivated them to get started or continue on their low-carb lifestyle, a 405-pound Canadian man made an incredible impact on me when he sent an e-mail with his testimony about how my book had inspired him to get serious about dealing with his obesity.

Here's what he wrote to me in that e-mail:

Dear Mr. Moore,

I have just finished your book and would like to thank you for writing it. Your story has motivated me to do something about my weight (405 pounds) once and for all. I have thrown out all carb-rich food in my house and replaced it with healthy low-carb foods instead (fish, lean meat, eggs, cheese, etc.).

I intend to follow your advice to the letter (nutrition and exercise). I figure, if I adopt the same eating lifestyle (see? I read the book I'm not using the word 'diet') and do the same workout I should reap similar results.

A quick question, I know that the low-carb lifestyle does not count calories, but did you in any way reduce your food intake during that period? Can you tell me how many calories you ate per day?

Again, thank you sir!!!

WOW, what a great compliment! I was so thrilled with his feedback that I happily replied to address the issues he raised in his e-mail to me:

CONGRATULATIONS to you for making the best decision of your life regarding your health — to start livin' la vida low-carb! You will be so pleased with the results I am quite sure of that. :)

When it comes to calories, I didn't count 'em and still don't. Never have and probably never will. It reminds me too much of being on a "diet." And you know how much I HATE those.

I also did not portion control during my weight loss. Your body naturally regulates that as long as you aren't gorging yourself on every meal. Be smart about it and allow the protein and fat you are consuming to send you the signal when you have had enough. You'll know.

Don't try to mimic exactly what I did because it may not work for you. But be sure to follow the low-carb plan you have chosen (I did Atkins) and stick to it for the rest of your life. YOU CAN DO THIS!

THANKS again for writing and I wish you only the best as you begin livin' la vida low-carb. I'm always here for you if you have any questions or need encouragement. God bless you!

My reader was kind enough to even post a book review at Amazon.com for me. THANK YOU! By the way, if you've read any of my books and would be willing to help me out with a book review at Amazon, then I'd be very appreciative if you would just take a moment to submit one for me. That would be awesome and thanks in advance!

I am so proud of readers like this and I'm humbled to know that I played even a small role in their decision to make this decision to start low-carb living. Whatever you do, don't ever give up on this at anytime, no matter how hard it may seem. Just push forward and keep going because it is the best feeling in the world to have the weight lifted off of your body and you are free to be the man God intended you to be physically. I'm still getting used to it myself and I've kept my weight off for five plus years!

The positive impact of my writings quickly spread across the Internet when I first started blogging as other web sites starting sharing about it with their readers. And once people found me, they shared their love and appreciation for what I was doing.

Hi Jimmy,

I happened to be at another web site and noticed your blog. Wow, you are an inspiration and thank you for speaking for the low-carb lifestyle.

I'm restarting low-carb today. I followed Dr. Atkins' diet about 4 years ago and lost about 25 pounds (total weight loss was 32 pounds — 7 with Weight Watchers in one whole year and the rest in 5 months on Atkins). Unfortunately I didn't keep it up and gained back most of the weight lost.

After trying various weight loss plans for the past 4 years (shame on me) I have finally, finally, finally decided to go back to Atkins. I currently weigh 183 (at 5'5") and want to weigh 135-140 in one year's time. I know this time it will be a bit more difficult since going back and forth makes weight loss much harder to do but with God's help and my determination I will succeed.

Thank you for your blog. I'll certainly be reading it daily to keep me on track.

YOU CAN DO IT, I KNOW IT! Believe in livin' la vida low-carb so strongly that you cannot help but be a success and watch it happen for you. That's what got me down from my high weight of 410 pounds! And here is what another woman wrote in an e-mail about the effect of my blogging on her weight loss efforts:

Dear Jimmy,

The reason for my email is just to say Thank You. I just finished reading the letter you wrote to Dr. Phil on your blog and I have tears in my eyes. I did lose some weight last year, about 40 pounds on the Atkins diet but I stopped and I know I need to lose more.

I'm 26, 5'9" and my weight is 210 lbs and I know I should lose more but I felt like I couldn't. And yes I am happy I lost 40 pounds but I'm still not where I want to be. And I thought I could never get there.

This year I decided I'M GOING TO LOSE MORE. So I've been on my diet for four days now, and as I'm sure you know it's been hard. But I want to reach my goal finally of 165 lbs.

And out of the blue I don't know how I got on to your blog page but I did. And reading your letter, when I read how much you lost and how you have kept it off. You have inspired me so much that is why I want to thank you. I know I can do it.

And I will continue to read your story and I am going to buy your book. And the day I reach my goal I will e-mail you again letting you know that I DID IT!

And you WILL do it! It sounds like you have a great plan in place and I just want to encourage you to press on, keep your head down, and trudge forward no matter what. Even if the plan seems to be stalling, just keep smiling and act like it is working like a charm. In the end, you will be SO glad you did and you WILL reach that 165-pound weight loss goal of yours. It truly warms my heart to hear so many people tell me how I have helped inspire them to begin losing weight. WOW, what a neat thing that is to me! I have been so blessed by this entire weight loss experience that I feel obligated to tell the whole world how livin' la vida low-carb changed my life forever!

Here's another e-mail from someone who commented on the videos my wife Christine and I regularly post at YouTube (YouTube.com/livinlowcarbman) as well as my podcasts:

Dear Jimmy,

I really want to thank you and Christine sincerely for your inspirational work every week. Since I started a low-carb diet at the end of July this year, I've been listening to your podcast show and I look forward to every entertaining episode. It's good to hear your practical advice and upbeat attitude, and I feel sure God put your show in my ears for encouragement on the low-carb journey He's leading me on.

There are three things in particular that you've helped me with in a big way. Can you hear me yelling "THANK YOU JIMMY" all the way from San Diego?

First, I appreciated all the interviews with bariatric doctors from the convention (with the really long name I can't even try to remember). There was so much helpful information in those that I needed to hear and didn't hear from my doctors.

Second, it gave me so much joy to hear you speak about how your relationship with Jesus helped you in your weight loss success...in a whole episode! I applaud that so much; you put yourself out there to give the Lord some credit and give that testimony, and you're absolutely right. (He's the only one who could get ME to go on a diet...ha ha)

Third, your exposure of the Kimkins diet was the voice of truth for me and 3 friends who had all been on that diet. Thankfully, all of us were modifying it a lot already, but now we're completely off thanks to your vigilance.

Jimmy, I trust you. I'm glad you're out there for us. Please keep up the GREAT work and God bless you and your lovely wife!

And the appreciation for my work just keeps rolling in all the time:

Hi Jimmy,

I am 51 years old and live just north of Sydney, Australia. I have (had) Type 2 diabetes and all the associated metabolic syndrome issues. I was told by my doctors that I, like you was a dead man walking. Having tried all sorts of diets in the past, I was getting desperate to the point of starting to consider bariatric surgery.

It was in my search for some info on bariatric surgery that someone posted a very small comment (as they often are) about your blog. From there I devoured your low-carb message like a meat starved homo-sapiens. I also took your message about going and reading Dr. Atkins' book before starting on the plan — did that and more (I think I ate the pages out of that book too).

I then immediately went on a low-carb Atkins diet. Induction was easy after reading the problems bariatric surgery patients had to deal with after their operation. That was 2 months ago. So far I have dropped about 20 pounds from a starting weight of nearly 300 pounds and I've already come off ALL of my diabetic medication (when you tell people that it gets them interested). My blood sugars now are totally normal which is amazing without the use of any drugs. I feel fantastic and can't believe the difference low-carb has made in my life.

As I said you probably saved my life. Thank you for that. My wife (also on the diet now) thanks you, too. But I had to know more, especially after your YouTube video on gluconeogenesis (I loved that episode). I am a trained chemical engineer with a background in biochemistry. Not content to just accept the obvious answer, I have been on a quest for knowledge. Not only about biochemistry and diseases but anthropology, evolution, traditional diets, supplements — you name it I am studying it.

Got a lot to go before I can present a completely integrated document on all this but when I do I would like to give you a copy of my research and to any others who may well be interested like I am. Thank you again so much Jimmy for opening my eyes to the truth.

* * *

Hey, Jimmy! I spoke to you a few months back about the difficulties low-carbing and trucking. Well, I'm happy to give you a little progress report: I'm down from 376 to 314 now — 63 pounds lost! And according to my training journal, I didn't even start Atkins until sometime in mid-to-early August! I feel tons better, and quite frankly I look it, too! I'm down from a size 56 to a size 48 so far.

I've been working out with Lifeline Fitness TNT Resistance Cables and man I feel almost like I'm 25 years old again! It's exhilarating to step into the shower and see my deltoids, biceps, triceps, and back muscles starting to reform (I used to be a bodybuilder in my early 20s before trucking)! I must admit to altering the diet slightly — I binge. Yeah, I know, but I went super strict carb first month, and progress staled out quick. So, I had a lapse of judgment, and binged. Two days later, I discovered that whereas in the previous two weeks I'd lost nothing, since I binged, I'd lost 3 pounds! So, when I'm home every 2 or 3 weeks, I binge for that day or 2.

It's not enough to replenish my body's sugar stores (when I was bodybuilding the logic was it took 72 hours of heavy carbing to reload your sugar stores after competition diets), but it does 2 things: 1) it helps me with that monkey of all those foods you know I love, and 2) I don't crave those foods insatiably like I used to because I know I'll get to try them when I get home. And besides, those foods taste good at the time, but I've actually found that my cravings have decreased sharply!

Wow, dude. I'm totally impressed with the results. Thanks for your web site and your tips for me at the time! My goal weight is 205 — I was last at that body weight when I was 23 when I was at 3-6% body fat. I'm dying to know what it'll be this time, and how I'm gonna look. YOU ROCK, JIMMY! Don't let anyone tell ya different!

* * *

I check your blog everyday and I just wanted to let you know how much you've helped me. At the start of 2008 I weighed 340 pounds and today I weigh slightly under 240. Yours was one of the first web sites I found when I was Googling "low-carb dieting" in December 2007 and through your posts and the information you've lead me to, you've probably been the single biggest help and inspiration to me with this. Well, I just wanted to say thanks. I'm a little embarrassed now that I haven't even submitted this before!

* * *

Dear Jimmy,

First, I'd like to thank you for your blog. It has been a wealth of information for me — and very entertaining. Allow me to introduce myself. I am a physician (pathologist), who stumbled onto low-carb sort of accidentally. My wife had read and recommended to me the book SUGAR SHOCK! I read it also, and thought I would try to eliminate sugar — but simultaneously decided to increase the fat in my diet (replace the calories in sugar and simple carbs).

I was startled at how much better I felt the very day I made the switch. Because I felt so much better, I decided to continue the changes, progressively decreasing the carbohydrates, and increasing the fat. I was also surprised when I spontaneously lost 10 pounds (I didn't have much to lose), my blood pressure dropped, an inflammatory skin condition that I have had for years cleared up (seborrheic dermatitis), and recurrent canker sores that I have suffered from cleared up.

As a physician, I was trained to be somewhat skeptical of dietary treatment of physical conditions, especially diets that claim to solve multiple problems but I cannot deny the changes in myself or others that I have observed following a low-carb diet. Since then I have tried to follow the research of low-carbohydrate diets on diseases of civilization. I have read Gary Taubes GOOD CALORIES, BAD CALORIES book and consider it a masterpiece.

* * *

I know a friend of mine who I turned on to your blog a long time ago and she reads your stuff religiously. She used to weigh 400 pounds and I was the one who suggested low-carb to her. She was hungry and depressed on other diets and would always gain it back — whereas I've stayed low to moderate-carb for a long time and even do it vegetarian-style now and still have success over the long run.

Anyway, my friend lost 200 pounds AND WAS THRILLED she could LIVE AGAIN. People were not making fun of her at every turn and she could walk for the first time in a long time. But she fell off a few times gaining back some weight, but each time she starts up again doing it the same way.

She continues to read your blog and menus every day and is so encouraged by your outlook and determination. In fact, she has said to me that it gives her a jump start every single day.

* * *

Thank you, Jimmy, for being there and facing all the really tough subjects face on. You have definitely helped me stay on track over the last several months.

* * *

I found your book by mistake while looking on the Internet. I ordered it and couldn't put it down. I was on a low-carb diet about 5 years ago and lost weight but went back to eating my old ways. Potato chips and chocolate. I can't believe how much sugar you ate and stayed healthy. I am now 40 lbs. overweight and don't like it. Since reading your book, I started again 4 days ago. I want to keep this up this time. My family and friends are not very encouraging. I was wondering if every now and then, you could send me some words of encouragement.

* * *

I love your web site and appreciate very much what you are doing. I am just dropping a line to let you know I am a devout follower of yours and am better physically and mentally for it. Please never quit what you're doing for us low-carbers out here. Your impact is tremendous.

* * *

I have really enjoyed your blog and have been living low-carb for a little over a month now. Wow! What a difference! I am so happy that there is somewhere to go that provides insight, cooking tips, and general positive messages.

My husband and I are both eating this way and it has truly opened up an exciting new world. I can't shut up about it and am even chronicling my journey in a book that I am writing. I would love to send it to you when I am finished. This change has been a long time coming, but with all the information out there and my deep desire to make life better, it is a snap judgment. There is no return and that's a good thing.

* * *

Please let me start off by saying what a HUGE FAN I am of your dedication and effort regarding low-carb living and all of the many lives you touch by reaching out and educating. I am sooo impressed by your genuine care for all those whom you respond to, with your sensitive replies and obvious passion for this way of life.

* * *

I'm sure you get thousands of e-mail messages like the one I am writing, but I just had to send a thank you to you. I am e-mailing because I've been living the low-carb lifestyle for about 2 months now. I've had my ups and downs, made a few mistakes, but have used my mistakes to learn from and have kept going, and I'm doing great. I want to lose weight, but what is even more important to me is the healthy feeling my diet gives me!

I just wanted you to know how much your website has meant to me during my change to this lifestyle. When I need inspiration, I turn on the Internet, and there you are as well as all the other wonderful people who write with awesome, inspiring words. I read for a while, and am re-inspired about my lifestyle choice. I live in a village of 14 year-round residents in the Arctic and we don't have any stores, television, or any services. Heck, we don't have electricity either (we use the sun in the summer and a gas generator in the winter when we want power and have a battery system for lights) or running hot water, and we only have outhouses!

Once in a while, I get to the nearest store (280 miles south of here, a 7 hour drive on a mostly unpaved road) and for a while I was buying low-carb bars that had maltitol in them to help me stay on my diet. I still have and may always have hankerings for sugar and chocolate, despite my diet having freed me from my true sugar addiction. Using those bars with maltitol helped me get through sugar cravings, but left me feeling really ill for two days after each bar and they stalled my weight loss. I was at my wits end and didn't know what to do, when I found your site.

Before logging on to your blog, I knew nothing about alternatives to maltitol, until I read about ChocoPerfection bars. I am so thankful you put that information out there on the web! Thank you so very much!!! Our average temperatures in the winter range from 20 below zero to 50 below zero, so it is hard to get outside to exercise and the lack of light is a challenge. Having a sweet treat that isn't high-carb and doesn't have sweeteners in it that make me ill, is a lifesaver here in the Arctic!

For all those low-carbers out there who are annoyed with rain or 40 degree temperatures, take heart, you can do it!!! I am here to say, that with great tools and inspiration that Jimmy's website provides, I am livin' la vida low-carb in the Arctic in the winter (it's 20 below zero and dark as I write this) and lovin' it!!! Thank you so very, very much for your absolutely wonderful site, you and everyone else who has shared on your site, you are all such a huge inspiration!

WOW! Now that's some testimony of being committed to the healthy low-carb lifestyle no matter what. Gee, I wonder what a ChocoPerfection bar feels like eating at 20 degrees below zero?! On second thought, I wouldn't want to know.

* * *

Please let me tell you what an inspiration you are to me. I'm struggling with low-carbing, but I know it's the right way for me to eat. Your excellent podcast interviews are giving me the confidence to feed my husband a low-carb diet. He is totally disabled and I am responsible for making his decisions. I have to tell you, it is the only way to humanely keep his weight down (important because he is in a wheelchair) because he loves to eat. It's been hard to have confidence deciding this for someone else when there really isn't support for this way of eating.

I enjoyed your book very much and I'm looking forward to another one. The podcasts are wonderful. They inspired this old 44-year old lady to figure out how to use her iPod Touch so she can listen to something worthwhile while she is at the gym and doing housework. My biggest problem is that I don't know how to get my two oldest children (both overweight and following in their genetic predisposition to become diabetic) to take the time to listen to the low-carb message. My baby does low-carb and she is a slim, energetic, and smart 21-year old who recognized that she has a metabolic problem.

Thank you for sharing and may God bless you with strength and wisdom to keep helping people.

* * *

Your story has inspired me to begin once again. I have used the Atkins diet once before and lost 80 pounds, but I got slack and thought "Oh, this one time will be fine..." Well the rest is history. I put back the 80 pounds plus another 10!

I stand today at 380 pounds and I am so sick of being this way. I know there is a thinner person inside screaming to be set free! Like your story before low-carb, I too can sit down at night, after the rest of my family has gone to bed and consume a whole pack of cookies, cakes, brownies — whatever! It's like an alcoholic or drug addict needing a fix.

I am a busy person with 2 jobs, one being a professional singer and I know my weight is standing in my way of accomplishing all the Lord has in store for me. I am serious about getting healthy this time no matter what. I have great wife that needs me and a 9-year old daughter that needs her daddy to be around for her and eventually her children.

I will continue to look to your web site daily for inspiration and look inside myself and from the good Lord above for strength. I don't know why I'm writing all this, I just need to let it out. Please continue your good work and any suggestions you may have along the way, I will welcome them.

* * *

Just wanted to tell you, I love your blog and I've been a faithful reader since I stumbled upon it in 2007. Keep up your EXCELLENT work. You just don't know how many people you help with your blog, especially me!

* * *

After months of reading your blog and listening to your podcast, and finally losing 10 of the 30 pounds I want to on low-carb, I feel I must communicate with my thanks for all your hard work.

Every day I check maybe a dozen low-carb blogs, and it dawned on me that I found them all, one way or another, through yours!

I don't have the most supportive family when it comes to low-carb living, so I've had to hang out with the online low-carb community for information, news and just virtual moral support.

Through you I found Fred Hahn's blog, for instance, and changed my workouts, which have changed me in dramatic ways. I feel better and stronger than I have in years.

Listening to one of your podcasts the other day, I realized that Livin' La Vida Low-Carb was the portal to important changes for me. So I thought I'd add my small communication to the many fans you must already hear from daily.

I laughed recently because of a couple of references to people who have lost weight on low-carb despite being of advanced age — like, in their 50s. I'm 56 but thanks to low-carbing for the past few months (yes, it's been slow), I feel years younger. (Having ADD helps.)

Keep up the great, important work, Jimmy.

* * *

Hi Jimmy. I just wanted to send you a quick note of thanks for all the information you put on your blog. A few years ago I did DANDR and lost 80 lbs (still had 120-ish to go to reach goal). I put nearly all of the 80 lbs back on and was debating doing low-carb again when I stumbled across your site. Why the low-carb debate? Well, I love the results, but really hate the plan.

Anyway, watching you and the gals at FitCamp was so inspirational and motivational that I became jealous that I was only 45 years old and couldn't move like that. I think what really got me was watching ya'll playing freeze tag and dodge ball. I wanna play!!! At any rate, I started back on low-carb (modified DANDR, if you will) one week ago yesterday and already notice a difference.

So anyways, thank you for helping a stranger out. :) KUTGW!

* * *

I just wanted to thank you for your web site and everything you are doing for all us low-carbers. I've enjoyed your videos on YouTube, have listened to your podcasts and read your web site daily. It's helping a lot. I was very touched that you emailed me and were so encouraging. I just wanted to pass that on. Thanks again!

* * *

I'm sure you get countless emails every day from people who want to thank you for everything you do on your blog and podcasts. I wanted to send my own, though, because you continue to do an exceptional job and deserve so much praise.

I found your blog a few weeks ago when I started Protein Power, and since then I've been exploring your archives. Your writing is not only thoughtful, humorous (at times), serious (when it needs to be), and engaging, but your diligence in linking every blog to other blogs is amazing. That alone makes your blog deserving of the awards you've won. Thank you for being so dedicated to your readers. We really admire you and get so much inspiration from you! Keep it up!

I could undoubtedly fill several books worth of e-mails like these that have crossed through my inbox each and every day since I started blogging and it never gets old knowing you are making a positive difference in the lives of real people. These keep me going when those people from the previous chapter try to get me down.

With so many people working their fingers to the bone trying to take care of their family, it can be difficult to try to get a handle on your weight and health. Most people use their busy lifestyle as an excuse for why they can't grab control of their life and take care of it themselves. That is so sad to me. Thankfully there are some who are working themselves hard, but are also doing something about sticking around for as long as God would have them here on Earth. Such is the case of a gentleman who found my blog after losing 100 pounds in one year.

He had sort of gotten lazy with his eating habits and the "Livin' La Vida Low-Carb" blog helped him realize he needed to get serious again to lose that final 50 pounds. Here's what he wrote to me in that e-mail:

I appreciate all the work you are doing to promote the low-carb lifestyle. I have been livin' la vida low-carb, as you put it, for about a year now and have lost 100 pounds. I have about 50 more pounds to go to reach my goal.

Since the first of the year, I have been a little wishy-washy in my weight loss journey. I had basically just maintained what I lost last year until I found your blog a little over a month ago and was inspired to really get back in the swing of things. I have done well over the past few weeks and I feel like I am well on my way to reaching my goal!

I also wanted to let you know that I appreciate the fact that you are not ashamed to share your faith on your web site. I am married and have 4 beautiful children. We are also a Christian family. I play the piano at my church and my wife homeschools our children.

In addition to being a husband, dad, musician, and full-time Purchasing Manager, I am also a licensed realtor. Yes, I am "burning the candle at both ends" so my wife can stay home with our kids and teach them in a Godly environment.

I said all that to say this — had I not started living the low-carb lifestyle, I'm afraid that candle might have already gone out! When I decided to get serious about losing weight and becoming healthy, my blood sugar was in the 400s and my eyesight was declining rapidly.

I realized that if I didn't change my eating habits and lose weight that I might not be around to raise my children and provide for my family. Today, my blood sugar is normal and my eyesight is back to 20/20! Praise the Lord! Thank you so much for your encouragement and support! Here's to our success!

I LOVE hearing from my readers who want to share with me about the changes they have made in their diet to lose weight and get healthy, so feel free to write to me anytime at livinlowcarbman@charter.net. Share your success story, your frustrations, your questions, your feedback and anything that's on your mind. Although it has gotten more and more difficult as the popularity and traffic at my blog has steadily increased over the years, I am still committed to personally writing back anyone who takes the time to write to me. It's the least you deserve for spending a few moments of your time writing to me.

Coming up in the next lesson, we're gonna hit on a major livin' la vida low-carb concept I've briefly discussed in previous chapters that unfortunately many of the current health "experts" still don't have a clue in the world about. They tell people to eat lots and lots of carbohydrates because they say your body needs them for energy. But as you will soon find out, nothing could be further from the truth.

LESSON #16
The body has no dietary need for carbohydrates — NONE!

"We used to think of gluconeogenesis as a kind of last ditch source of glucose after glycogen is exhausted but it is now clear that it goes on all the time and is part of normal glucose metabolism: gluconeogenesis, glycolysis and glycogen synthesis and breakdown are really one process that is continually re-adjusting itself in response to a changing environment."

— **Dr. Richard D. Feinman**, Ph.D., professor of biochemistry at SUNY Downstate Medical Center in Brooklyn, New York and Founder of the *Nutrition & Metabolism* journal (NutritionandMetabolism.com) and The Metabolism Society (NMSociety.org)

As a never-ending student of the low-carbohydrate nutritional approach, I have to admit I don't always understand every little detail about how and why this way of eating works so well metabolically to help people manage their obesity, diabetes, and other health-related issues. But that doesn't mean I'm just gonna throw my hands up in the air in disgust and give up trying to absorb all the information I can about livin' la vida low-carb without trying to become as informed a layperson as I possibly can. Instead, hopefully I can do my best to learn as much as I can about this remarkable way of eating and impart to you what I have learned in easy-to-understand language that will make it crystal clear why low-carb is the fantastically miraculous way of eating so many of us know that it is.

I want to introduce to you a vital concept in the wonderful world of low-carb that you may or may not have heard about before. I came across it for the first time in January 2006 at the Nutritional & Metabolic Aspects of Carbohydrate

Restriction conference put on by The Metabolism Society (NMSociety.org) that took place in Brooklyn, New York. I had no idea what it was back when I was losing weight on the Atkins diet in 2004. But the more I have found out about this incredible metabolic process, the bigger my smile has gotten for choosing low-carb as my permanent way of eating. Understanding this revolutionary concept alone about low-carb will arm you with so much knowledge that you will simply confound the enemies of low-carb living with your intellectual prowess — they'll be left speechless!

What is it? In a word, it's GLUCONEOGENESIS!

Glucosaywhatsaywhat?!?! Get used to saying it because it is a key concept in livin' la vida low-carb. Gluconeogenesis (Pronounced GLUE-CO-NAY-OH-GEN-EH-SIS), also known as GNG (that's easier to say anyway, isn't it?), is the body's way of creating its own glucose, or sugar carbs in the body, out of the breakdown of proteins in the liver. It's a complex process that happens in the body, but it is something most people who try a low-carb diet have no working knowledge about. Although opponents of low-carb programs believe you are depriving your body of important dietary nutrients when you don't eat the large amount of carbohydrates that are so heavily recommended, gluconeogenesis blows that theory out of the water because actually your body can make its own carbs from the protein you eat.

Did you know this? I dare say not many people do, including those who are following a low-carb nutritional approach and have this process happening inside of their bodies every single day. Should gluconeogenesis be a part of any discussion of healthy dietary methods and which macronutrients are absolutely necessary for people to consume for energy? I sure think so! During gluconeogenesis, blood glucose levels in the body are normalized and maintained when the glucose is created as the protein passes through the liver. During those times when the body is not taking in any food (i.e. while you are sleeping), gluconeogenesis goes to work in this "fasting" mode using amino acids, lactate, and glycerol to begin creating the sugar the body needs and it is controlled by hormones such as cortisol and insulin to maintain proper levels of glucose.

After about one day of fasting, all of the glycogen in the liver is depleted and gluconeogenesis begins in earnest using things such as lactic acid and protein to create glucose for the body. The exciting part of gluconeogenesis is that it sets your body into fat-burning mode (WOO HOO!), or ketosis (the state your body enters into when you are on the Induction phase of 20g carbs daily for the first two weeks of the Atkins diet), where excess ketone bodies are released into the blood system, brain, heart and muscles for energy.

Isn't this an incredible process? Once you grasp the concept of gluconeogenesis, you are light years ahead of most people in understanding better about the low-carb lifestyle and what makes it so special in the realm of diet, health and nutrition. More importantly, you will have the scientific facts to throw back at these naysayers who tell you that you "need" to eat carbohydrates for your body to function right. As my wife Christine would say, "Bullfunky!" No you don't. With gluconeogenesis working for you, your body could never take in another carbohydrate ever again and you'd still survive just fine.

That's the amazing process of gluconeogenesis defined!

Awwww, but Jimmy, don't you know that we just can't survive without carbohydrates in our diet because they are our body's major fuel source? Have you heard that one a time or two from people since you started eating low-carb? I'm sure you have (and if you haven't yet, you will!). In fact, you'll see this idea promoted by health columnists and experts in the media all the time.

I remember one column that appeared in the *UK Mirror* by one of these current health "experts" named Madeleine Bailey. She claimed not only do people need to eat high-carb foods such as pasta and bread because she contends these foods aren't the reason for weight gain, but she also portends your health will IMPROVE by consuming a very high-carb diet.

She hit the ground running with her column by stating her position about what she thinks about carbohydrates right off the bat.

"Let's get one thing straight: carbs don't make you fat. End of story."

While it is certainly true the mere consumption of carbs alone will not necessarily cause you to gain weight, you can't just say that's the end of the story when there are so many other complexities involved, including those of us who have a problem with insulin and blood sugar when we consume carbohydrates.

She goes on to explain in her column about how there are more calories in fat than in carbs, but again, that's not the whole story. Bailey was simply repeating the "calorie is a calorie" argument that most of us low-carbers don't necessarily adhere to because the quality of those calories count much more so than the quantity. I'll repeat this concept again and again because it's important. The quality of calories count so much more so than the quantity.

In fact, many people who are livin' la vida low-carb, myself included, don't even pay attention to the number of calories or portions when we are starting off on this way of eating because we just eat healthy, delicious and nutritious whole low-carb foods that keep our hunger at bay, give us lots of energy, and keep us satisfied and fulfilled throughout the day. Calories whether they come from fat or not are automatically regulated.

But for Bailey, she thinks just the opposite is true and she even asserted in her column that eating more high-carb foods like rice and pasta without any added fats (which she says are bad for your heart) will have you eating fewer calories and less fat.

I don't know where you are getting your information from, Ms. Bailey, but recent studies have shown fat consumption in combination with a low-carbohydrate diet has been found to lower blood pressure and cholesterol while improving heart health. Plus, my own experience with eating foods like rice and pasta is that I am much hungrier within an hour of eating them to the point that I absolutely have to eat something else to take care of my growling stomach. Eating carbs doesn't fill you up, but eating more fat and protein does which is the secret behind why low-carb weight loss works so well. You're just not hungry all the time like you are on tasteless, high-carb, low-fat diets.

Not surprisingly, Bailey quoted a registered dietitian who said to burn off more calories than you take in, or you'll gain weight. Yeah yeah yeah, we've all heard that long-standing, but incredibly flawed statement for so long about "calories in, calories out" that most people now believe it is the gospel truth. But alas it has been proven otherwise by solid research and for good reason. There are metabolic advantages associated with eating a low-carb lifestyle that can turn your body into a lean, mean fat-burning machine.

Don't try telling any of that to Bailey, though, who obviously doesn't want the facts to get in the way of her low-fat, high-carb agenda. She puts forth the notion that the body needs carbs as the chief source of energy and that restricting your carbohydrate intake as you do on low-carb plans such as the Atkins diet actually makes you lethargic. She adds that any subsequent weight loss on the low-carb lifestyle is actually no more effective than a low-fat diet over the long-term.

Some people are under the assumption that if you don't eat carbs, then your body will simply shut down. That's so shortsighted. Now, if you stopped eating any food at all, then I would agree that the body would not last very long. But why are fat and protein getting the short shrift of the macronutrients? The truth of the matter is fat and to a lesser extent protein become your fuel for energy when you begin livin' la vida low-carb. That's so hard to explain to people who have been indoctrinated with the "fat-is-bad" mantra that has been hammered down our throats for three decades that we've become completely fat-phobic. But eating fat, even the much-maligned saturated fat, is extremely healthy for you.

Honestly, those first few days on low-carb are indeed hellacious as I describe in my personal experience about beginning a low-carb program in my first book. Let's just say it wasn't a pretty picture when I first started, but it got much better for me in less than two weeks. Then, as my weight began pouring off my body like never before, guess what happened to my energy? Was I moping around like some Ichabod Crane weakling? HA! Not even close.

Like so many other people who have been on low-carb, my body has never felt this healthy, vibrant and alive as it does today. I eat around 30-50g carbs per day which Bailey believes should have me falling flat on my face. But this has not happened.

In fact, I know I could run circles around people like Bailey because I am fit as a fiddle thanks to my low-carb lifestyle. Oh, and by the way, in case you can't add up the years since I began my low-carb plan, it's over five years and counting towards the rest of my life! I wouldn't even think of eating any other way — and gladly so!

Nevertheless, Bailey says eating carbs, such as oats, brown rice, whole wheat breads and pastas, can help "keep you slim" because you stay fuller longer. I think I've pretty well established how incredibly incorrect such a statement is in light of the science showing fat and protein are much more satisfying.

Here are a list of reasons why Bailey says you need carbs and my explanation about what make these dead wrong:

1. For energy

Bailey's belief that carbs are the main source of energy for the body explains why she thinks this is a reason to eat more carbs. She even pokes fun at us low-carbers for feeling "tired, weak and irritable" because we allegedly don't eat enough carbs. What I have found since I stopped eating so many carbs is that my energy has increased dramatically and eating a lot of carbs brings me down. In fact, I no longer have all the extreme blood sugar highs and lows that consuming sugar and other excessive carbs kept me on all the time. I'm a happy and jovial man because of the changes low-carb has made in me both physically and emotionally.

2. For heart health

I actually agree somewhat with Bailey regarding this point inasmuch as eating fiber, which is a carbohydrate that you don't have to count in your net carbs, is an important part of keeping your body functioning well as part of your healthy lifestyle. This is a message low-carbers preach until they are blue in the face. But you also must start eating more fat and less sugar (CARBS!) if you ever hope to protect against obesity and your heart from a cardiovascular event.

3. For regularity

Again, this is referring to the healthy carbs from fiber to help, as my brother Kevin used to always say, "Make sure everything comes out alright." Or as I put it in a blog post once, you need to allow your bowel to shake, rattle and roll!

4. For lowering cancer risk

The assumption that eating a non-specific amount and kind of fruits and vegetables will fight diseases like cancer is the premise behind high-carb, low-fat vegetarian diets. It just assumes that if you eat low-carb that you don't eat ANY fruits or veggies at all. Then somebody needs to come look inside my fridge right now which is loaded with fresh strawberries, blueberries, spinach leaves, green beans, spaghetti squash, cauliflower, broccoli...need I go on? Low-fat and vegetarian diets don't own the exclusive rights to enjoying the benefits of eating fruits and vegetables because they are just as important for me on my low-carb lifestyle and will help keep the cancer bug away just as well (which I thoroughly addressed in an earlier lesson).

5. For making better choices

This is the bottom line — What are you putting in your mouth? Bailey believes you need a carbohydrate/fat/protein ratio of 50/35/15, but that your carbs need to be the "right" kind. The stark reality of this cannot be ignored, though. If half of your food intake is carbohydrates, then you'll never be able to experience stabilized blood sugar levels regardless of the "right" or "good" carbs.

But even within the context of "good carbs," there can be poor options for people to consider. I applaud Bailey for pointing out such "baddies" regarding carbs including the highly processed "white bread, cakes and biscuits."

"Eat too many of [the bad carbs] and you'll end up on a rollercoaster of highs and lows, and in the long-term you could be increasing your risk of diabetes."

Well I do agree with that. While the point of her story was to try to ease people's anxieties about eating carbs again since half of Americans are now consciously lowering their carb intake, Bailey totally misled her readers into thinking a big bowl of pasta is actually good for them to eat.

People don't need carbs. I suggest you read up on all the latest studies showing how healthy and effective livin' la vida low-carb is for people needing to manage their weight and disease (check out NutritionAndMetabolism.com for all the latest cutting-edge research on carbohydrate restriction). It will truly astound you. Now that's some low-carb food for thought!

A common topic of feedback that I receive from time to time centers on my qualifications to blog about the subject of diet, health, and nutrition. I've answered this charge by basically asserting very clearly that I am just a layman using my First Amendment right to free speech to share the personal lessons I have learned from losing nearly half my body weight and restoring my health. Apparently, that explanation wasn't good enough for a registered dietitian named Adam Goff.

Flexing his educational muscles at me and my blog, this gentleman berated and ridiculed the work I am doing claiming my assertions about the dangers of excessive carbs is wrong and deceptive. Oh brother! Why would I ever expect a dietitian to understand livin' la vida low-carb? It goes against everything they've ever been taught about healthy eating, so they'd have to admit they were wrong if low-carb living were to ever be embraced as a viable method for weight loss and improving health.

The evidence is growing stronger and stronger about low-carb diets in the research community, but dietitians like this Goff fella don't want to have any part of it. He's not the first one who has challenged me and he won't be the last. But I'll just keep doing my part to spread the positive message of the low-carb lifestyle.

Incidentally, here's what Goff wrote to me on my blog:

I wish I had never clicked through to your blog and here's why. While I am glad to hear that you made a conscious decision to change your eating habits in an effort to lose weight, I am insulted by the tone you take on your blog.

I am one of those "well meaning health 'experts'," and I did not spend four years and $60,000 dollars on a degree in dietetics just to be put down and contradicted by some previously overweight gentleman who read a book.

Contrary to your OPINIONS, complex carbohydrates are essential to a healthy diet. Completely removing anything from one's diet is a bad move no matter which way you cut it. I am all for eliminating simple carbs from one's diet, but despite what you preach, complex carbs are the body's preferred source of fuel. Period.

Do you honestly think that we in the field of nutrition just make this stuff up? You may have lost the weight you so desired but I would love to see how your body will hold up 30 years from now continuing on the road you're on. The fundamental key to weight loss is not the elimination of any food group but is the overall restriction of calories and an adherence to a proper exercise program.

I can only hope that people seek alternative sources for information than relying solely on your blog.

Adam Goff, R.D.

THANK YOU for sharing your feedback, Mr. Goff. But I do have a few corrections and responses to make about your charges against me. While I am happy you found my blog, you need not be "insulted" by anything I have written. My job is to provide information presented in an engaging and entertaining way to help others make decisions about what to do for their own health. Sadly, we don't have enough of that happening with the same old tired high-carb, low-fat diet message that has been proven to be incorrect.

What we need are more dieticians like yourself to begin acknowledging the tidal wave of changes in the science that has been happening in recent years rather than resting on the knowledge you have always thought to be true about diet and health. A little self-research would go a long way for anyone like yourself who is supposed to be educated in nutrition and medicine. While I may not have the educational background in nutrition that you do, Mr. Goff, I am a tenacious researcher absorbing information like a sponge and then making it palatable to the common man. That's what I've been doing for over five years and I'll keep on doing for as long as I have a platform to reach people.

Incidentally, I've met some truly remarkable leaders in the world of diet and weight loss too numerous to name them all. But Dr. Jonny Bowden (JonnyBowden.com) is one who certainly comes to mind right away as one who understands there is more to nutrition and health than a monopolistic approach as is advocated by too many of the current health "experts." Although you spent tens of thousands of dollars on your dietetics degree, that does not give you more of a right to speak on the subject of diet than me. Similarly, I wouldn't disqualify what you have to say about government and politics just because you didn't earn a Master's degree in Public Policy like I did (costing me $50,000 to earn, by the way).

You may not have enjoyed being "put down" as you claim I did to you, but you did the same thing with the snide "some previously overweight gentleman who read a book." Believe what you want about carbs, but the body recognizes them as sugar. This is a nutritional truth that I wish more dietitians would communicate clearly to the general public. The idea that the body "needs" carbs is just plain wrong. You don't need carbohydrate in your diet at all to survive thanks to gluconeogenesis. That's how our ancestors lived and it's how we can live today.

I'm not completely removing anything from my diet, and I never do get rid of all carbs. While some low-carbers may eat that way, even for a short time, most low-carb diets include between 20-100g carbs daily depending on their individual tolerance level. That's significantly lower than the average American consumes, but still doesn't eliminate them entirely as you claim.

Fat becomes your "fuel" on a low-carb diet — both the fat that you consume as well as that stored body fat that people want to burn, baby, burn! For carbohydrate addicts, this way of eating is the answer to their obesity problem and getting their health in order once and for all. Again, I wish people like you would even consider for a moment the tremendous good a low-carb diet can produce in the health and weight of so many people.

Where else are people going to learn the truth about low-carb living if they don't read it on blogs like mine, Regina Wilshire's "Weight of the Evidence" blog (WeightOfTheEvidence.com), Dr. Mike Eades' blog (ProteinPower.com/ DrMike) and elsewhere? The answer is nowhere! Low-carb has stood the test of time for millions of years and will continue to do so. I know one thing for sure — I'll be much better off 30 years from now than I ever would have been had I remained at 410 pounds!

I've never claimed my blog to be the only place for people to get their information about diet and health. In fact, oftentimes I will provide links to many reputable books and places on the Internet for people to do their own research for themselves (as I have done throughout this book, too). Knowledge is power and I am merely attempting to be the spark that gets the fire started for some. Mr. Goff, you might want to read my books and blog a little more closely to learn more about why I believe what I do about livin' la vida low-carb. I wouldn't think of ever eating any other way! This is the best diet I have ever found because it changed my life forever for the better!

Despite criticism from people like that dietitian I just discussed, my favorite part about writing is to see what kind of reaction people will have to what I've written. Nothing is more boring than the same old thing you read everywhere else, so I like to mix it up a bit every once in a while by writing about topics you may not see elsewhere. And just because I write about a subject doesn't necessarily mean I fully embrace it as a concept myself. Unfortunately, there are some people who think if I write about it, then it must be a part of my core beliefs.

One example is a blog post I wrote asking the question "Is a Zero-Carb or Even a Low-Carb Diet Healthy for a Pregnant Woman?" It was merely a question of curiosity that was worthy of discussion within the context of what I write about on a daily basis. In that column, I took great pains to leave my personal opinion about zero-carb diets out of it and I simply reported what real low-carb experts like Dr. Barry Groves, Dr. James E. Carlson, and others had to say about the subject. It was a fascinating concept that hopefully got people to think. However, it did more than that.

Based on all the comments I received about it, this post really fired people up! And that's fabulous because my job is to present information in an engaging manner so the brain juices will start to flow and a conversation about that particular topic will begin in earnest. But something rather odd happened as this particular column was being discussed — some of my readers made the leap of faith that because I wrote about zero-carb and pregnancy that I somehow believe eating that way is healthy.

I'm not sure where this came from because never once did I ever express what I believe about zero-carb diets in that particular post. Sure, I've interviewed a zero-carb advocate before at my podcast show, but does that mean I personally support such a nutritional approach? Well, I thought I made the answer to that question pretty clear when I distinguished the difference between "low-carb" and "no carb" in a previous blog post. When you've written as much as I have, then I suppose some views get lost in the shuffle and people miss them.

What's really funny is this uproar over the zero-carb diet happened as if it was something new within the realm of discussion. It is not. These people who support zero-carb have been out there for YEARS touting this as their diet of choice and I first blogged about them in 2006. The "Zero Carb Path," as the supporters describe it, is something that is completely relevant to talk about since oftentimes the low-carb lifestyle is interpreted by the media and current health experts as eating zero carbs. You and I both know that is simply untrue which is why there is a distinction between the kind of diet that Dr. Atkins promoted, for example, and a "meat and water only" diet, for example.

Quite frankly, I'm surprised by the kind of hysteria that was unleashed following my column about being on a zero-carb diet while pregnant. I was merely asking a question that I'm sure was on the minds of other people, too, and that's really all I did — ask the question publicly. That doesn't mean I endorsed one side or the other or expressed my opinions about it. I merely reported the story and let people come to whatever conclusions they wanted about it.

For your benefit, here's that aforementioned column that I wrote that opened the floodgates in the comments section of my blog and accompanying web sites:

"Is A Zero-Carb Or Even A Low-Carb Diet Healthy For A Pregnant Woman?"
Posted on September 30, 2008

Sometimes the most interesting topics of discussion for me to blog about just sort of happen. Such is the case with what I am about to share with you today. It all started when one of my moderators at my "Livin' La Vida Low-Carb Discussion" forum (LivinLowCarbDiscussion.com) named Charles, an avid zero-carb advocate, posted his thoughts based on the research he has conducted in response to another member who had recently become pregnant.

The pregnant forum member wrote:

I've read everything I can find about low-carbing during pregnancy, including the standard medical advice (eat according to the Food Pyramid). Practically all the studies that found negative effects of ketosis were done either in diabetics (in ketoacidosis), or women who were burning ketones due to starvation. Obviously, neither of those is equivalent to a woman on a low-carb diet.

The general opinion is there isn't enough research done to know if ketones are safe for the baby so it's best to avoid them. Which is all well and good unless you are one of the many women who need to stay at a very low-carb level to avoid gestational diabetes and the sugar high/crash rollercoaster. Given a choice between the known negative consequences of gestational diabetes (on mother and baby) and the theoretical consequences of ketones on the baby (since ketones obviously don't harm the mom), I would take my chances with the latter.

The pregnant forum member detailed that she realized the alleged risks involved with continuing on a ketogenic diet during her pregnancy and was willing to take her chances based on her own decision. In fact, she had been pregnant consuming a low-carb diet in the past, so the presence of ketones while she was pregnant before didn't negatively impact her. This is when Charles chimed in and agreed that a zero-carb diet during her pregnancy should not negatively impact the health of her baby. In other words, he was reassuring the pregnant forum member of her decision regardless of what she ultimately decided to do.

She responded to Charles' comments with the following:

The way I'm eating now is still very low-carb; it's still very much based on fatty meat. I just let myself have some veggies, cheese, cream and the occasional berry or small piece of fruit on the side. It's not because I think zero-carb is unhealthy; it's because I think this is a carb level I can sustain throughout the pregnancy. I think if I ate zero-carb for a few months during my pregnancy but was unable to stick with it (because I couldn't tolerate red meat, say, which happened for a while during my last pregnancy), the consequences would be worse than just starting off at a slightly higher carb level to begin with. I do hope to go back to zero-carb after this baby is born and hopefully get adjusted enough to it that my next one can be a zero-carb baby, but I just think it's too drastic a change to implement in the middle of a pregnancy.

Unfortunately, this didn't sit too well with someone who read this thread in my forum and decided to sign up at my forum as a pretend character named "Ogg." This person claimed to be on the "Yak and Water Diet" because it was the healthiest way to eat. From the very beginning, I realized this person was trying to make some kind of a point, although it was never clear what the root issue really was. After a few days of ridiculous and nonsensical posts about this miracle diet of just yak and water, the truth came out: "Ogg" didn't like that Charles was recommending a zero-carb diet for pregnant women.

Of course, the person behind "Ogg" never came to me to express these concerns beforehand, so I had no way of addressing them. Finally, I did hear directly from this person who was concerned I was promoting the killing of babies by allowing such advice to be shared on my forum. She castigated me and my Christianity for allowing my moderator Charles to provide medical advice without a medical license. I assured her he was not offering any medical advice, but simply sharing from his own personal research, experiences, and what respected low-carb doctors like Dr. Barry Groves and Dr. James E. Carlson have both said previously regarding low-carb diets and pregnancies.

She said she didn't have a problem with "low-carb and pregnancy," but rather a zero-carb diet and pregnancy. Since I have the ability to contact Dr. Groves and Dr. Carlson directly, the woman formerly known as "Ogg" requested that I ask them the following question:

"Is it safe for unborn and newborn babies if their Moms to eat nothing but store bought meat, animal fat and water — and nothing else — for the entire duration of the pregnancy?"

It sounded like a fair enough question to see what the good doctors thought. So I first posed the question to Dr. Groves, author of the book *Trick And Treat: How 'Healthy' Eating Is Making Us Ill*, because he dedicates an entire chapter to the subject of ketogenic diets for pregnant women.

Here's what Dr. Groves wrote in response to my e-mail query:

Why would being pregnant change anything? Do you see a pregnant lioness eating grass during pregnancy rather than antelope? Of course not. Do rabbits decide that grass is a bit restrictive for a growing rabbit fetus and eat mice instead when they are pregnant? The amount a pregnant woman eats may increase — she really is eating for two, after all, and it may be necessary for her to pay more attention to the quality of the food she eats. But the idea that her diet should change radically during pregnancy is absurd. All of us, whether pregnant or not, should eat good quality food all the time. And every nutrient we need for a long healthy life is to be found in a diet of fatty meats. How else would peoples such as the Inuit and Maasai have survived and been so successful?

From his well-worded response, you could say that Dr. Groves believes a zero-carb diet for a pregnant woman is perfectly fine. But what about Dr. Carlson, author of the book *Genocide!: How Your Doctor's Dietary Ignorance Will Kill You?* Does he agree with Dr. Groves that a zero-carb diet that has "Ogg" so concerned about the babies is worth bellyaching over since the longest chapter in his book is how a pregnant woman should absolutely be eating a low-carb diet for the best health for themselves and their baby?

Here's what Dr. Carlson said in his response:

Yes, doing low-carb during pregnancy is safe, as long as you are working with a doctor who is familiar with it. I have had the privilege of working with hundreds of pregnant women who began or continued their low-carb lifestyle throughout their pregnancy. If a woman had gestational diabetes, pregnancy induced hypertension (commonly referred to as PIH), preeclampsia, had prior macrosomic deliveries, or was obese; these women must start a low-carb regimen. The babies delivered to the women consuming low-carb diets were healthy, appropriately sized newborns. I have worked with obese women who were told they were going to have the same complications by their OB/GYN doc, only to see no complications and again healthy babies born at appropriate weights, all due to a low-carb lifestyle. The OB/GYN docs are utterly amazed at the progress and success of the pregnancy, but their amazement is due to the fact they do not understand low-carb.

I am a little confused at the "store bought meat, animal fat, and water" statement. I would never suggest one only consume cattle and water. But if we go back to when we lived in an ice age, for tens of thousands of years, the only thing around to eat were fat animals. We also need to understand that our ancestors did not just eat the meat. Not to gross anyone out, but we also consumed all the organs as well. Yes, the heart, liver, kidneys, stomach — well, you get my point. A low-carb lifestyle is more than just cattle, fat and water. It also includes too many other food sources to list, but a few more would be fish, chicken, green leafy veggies, small servings of berries. One can avoid red meat altogether and still consume enough protein. Remember, a developing embryo needs protein, fat and cholesterol for proper growth. Even in an adult, the percentage of carbohydrate represents only 2% of our biological makeup. Two percent. But the vast majority of people out there consume very little protein and fat, with the majority of their food consisting of carbohydrates.

I hear Dr. Carlson saying that a low-carb diet is indeed recommended for pregnancy, but perhaps going zero-carb isn't necessarily the answer since there are other food sources for pregnant women to eat for variety and healthy nutrition for their baby. He doesn't come out and say that a zero-carb diet is bad, per se, but it does not appear he promotes such a diet for childbearing. Is this becoming clear as mud for you right about now?

When I posed this question to popular low-carb blogger and friend Regina Wilshire from the "Weight of the Evidence" blog (WeightOfTheEvidence.com), she said it's probably "not a good idea" because it can be "risky." And she's not alone. Judith E. Brown, RD, MPH, PhD, Professor Emerita of the Division of Epidemiology and the Department of Obstetrics and Gynecology, University of Minnesota, responded to this "crazy" notion of a zero-carb, carnivorous diet with great concern. You'll notice much of what she states is rooted in the traditional dietary approach, but that's to be expected.

The short answer to the question about consumption of a meat and water diet during pregnancy is don't do it. A balanced and adequate diet, such as that recommended at MyPyramid.gov, is the nutritional path to a healthy mother and newborn. Both women and their growing fetuses need a wide variety of nutrients, and these are not supplied by diets limited to a few foods like meat and water. It is recommended that women consume at least

175 grams (700 calories) daily of carbohydrate to provide the fetus with a continuous supply of glucose, and to avoid ketosis. Although it is true that the fetus can use ketone bodies to some extent, it is not their body's preferred source of energy. Excess use of ketones is harmful to fetal growth and development.

This wasn't a surprising answer from a mainstream prenatal care expert, but it does give you the kind of response you'd expect to hear from a trained professional in this arena of medicine. But is she right to recommend such a high-carb diet? Or is Dr. Groves right stating zero-carb is perfectly fine during pregnancy? Or does Dr. Carlson have a point staking claim somewhere in between leaning towards a low-carb, not zero-carb approach? The question still looms as a big fat question mark.

Well, what does Charles think about "Ogg" and her question — "Is it safe for expectant Moms, unborn babies, and newborn babies to eat nothing except store bought cattle, cattle fat and water — please read that again — nothing except store bought cattle, cattle fat, and water — and nothing else for the entire duration of the Moms' pregnancy?" I decided to ask him directly.

And here's what Charles had to say:

Yes, as long as the woman is ketoadapted and successfully adapted to the zero-carb regimen for at least six months. I don't think it would feel particularly good for the woman if she began a zero-carb diet mid-pregnancy; however, if she was already on a low-carb diet of 30 grams or less, then she could transition to zero-carb even during pregnancy if she chose to. This seems controversial because the conventional wisdom is that a meat-rich, plant-poor diet will result in nutritional deficiencies.

The nutritionists of the 1920s and 30s didn't know that animal foods contain all of the essential amino acids and they do so in the ratios that maximizes their utility to humans. They also contain twelve of the thirteen essential vitamins in large quantities. Meat is a particularly concentrated source of vitamins A, E, and the entire complex of B vitamins. Vitamins D and B12 are found only in animal products and we can get sufficient vitamin D from sunlight on our skin. Because those on zero-carbohydrate diets do not suffer deficiency diseases nor suffer from chronic disease, this indicates that they are consuming what is by definition a healthy diet.

A zero-carb diet of beef, beef fat and water will produce no fat storage and all of the available energy will be utilized by the body. There will be no nutrient deficiencies because refined and easily digestible sugars and starches will not be consumed. Therefore, I argue that such a diet would be safe for any nursing or expectant woman. The Native American of the Great Plains, the Inuit, the Masai, etc. — cultures that consisted of primarily zero-carb, high-fat diets — all have babies and they are completely healthy without food from vegetation. Myself and many others consume an all-meat diet which results in great health. If a woman is healthy while she consumes such a diet, why would anything change once she became pregnant?

And thus we have come full circle on this question again. Charles is convinced based on the evidence he has presented many times that a zero-carb diet is the way to go for pregnant women. Do you buy his theory or do you have evidence that disproves anything he has shared? Are you as concerned about this kind of dietary advice being given to pregnant women as "Ogg" is? Is a zero-carb or even a low-carb diet healthy for a pregnant woman to consume? This one should be a real doozy of a discussion!

Okay, so that's the post that attracted all the criticism. You'll notice that not once did I provide any "advice" that a zero-carb diet is "advisable" for a pregnant woman to be on as some claimed I was doing. They even called for one of the web sites I write for (Examiner.com) to force me to remove the column and cease writing for them altogether because of this. And still I am called unstable!

With all that said, because there have been some misconceptions about where I stand on zero-carb diets and the notion I've put forth in this chapter about the fact that there is no dietary need for carbohydrates, let me be crystal clear about my position on low-carb versus zero-carb diets. I do not support a long-term zero-carb diet for health or weight loss. My personal belief is that you cannot possibly get all the nutrients your body needs eating just meat that you purchase from your local grocery store.

There are great advantages to adding nutrient-dense foods like eggs, nuts, green leafy veggies, berries, and more that people who follow a zero-carb diet are missing out on. Plus, there's the sustainability factor. Can you live a completely carbohydrate-free diet for the rest of your life? If people think low-carb is "restrictive," then think about how bad a zero-carb diet would be to follow forever and ever amen. Yikes! Not for me and I wouldn't recommend it as a preferred method for weight or health management. Besides, even those supposedly "no-carb" foods like meat have carbohydrates in the form of glycogen stores in them, so it's really a misnomer for anyone to claim they are eating a truly "zero-carb" diet in the first place.

For the record, let me repeat: I do not support a long-term zero-carb diet for health or weight loss. But it's not just me who disagrees with zero-carb. I went out into the low-carb community to get a sampling of familiar names to express their thoughts and reactions to what some would describe as a rather extreme version of the healthy low-carb lifestyle that so many of us enjoy. You'll notice many of the responses explain that a zero-carb diet in modern society is vastly different from what a zero-carb diet from primitive groups like the Inuit consumed and that there really is no such thing as a truly carbohydrate-free diet in the 21st Century.

The simple question I asked them was this: "Is a zero-carb diet healthy or not?"

Here's what they told me:

DR. JONNY BOWDEN (JonnyBowden.com)
"I think it's a pretty theoretical question. Even the Inuit living on walrus blubber and seal meat probably got some carbohydrates in their diet, and even a lion living on zebras and hyenas gets some carbs (in the entrails of their prey, who themselves graze on grass). But as a practical matter, I think it's not very advisable. There's too much evidence for the health properties of the plant phenols, polyphenols, flavonoids, vitamins, minerals and fiber found in abundance in vegetables and fruit.

I know there are people who seem to do pretty darn well with minimum amounts of these foods, but I suspect they are genetically or metabolically adapted to these diets more than the rest of us. Personally, I wouldn't choose a no-carb diet, though I wouldn't doubt that you could survive on one (which you, by the way, could not do on a zero-fat or zero-protein diet!). I think the good stuff in vegetables and low-sugar fruit is just too good to leave off the menu, and I think you can get all the benefits of low-sugar eating and still include plenty of vegetables and berries."

KENT ALTENA (BOWULF) (Network-Admin.net)

"I actually made a YouTube video on this topic recently and here is a summary of the video: 'I am pretty convinced that for most people going zero carb is an unnecessary step. Sure there are some very metabolically resistant and/or people suffering with hyperinsulinemia. For the most part, most people should be getting their veggies in and not fearing adding back a reasonable amount of carbs. Trying to discover what the magic number per day can certainly be trying, but your health will appreciate it. Thinking zero carbs is the answer also misses number of things: phytonutrients without getting more chemicals, fiber-rich vegetables, and carbs present in other non-veggie sources, like nuts, eggs, or cheese. Unless you are really hyper sensitive to carbs, enjoy the variety of nature and food selection.'

I think eating zero carb CAN be healthy, but it requires a level of vigilance and dedication to get adequate levels of nutrients that a standard low-carber does not have to be as concerned. The meat and other items they eat can have the vitamins within the fat they eat like the Inuit used to get from blubber and organ meats. More than likely though modern zero carbers will need to be vigilant to supplement their diet with other items. Therefore, I would only recommend the diet to only those who are really metabolically resistant. I think you can see that in Dr. Atkins' reticence in promoting the fat fast."

JUDY BARNES BAKER (CarbWars.blogspot.com)

"It should be possible to live entirely without plant foods, since many of our ancestors did and some societies that exist today still do, but that is not the same as living on a diet of nothing but muscle meat from domesticated animals. The Arctic explorer, Vilhjalmur Stefansson, proved in the early 1900s that you could be healthy on a diet of meat, fat, and water. He and a companion had themselves locked into a hospital ward and were fed a diet that consisted of 80% fat and 20% animal protein for one year and suffered no ill effects. However, he believed that you needed to eat some of the meat raw (or at least rare) and include organ meats. He pointed out that during his time living with the Inuit, he had eaten whole fish, including the bones, organs, tails, and heads.

Also, some non-plant foods do have carbs, oysters, scallops, liver, and eggs, for example, so a diet without plants is not necessarily a zero-carb diet. Does this mean some carbs are necessary? Probably not, but some variety might be. I think we all agree that the starch and sugar in plants are not essential for humans. The argument that there are other necessary elements in fruits, vegetables, and grains was refuted by Gary Taubes in Good Calories, Bad Calories. He said that it is the anti-nutrients in grains that cause us to need additional vitamins and minerals.

So, I guess my answer to your question would be that, in my opinion, you could live without plants and be healthy, pregnant or not, IF you had access to a wide variety of fresh, natural, unprocessed meat and fat, fish, and crustaceans and good, clean, mineral-rich water, all hard to come by where I live. Otherwise, including a few berries, nuts, and green vegetables might be prudent."

LAURA DOLSON (LowCarbDiets.about.com)

"Zero-carb is not a good idea, and in fact is almost impossible for very long, as the number of foods that contain no carbohydrate at all is quite small. I've spent quite a lot of time designing low-carb menus that have all the essential nutrients in them. Although it is possible at 20 grams of net carbs, it is not at all easy. Just adding 10 or 15 more grams makes it much more attainable. If you want to make it easy, go to 40-50 grams per day, which means you can also get a wider variety of phytonutrients as well. I realize that there are some people who are extremely sensitive to carbohydrate and cannot tolerate this much, but in my experience most people can, especially if most of the carbohydrate comes from non-starchy vegetables. (For example, spinach and other greens have carbs, but they are so wrapped up in fiber that most people will not experience a blood glucose impact at normal amounts.) To eat zero carbs is to seriously restrict the range of nutrients you can eat, and not a good idea."

DR. MARY C. VERNON

"First, of course, nothing I say should be taken as medical advice for any one person. That is a complex matter and requires individual consultation. That said, I believe there is quite a bit of historical information regarding very low-carb diets. Meat has some glycogen, so even it is not completely zero carb. The Inuit were able to prosper in extremely tough climatic conditions eating very low-carb diets. They were able to have children and breast feed them.

However, their zero carb diet might not translate to the Western world, because they ate things that are not favorite items in our culture and they ate at least some of these things without cooking them. So, we have historical information that this very low-carb diet can be done, if done in the way the Inuit *developed and practiced it. The European explorers who followed the Inuit example did fine. Those explorers who did not follow the Inuit way but ate as they were accustomed were not as successful. The person who has studied this in great detail is Dr. Steve Phinney. I learned most of what I know about this from him."*

DR. JEFF VOLEK

"With normal foods it would be very difficult to achieve zero carbs. Even meat, eggs, cheese have some albeit few carbs. Sure you could survive; gluconeo-genesis is more than adequate to maintain obligatory glucose needs. Although I'm a hardcore omnivore, meat at every meal with absolutely no other nutrition sounds incredibly monotonous and I suspect not optimal for health."

DR. RICHARD FEINMAN (MetabolismSociety.org)

"This question is actually of some interest because, as you write, people get the idea that, because there is no biological requirement for dietary carbohydrate, zero carbohydrate diets are recommended. In fact, I don't know anybody who recommends a zero carbohydrate diet but the question points up some of the confusion in the whole field. What you really want to know about a diet is the immediate effect on the plasma distribution of macronutrients. So a zero car-bohydrate diet, of course, does not mean zero glucose in the blood.

Obviously, in the absence of diseases, you can survive for a long time with zero carbohydrate. That's what you do when you're starving. As far as we know, most of the undesirable effects of starvation reside in the absence of protein, total amount and availability of essential amino acids and, to a lesser extent, essential fatty acids. The other side of the coin is high and low-fat where if carbohydrate is low a high fat diet may have lower total fat in the plasma than a low-fat. The point is the limitations of 'you are what you eat' and it is not obvious, in terms of blood glucose that zero carbs is so different from low-carbs. In general, more information is needed than the level of one nutrient to predict the effect of a diet.

A side issue is that it is probably impossible to get a zero-carb diet with normal food. Even meat has some carbohydrate in glycogen and cell material. When you brown meat in frying, the brown part is a reaction between the carbohy-drate and protein in the meat. The browning reaction is called the Maillard re-action and is chemically similar to the reaction of glucose with proteins, under conditions where there is high blood glucose, to produce so-called advanced glycation products (AGEs), the best known of which is hemoglobin A1c."

GARY TAUBES

"It does seem a bit extreme going to consume meat and water only, and as Dr. Carlson points out, muscle meat might not be sufficient to provide all the vitamins needed, if that's all that's being consumed. So, yes, why limit it to store bought meat and nothing else, other than to set up a hypothetical situation for discussion? Finally, one minor point: even a diet of meat and water is not zero carb. There will be a few percent carbohydrates from glycogen stored in the muscle."

JACKIE EBERSTEIN (ControlCarb.com)

"There were only two circumstances when Dr. Atkins used a diet below 20 grams of carbs. One was the fat fast for limited periods used while attempting to break a plateau. The other was 0 carbs for 3 days before a patient visited the office to measure ketones on our breathe analyzer. The purpose was to determine how ketone-resistant a person was. In both of these circumstances patients were following their supplement program to avoid a lack of nutrients.

Dr. Atkins did not believe there was any benefit to less than 20 grams. Since he considered the program a permanent lifestyle the idea of avoiding all vegetables and the other foods that make up the 20 grams on Induction simply does not make sense in the long run. He wanted the plan to have as much variety, palatability, texture and phytonutrient content as possible and still get the job done.

It is vitally important to remember that weight, blood sugar and insulin balance as well as the nutrient intake of a woman in the months before pregnancy has an impact on the baby. I discussed some of this in this column I wrote. There is no reason why a pregnant woman can't have a healthy and successful pregnancy as our patients did with an individualized low-carb plan under appropriate supervision."

MARK SISSON (MarksDailyApple.com)

"This is an interesting question with lots of variables to consider. As you know, I am not of the zero carb camp. I am a low-carber. My optimum maintenance range is 100-150 grams a day. My weight loss recommended range is 50-100 and my 'aggressive, short-term, hit the weight-loss hard' range is under 50. It's almost impossible to be zero carb if you are eating healthy fats (including nuts, seeds) and all manner of animal flesh. It's clear that we CAN live without directly eating carbs.

The question is whether a pregnant woman raised her whole prior life on carbs can gestate a healthy baby without any. I wouldn't recommend it (not that it can't be done) given the types of protein/fat-only foods normally available. Veggies need to be included at some level to provide vitamins and minerals that can't all be obtained from 99% of available protein sources. Even Inuit eat plants in summer and animal stomach-contents otherwise.

While gestational diabetes is a possible problem at typical carb intakes, I don't think it's an issue in an exercising mother at 150g/day. My main goal in suggesting that some carbs are advisable would be simply to promote insulin sensitivity during development. The idea is that unless the child were to continue on with a life of zero carb, it might be less-than-optimum to set him up that way (that's just intuitively)."

FRED HAHN (SlowBurn.typepad.com)

"We know that a low-carb diet is healthful. Study after study and client after client has shown that this is so. Jimmy brings up a good question — can a ZERO carb diet be healthy or does it lack essential nutrients for 'optimal' human health? Well we know what Dean Ornish, Gary Null and others of their ilk would say. They'd say you'd be dead in a year from heart disease. Of course the Inuit peoples would prove this wrong. And you can't say 'Waitaminnut! The Eskimos had generations to adapt to this kind of diet.' Why? When the British arctic explorers (Amundsen and crew) in the early part of the previous century ate what the Inuit ate for years they experienced robust health. Only when they switched back to eating to their local fare upon return to England did their health begin to suffer. So we know that going Eskimo does not kill us and can in fact improve our health.

But will going really low-carb to the point of zero carbs make us loco? Will it rob us of essential nutrients? The answer is tricky and it depends. If we are eating organ meats, bone marrow, etc. along with the rest of the common cuts of an animal there are few micronutrients we are not getting. But we usually don't. So getting some of the micronutrients like vitamin C from an orange or green peppers might be a wise idea. Personally I eat an extremely low-carb diet and enjoy robust health."

NINA PLANCK (NinaPlanck.com)

"Interesting debate. I don't see the merits of zero-carb for pregnant women in part because steady blood sugar is so important and carbohydrates can be

part of that. There are times when pregnant women will not be in the mood for protein, fat, and salt — vital as these nutrients are. There's nothing wrong with a peach or a sweet potato because there's a lot of good in them. But the ideal quantity of white flour and white sugar is undoubtedly zero, so if you can curb your addiction to carbage your baby will be much better off, and so will you."

DR. NATHAN ELIASON

"It is probably just fine to have the mild ketosis associated with a very low-carbohydrate diet during pregnancy. As you are aware, you can have a fairly low-carbohydrate diet in which you are not in ketosis which almost surely is fine during pregnancy. On the other hand, a high-carbohydrate diet likely will lead to complications which we see more and more frequently (macrosomia, neonatal hypoglycemia, gestational diabetes). The complications of having a baby which is too large are very real. However, we will surely never know for sure if a ketotic low-carbohydrate diet is safe, and probably never know if a relatively low-carbohydrate diet is safe because of the very real legal risk that obstetricians run. Unfortunately, it is far safer for them to recommend the 'standard' high-carb, low-fat diet than to allow for anything outside of the standard."

DANA CARPENDER (HoldTheToast.com)

"Is a zero-carb diet healthy? For what values of 'healthy?' We have reason to believe that the Inuit (Eskimo) lived on a nearly carb-free diet during the winter, and they apparently didn't suffer scurvy or other nutritional deficiency diseases. This is evidence that given the proper balance of animal foods, carbohydrate foods are inessential. On the other hand, the Inuit were eating a VERY different diet from your modern low-carber. They ate game and wild-caught fish, not animal foods from domesticated animals that had been raised on a commercial diet. They ate a diet so high in fat many of us would find it unappealing. They ate parts of the animal many modern Americans won't touch — liver, brains, kidneys, marrow, all of the organ meats (some of which, I might add, do contain a bit of carbs — liver especially.) And they ate much of their meat, fish, and blubber raw — and aged it well first. It is impossible to extrapolate from the effects of such a diet that a diet consisting solely of the animal foods available in your local grocery store, and familiar to modern American palates, is healthful, much less ideal."

As you can see from this cross-section of the best and brightest in the low-carb universe, most of them are very skeptical that anyone trying to follow a zero-carb diet in modern-day life is probably missing out on key nutrients in their diet because zero-carb today isn't the same as it was thousands of years ago. That's why you don't see me mention anything positive about "no-carb" or "zero-carb" diets in my books, on my blog, podcasts, YouTube videos, or forum. It's just inappropriate since the original purpose of my "Livin' La Vida Low-Carb" platform was to talk about "low-carb" living and how it can positively impact your weight and health. If you have questions about Atkins, Protein Power, or any of the other established low-carb diets and want to talk about them, then that is what my mission is all about.

Although your body doesn't have any dietary need for carbohydrates like it does fat and protein, that doesn't mean you have to cut them out entirely. Getting adequate amounts of non-starchy, green leafy veggies, nuts, seeds, berries, and other such low-carb foods is an excellent way to make your diet nutrient-dense and diverse enough to be easily assimilated into your healthy lifestyle change. Livin' la vida low-carb isn't as impossible as some people think it is. You just have to be armed with the knowledge about what you're putting in your mouth before you start eating. And reading this book is making you light years ahead of most people in this regard.

Coming up in the next chapter is one of the hardest lessons I have learned over the past five years of putting myself out there so prominently online. It taught me a very difficult lesson that not everyone who is on the Internet has as noble a purpose as I do regarding those they come into contact with each day. There are real opportunists out there whose only desire is to manipulate and bilk people into paying them money under fraudulent pretenses. It's very serious business and it happened to me soon after I started blogging. Get the full details about what happened to and how to avoid having it happen to you in the future.

LESSON #17
Opportunists on the Internet like Heidi Diaz from Kimkins lurk online

"The attractiveness of low-carb living makes it an eye-catching keyword for criminals who think they can make a quick dollar on its popularity. When coupled with other dieting catch phrases, this combination can be downright dangerous. Scammers like Heidi Diaz pairing things such as 'low-fat' AND 'low-carb' pose a very attractive 'best of both worlds'-type of scenario which, unchecked by medical backing, can produce devastating results. When these people hide behind the electronic curtain of the internet, it provides a unique and dangerous facade for the potential dieter."

— **Christin Sherburne**, former Kimkins member *Woman's World* magazine cover girl in June 2007 and active low-carb blogger at The-Journey-On. blogspot.com

I've been putting off writing this particular chapter for months because quite frankly it's not a pleasant time in my life that I'm very proud of. But, as with all things in life, there are even lessons to be learned even when you royally mess up. People who go through life perfectly without ever falling down or failing at anything are few and far between. Most of us have had it happen to us many times during our lives and it is our response to these adversities that determines whether we grow from the experience or allow it to stand in the way of moving forward. I've chosen the former in regards to my association with a diet known as Kimkins.

A lot has been made about my supposed collaborative business relationship with the founder of this online diet named Heidi "Kimmer" Diaz. I wanted to take this opportunity to tell my side of the story in this book while warning you against other Internet opportunists out there who are lurking online waiting for the next victim of their devious money-grabbing schemes. I suppose I was a bit naive to think that everyone in the weight loss and health community on the Internet would have the same good intentions that I did about helping people when I first started blogging in April 2005. However, I learned very quickly just how untrue that really is.

My initial encounter with the Kimkins diet happened when I was approached by a woman named Catherine MacDonald who contacted me in early 2006 about a new affiliate program she was recruiting bloggers to be a part of. At the time, my blog readership had grown to such a respectable level of visitors after one year online that companies were becoming interested in supporting the work I was doing through sponsorships to help compensate me for the time I invested into writing. While I had tried a few other affiliate relationships prior to this one, I was intrigued by what seemed like an exciting new low-carb plan.

My philosophy has always been to find the proven plan that works for you, follow it exactly as prescribed, and then keep doing it for the rest of your life. If Kimkins was a low-carb plan that someone wanted to do, then there seemed to be enough people succeeding on it according to the posted success stories on the web site replete with stunning before and after photos to start telling people about it through this affiliate relationship where I would get a portion of the sales generated whenever someone purchased one of the lifetime memberships. It sounded like the perfect thing for my low-carb blog and readers.

Beginning in the summer of 2006, I started promoting the Kimkins diet on my blog as another option for people who were interested in livin' la vida low-carb with regular posts highlighting the many success stories that appeared at the Kimkins web site. I became active on the Kimkins support forum where I met so many wonderful people who were looking for hope and encouragement in their weight loss efforts and Kimkins seemed to fit the bill for them perfectly.

This was right about the time when I first "met" the woman behind the diet who simply referred to herself as "Kimmer." She shared what seemed to be an unbelievable story of success by following her Kimkins diet plan to the tune of an amazing 200-pound weight loss. That was quite impressive and gave Kimmer instant credibility to everyone she came into contact with. I lauded her accomplishment on her forums where she provided answers to questions about her diet that people were posing to her on a daily basis. All in all, things looked to be on the up and up about this web site and its founder.

Just months after the new Kimkins web site came online, Kimmer suddenly fired her affiliate manager Catherine in a very open manner through various open exchanges (this was my first red flag!). I later found out that Kimmer accused Catherine, who did virtually all the footwork by setting up the Kimkins web site and marketed the affiliate program to hundreds of bloggers just like me, of keeping more money than she was authorized to by Kimmer from the affiliate sales. So my one and only contact about this affiliate relationship was now gone just months after recruiting me and Kimmer immediately took over with the promotion and marketing of her web site.

It was through my direct e-mail contact with Kimmer in October 2006 that she revealed her true identity to me as Heidi Diaz. I saw that name on the affiliate checks that she mailed to me and I thought it was strange that she'd call herself Kimmer online. In fact, most of her contact with me was from her "Kimmer" address until one day I received an e-mail after I conducted a blog interview with her that showed it was sent from "Heidi K. Diaz" which she joked was her "secret identity."

Yep, you read that right! Kimmer told me she was REALLY Heidi Diaz which becomes extremely important later on in this sad story because she vehemently denied it in my May 2007 podcast interview with her when she outright lied and told me that was her cousin's name. More on that in a moment.

In early 2007, there were rumblings starting to happen on popular low-carb forum web sites like Low-Carb Friends (LCF) as well as some newly-formed "anti-Kimkins" blogs about how there seemed to be some major discrepancies with what "Kimmer" was claiming about her diet and what was really happening. To be honest, I didn't even know about the wildly-popular "What's The Fascination with Kimmer?" thread on the LCF site or these new blogs that set out to expose the truth about Kimkins until several months later. I was still running my blog posting articles about low-carb living while interspersing the content with information about Kimkins which I didn't have any qualms with at the time.

In March 2007, a representative from *Woman's World* magazine contacted me about doing a story on the Kimkins diet and she wanted to know if I had contact information for Kimmer. I was excited to be able to share this information about the diet possibly being featured in such a major woman's weight loss publication. To be honest, I didn't really think much would come of it after I passed on the contact information to Heidi. Boy was I wrong when I saw that Kimkins was not just discussed in the magazine, but actually appeared on the front cover feature story highlighting the weight loss success of a woman named Christin Sherburne (who wrote the quote that appears at the beginning of this chapter). You'll learn more about Christin's role in the Kimkins story coming up.

It wasn't until I decided to try a version of the Kimkins diet for myself around April 2007 that I felt the real ire of the negative response some people were having towards the Kimkins diet. I wasn't sure what their problem was at the time because I tried the Kimmer Experiment (K/E) where you could eat unlimited amounts of lean protein which didn't seem to be too far off of what Dr. Atkins recommended in his books. Kimmer's suggestion to cut the fat seemed silly to me since I knew from my personal experience on the Atkins diet that you could eat fat without negative consequences to your weight and health as long as carbohydrates were reduced. And so I ate my unlimited protein along with fat to see what would happen. Predictably, I lost weight on it and shared my experiences on my blog. This was what brought out the Kimkins naysayers in droves against me and my blog.

At first, I didn't understand why people were in such a tizzy about this since it was a low-carb plan that was helping people attain the weight loss success they were longing for. I just chalked it up to people nitpicking for whatever their reason which is well-known to happen very often in the online dieting world. What I didn't realize at the time is these people were on to something big — and I mean REALLY big!

In May 2007, I finally convinced Kimmer to appear on my podcast show for an interview to answer the tough questions people were posting about her and her diet plan. It was a battle getting her to agree to an interview because she claimed to have agoraphobia and was allegedly too shy to do something like this. But she said she wanted to do this for me since I had been such a successful affiliate for her company.

Some of the complaints people had about Kimmer included the veracity of her personal 200-pound weight loss claim since nobody had ever seen her in person, banning members who had paid for a lifetime membership to the Kimkins web site, encouraging people to eat obsessively low levels of calories — as little as 400 calories daily along with taking laxatives to achieve weight loss, and the cover-up of some mysterious health complications that many Kimkins members were experiencing. All of this was fodder for discussion during my interview with Kimmer who I was beginning to have some serious doubts about. My hope was that the podcast interview would clear those doubts up. However, all it did was solidify in my mind that all the claims being made about Kimkins and Heidi Diaz were 100% true!

Prior to the podcast interview, the Kimkins story hit *Woman's World* magazine in June 2007 and all you know what broke loose. Overnight the web site went from a few thousand members to tens of thousands of members. The financial payoff for Heidi getting this front-cover feature was easily worth nearly $1 million in profits for her. And to think I was partially responsible for making this happen because I passed on contact information to "Kimmer" makes my stomach churn to this very day. Contrary to what some have said about me, I did not receive a large "finders fee" compensation check for doing this.

When I was able to share my interview with "Kimmer" in July 2007, I had no idea she was willing to share untruths so freely. From claiming she was that skinny woman in the red dress that was posted so prominently on the Kimkins web site and appearing as her forum avatar to promoting her diet as just another "low-carb plan," this was not some innocent little oversight by a woman who claimed to be "just a mom." Instead, it seemed to be a deliberate attempt to fool literally tens of thousands of people into thinking the Kimkins diet was the answer — including Jimmy Moore.

I encourage you to listen to Episode 94 of my podcast "The Livin' La Vida Low-Carb Show with Jimmy Moore" (http://www.thelivinlowcarbshow.com/shownotes) where I pull out excerpts from my 90-minute interview with the real "Kimmer" — Heidi Kimberly Diaz — where she made some rather eye-opening comments about herself and her diet that were subsequently proven false less than three months later. The answers she provided are juxtaposed with the truth that continues to be revealed to this very day. Heidi Diaz does NOT want anyone to hear about this, but the truth needs to be shared for the sake of those who are still involved with this diet program.

When I was speaking to Heidi/Kimmer during our interview, it was becoming more and more obvious this woman was buying into her own propaganda and making it up as she was going along. And when you stop and think about the fact that she was so easily answering all of my questions about her alleged triple-digit weight loss when she was in fact sitting there as a 300+ pound woman, it is sickening beyond the words I need to describe it. Oh yes, we're getting to that shocking part of the story.

During the interview itself, she had no problem answering the questions I posed to her confidently without any shyness whatsoever. This was the first time anyone heard the voice of Heidi Diaz up close and personal which would turn out to be a huge mistake on her part because it would end up revealing her true identity just a couple of months later when a television reporter caught up with her at her home to discuss the Kimkins controversy.

The week I shared this Kimmer interview with my podcast listeners, Christine and I had gotten away to visit some friends in Missouri to seriously reconsider my affiliate relationship with the Kimkins web site. Yes, I had made some money from telling others about this diet plan that I thought was an acceptable low-carb option, but now there was talk that people following this plan were being encouraged to lower their calories to obscenely low amounts (as little as 200-300 calories a day) while restricting their food intake to basically protein only. It was a recipe for disaster just waiting to happen and I couldn't stand idly by no matter how much it would negatively impact me financially.

And so, with great humility and deep regret for being duped and bringing my readers along for the ride, I penned the following apology blog post to my readers and all those who I had misled towards the Kimkins diet on Friday, July 27, 2007:

With time away in Missouri to rest, relax, and reflect on everything that's happened over the past few months, I've now come to realize that my blog has changed in many ways and is headed in a direction that I feel isn't in the best interests of the larger audience of readers who come here. Because of that, I think today is a good day to share some of my sincere regrets, what I have learned from those, and where I recognize I need to be refocusing on from this day forward.

In the last few months I have made some very real mistakes which have caused many people to question my intentions and motivations here at my blog. Admittedly, I was unwilling to listen to the criticism from those who were only trying to help me and I began growing frustrated to the point that my frustrations got the better of me.

Over the last few months there has been a growing concern from those in the low-carb community about my promotion of Kimkins. I had failed to openly disclose my affiliate relationship with that diet plan and I now realize I should have. Additionally, my insistence that Kimkins was just another low-carb diet similar to Atkins, Protein Power or South Beach as well as my posts encouraging readers to join me when I started what I believed to be the K/E option was overzealous to say the least. I apologize for not being more upfront about that.

More importantly, my refusal to properly review and then hold Kimkins to the same standard as other plans and approaches I've praised and criticized was a glaring mistake of omission for which I regret. My intentions were good, but now I can see why there were questions arising about me and my business relationship to Kimkins.

Call me stubborn, but for the life of me I could not see what the problem was; I truly believed I was indeed following K/E and honestly had not reviewed the other plans on the site. Now I know I should have.

While I've been on vacation in Missouri this past week, I've now taken the time with some gentle nudges from those that implored me to review all the plans, review the content that is publicly available (present and archived), and then review the historical content found on the Low-Carb Friends forum.

After doing that, I can now see why this issue with Kimkins has stirred up such a fiery controversy because most of the plans are a controversial approach to losing weight by encouraging fast weight loss without mention of the very real risks involved with doing so. I regret that I allowed my excitement about my renewed commitment to losing those last few pounds I wanted to overwhelm me to the point I lost my good sense.

I hope sharing this with you today will help us all avoid making similar missteps in the future. To be very honest, the thing that held my emotions so well was the strong sense of community I felt from those on the forums at Kimkins. It's something that I missed terribly since I was banned from Low-Carb Friends and I didn't recognize that until recently.

With the Kimkins forum, I felt a sense of belonging that often lacks when you're writing day-to-day on a blog. There's such a sense of community that I now recognize I can be part of if I join any number of online support forums by taking the initiative to do so. There are some truly GREAT people providing support out there.

In the past I did join Low-Carb Friends in part to be a part of a community and in part to promote my blog. In doing that, joining with an underlying agenda to serve my own needs, I missed the opportunity to really be part of a community and found myself quickly banished by the admins there. In my enthusiasm to promote my blog in the early days, I violated the terms of service and was rightfully banned.

Instead of doing what I should have done by apologizing to the admins and ask to be reinstated with the agreement I would not promote my blog within the forums anymore, I walked away disappointed and slowly allowed resentment to build. The January post I wrote at my blog about Low-Carb Friends earlier this year was inappropriate and uncalled for because it deeply offended many at that board. For this I am truly sorry and can only hope that, in time, those who make Low-Carb Friends their community for online support will find it in their hearts to forgive me.

I now realize that without Low-Carb Friends I would not have been able to review the historical posts that led to the creation of the controversial Kimkins web site. It is an eye-opening look at how many people were ill-advised and mistreated over months and years prior to the launch of the Kimkins web site that I started promoting last year. It is something I should have taken the time to read much sooner, something that should have been part of the necessary due diligence on my part before agreeing to support and promote what I believed was just another low-carb diet.

So first I must thank the admins and owner at Low-Carb Friends for maintaining the sticky thread "Ask Kimmer" because it has helped me begin to see many of the errors I've made in my assumptions about most of the Kimkins diet plans these past few months.

I also find myself once again in need of giving an apology to my readers here at "Livin' La Vida Low-Carb." I allowed the strong sense of community I felt with Kimkins to cloud my judgment and subsequent action to continue promoting Kimkins even in the face of numerous people pointing out problems that are clear as day even after my podcast interview with Kimmer.

Had I only stepped back and looked objectively at the criticism for what it was — again a way to help, not harm me — then the entire last year may have taken a different path. While I cannot change what I have done in the past, I can change what I do starting today and moving forward.

Today begins a refocusing back to the original purpose and mission of my blog — to educate, encourage, and inspire people about the healthy low-carb lifestyle!

I have always maintained that each person must find the diet that works for them, whether that's low-carb, low-fat, or whatever. If it works for you and you can do it over the long-term with your health improving because of it, then go for it and rejoice as you take control of your health! I very clearly do not agree with low-fat and low-calorie options as I lost most of my weight on the Atkins diet, but that does not mean they do not work, nor serve some well even in the short-term.

Because I do not agree with those dietary approaches, I focus on carbohydrate restriction and proper fat intake since research supports that as a healthy way to lose weight and find optimal health over the long-term.

In the past I have taken many others to task over their diets and I now regret I did not critically evaluate the full context of the various dietary plans for Kimkins.

I should have because, as many have repeatedly said, the plans are very low-calorie diets despite any specific requirement to count calories (in some plans like K/E), thus by design they are low-fat and low-carb because they are very-low-calorie in nature.

One of the most objective reviews I recently read was from my friend Carol Bardelli at the "Kudos for Low-Carb" blog. She provided a wealth of information about very low-calorie diets in that post that I encourage my readers to review to gain more understanding of why it's important to nourish our bodies as we lose weight. Also, Sherrie from the "Pinch Of..." blog made some very valuable points on this same issue as well.

As one poster on Low-Carb Friends has integrated into her signature, "It shouldn't be a RACE to get thin. It should be a Journey to good health." I couldn't agree more!

Therefore, you will notice I have made some necessary changes to my blog that reflect that sentiment to remind myself that part of finding what works for me and you finding what works for you means encouraging each other to also make good decisions that optimize our long-term health in the process. Livin' la vida low-carb is as much about improving health as it is weight loss.

You will notice that I have removed the banners promoting the Kimkins diet today as a matter of conscience. In the last week I have realized that I cannot try to "educate, encourage and inspire" my readers if I am associated with Kimkins, a web site promoting some plans which may indeed be unhealthy if followed over the long-term.

My focus has been on the best of the five plans (K/E) and I cannot say they're all sound and healthy ways to lose weight on your own. Because of this, I cannot encourage my readers to join the site knowing they may wind up following a plan that may do more harm than good in the long-term. Be smart about any diet plan you go on.

Let me also state clearly that I believe it is extremely important for people to research any diet before they begin and even talk with your doctor about not just the short-term impact, but also the long-term effects and potential health risks you may face.

While many believed I was making great big bundles of money from my affiliate relationship with Kimkins, let me just say that no amount of money is worth losing sight of the bigger picture to educate my readers with quality information, encourage them to find a way of eating to help them regain their health while losing weight, and inspire them to be their best while going through this process.

While I still believe it is possible to tweak things within some plans promoted by Kimkins, I also realize that this is strongly discouraged on the plan. If something is not working, then it's easy to say you're not working the plan. But, then again, as many of us know it's in the little bit of tweaking that we find our strength and confidence to make the diet our own over the long-term. That's what I did after Atkins, although I am sure the late great Dr. Robert C. Atkins would not object.

With that understanding now, I'm left questioning what I am really doing here and why I felt compelled to start making changes in my diet in the first place.

I now realize I find myself exactly where many other low-carbers land when they lose weight with a low-carb diet — a place where I am comfortable making modifications that make low-carb work for me over the long-term!

I could label it and say it's Atkins, or Kimkins, or South Beach, or any number of plans as recommended for maintenance, but that wouldn't be honest! The truth is, I'm doing what works for Jimmy Moore right now and it is simply a low-carb diet where I've started to also look at my fat intake to control calories naturally. That's all! I don't need to place a label on it to make it mine and I certainly don't need to convince my readers what they already know — finding the plan that's right for you and then DOING IT!

By opening up my mind to better understand what I am doing, what I can tell my readers is that I now truly understand that I have not been following K/E as recommended, nor could I. What I have done is merely modify and play with what I'm eating to find what will work for me now and that's simply been lowering carbohydrate, reducing fat slightly and paying more attention to carefully choose the treats I still do include to make the plan work for me.

For me, life without small indulgences like bread and chocolate here and there is not what I want. So, I'm still playing around with what will work for me and wish others well with what works for them. If that includes low-carb products, then great; but if not, that's cool, too.

Over the last few months, my promotion of and subsequent insistence that I am following the Kimkins K/E plan has caused a polarization within the various low-carb forums. I am deeply sorry for bringing much of this on myself, by both words and actions, by fueling the debate and ignoring many of the red flags and warnings people had for me.

We low-carbers are an ever-growing by leaps and bounds community online with brand new people looking for hope for their obesity and I am becoming more and more aware of that fact. With Kimkins, I saw an easy quick-fix and ran with it, unwittingly undermining my mission here to educate, encourage, and inspire others.

This too is something I hope my readers will forgive me for doing. As I go, I grow. I learn sometimes slowly along the way and can only hope that those who have spent time and effort to educate me, encourage me to take the time to really scrutinize what I'm doing, and inspire me to hold myself accountable, will understand that I am now listening, I am hearing you, and I am trying to make right what many have pointed out were errors on my part. I too am human, imperfect, and do make mistakes.

Where I've erred, I hope you can forgive me for that, too.

Along with the criticisms sent my way about Kimkins also came criticism for not clearly disclosing sponsor and affiliate relationships that allow me to maintain this blog freely to all who wish to read it. I strongly believe that those of us who write about low-carb need to be free to publish information that is lacking in the mainstream media, or even worse, manipulated or twisted in ways that cause confusion.

I've said it before, my purpose is to educate, encourage, and inspire.

I hope my readers understand that to write every single day like I do takes many hours of my time to do — time to research, review, read, gather information and then write my articles.

Over the last two years, the time invested in writing for my blog has grown from a few hours when I first began in April 2005 to now as much as 12 hours a day. It really has become more of a full-time job now and is something I cannot continue to do without a means to pay my bills and support my family.

I so passionately feel it's important to continue on with my blog that I sought out a way to support my family so I can continue to write. But I failed to disclose those changes along the way with my readers. I had a responsibility to do so, and am now making changes to insure you understand how I choose sponsors and how they're included here.

I do take seriously my real responsibility to choose wisely those whom are offering me opportunities to make my blog possible. Plus, I am keenly aware that not only are my readers a quality audience to many companies, but that my readers expect I will choose products and services from companies that are of the highest quality.

You'll now notice I have placed a conflict-of-interest disclosure that fully informs my readers that this blog is, in part, sponsored by companies who recognize the value of low-carbohydrate diets and respect my reader's dietary choice. They want to do business with us and it is my policy that I will only accept sponsors and affiliates whom I believe offer quality products or services, along with good customer service and responsiveness to needs of my readers. While we won't always agree about whom I've included, it should now be clear that banners on my blog are from sponsors and affiliates I have chosen to include after I've researched their offerings and am comfortable to offer something of value to many of my readers.

I've also clearly stated that when I am including a post that does mention a sponsors product or service, that is my opinion about the product or service and I have not been compelled by contractual obligation to promote the product or service to my readers within the text content of my blog. I want to assure my readers that none of the sponsors or affiliates they see on my blog have contracted with me to specifically mention or promote their products within the text content of my blog, nor will I enter into such contracts in the future. So, yes, when I am enthusiastic about a product or service, it is because I really am, not because I have to be because I'm being paid to say something I do not believe.

There is one small exception to this that I believe is a win-win for all of us. When a company that meets the standards to be included here offers a give-away or contest to my readers with no obligation, and I write about it, then it is the writing about it that brings it to your attention. You are never under any obligation to participate or enter, but I feel including it meets my goal to educate, encourage and inspire. In posts such as this, I will clearly state the nature of my relationship in the promotion.

Right now I can only hope my readers will forgive my past sins and understand that I didn't fully appreciate how important such disclosures are. I've taken many researchers to task because they did not adequately disclose potential conflicts of interest in studies, but I failed to hold myself to that same standard. I believe I am now correcting my own error of omission and hope you will continue to point out things if I fail to live up to my words in the future.

The last thing I feel it's necessary to address is the fact I've allowed my emotions to get the better of me at times when I should have "taken my medicine" like a man. Instead, I acted out and sometimes aggressively responded to criticism in ways I wish I could take back. Calling those who were critical of my words and decisions various names, including "haters and crybabies," was not only wrong, but failing to live up to the spirit of open-and-lively discussion and debate.

I closed the door to listen to some of my readers and realize how damaging that is to all of us, no matter what your view is on the controversy around Kim-kins. I hope today to reopen the door to those who have been turned off and welcome you back with open arms so we can work together to help each other on this low-carb journey.

In the future, I will be ever-mindful that we're all in this together. Some will agree with me, others will disagree. But all views are important and should be heard whether everyone agrees or not.

I will do my best to honor this commitment I am making today to temper my immediate reaction and try to give more thought to my replies in an effort to be a better writer and fulfill my desire to make the "Livin' La Vida Low-Carb" blog a place where facts are at the forefront and opinions, while still critically important in the big picture, are provided by me in the light of solid, reputable evidence and data that must be part of any substantive debate of ideas in the health arena.

I realize now that I focused heavily on the positive feedback, largely ignoring the negative. While it's important to stay positive, it's also very important to be open to hearing the negative to really understand the issues. It's constructive either way and that's how I will view it from now on.

Without that acknowledgment and respect for the fact we don't all agree about everything, we cannot make progress to educate others about the benefits of low-carb diets, encourage each other to be our best each day, nor can we effectively inspire those who want to know more to seek out and find more information, even with our faults.

So I am hoping today to begin anew on a path that will enable me to serve my readers and their best interests, to be cognizant of a standard of excellence I must hold myself to each and every day as I write about livin' la vida low-carb, and remember the all-important bigger picture — YOU, my readers, our com-mon goals and desires, our interconnectedness that makes us an online com-munity on the same path, finding what works for each of us along the way and our mutual agreement and understanding that for the long-term, good health is attainable with healthy low-carb living.

Each of us must be able to freely share what is working for us as well as the pitfalls and obstacles we may face along the way. When we share these things — both the good and the bad — with each other, we all grow in our understanding and help each other in the long-term.

And that, my friends, really is where my heart is — to help, both myself and my readers, learn how livin' la vida low-carb truly can benefit health over the long haul. It is a position I feel is strongly supported not just by the latest research, but also through my own experiences.

These experiences are ones I want to continue sharing with all the thousands of people who come to read here each day. Through that, I am sure there will be plenty of education, encouragement, and inspiration along the way. Even if someone decides low-carb isn't for them, then at least they will realize it is something that works for many who do make the choice to follow it as their permanent way of eating for life.

I ask nothing more from you than to please allow me to try to be the best that I can be by continuing to support my mission here to educate, encourage and inspire. I cannot change who I am as a person. I'm not suddenly going to be different or less outspoken than I have been, but I will be much more aware of the fact that we are all in this together, and without you my readers, I cannot fulfill my hopes and dreams to help others find their way to health like I did.

Working together, we can do that and more! So I hope you know from the bottom of my heart, I'm sorry. Please forgive me for my mistakes and help me as I continue to learn and write about a subject we all are enthusiastically passionate about — that's Livin' La Vida Low-Carb, baby!

That was one of the most difficult things I had ever done in my entire life writing that apology. But it was something I could no longer run away from and the time was right. I didn't blog for several days after the apology was published and I felt such a huge sense of release from a burden that had unknowingly weighed me down in the months leading up to this point.

The tremendous outpouring of feedback on my blog was mostly positive as many of my readers appreciated the fact that I admitted my faults in promoting what turned out to be a fraudulent diet plan by a woman who never lost the weight as she had claimed. At the same time, there was an immediate sense of betrayal by those who were still Kimkins believers and Kimmer herself distanced herself from me stating my denunciation of the Kimkins diet would have little bearing on her business. That was a laughable statement since I was the one who had sent so many people to her web site in the year prior. It was yet more confirmation in my mind that this was the right thing to do.

Although it was a hard decision to finally cut all ties with Kimkins and re-move every last vestige of references to the diet on my web site (which took me weeks to do!), I can honestly say it was the right thing to do in light of all that was being revealed about the person behind the diet. My only re-gret about leaving Kimkins was the people on the forum I left behind. They were the ones who kept me there because I appreciated the open dialog with such a loving and caring group of people. I had missed the unity from the community atmosphere until I created my new "Livin' La Vida Low-Carb Discussion" forum (LivinLowCarbDiscussion.com) a few weeks after leaving Kimkins.

The instant connection at my new forum between the members there from the get-go was magical because we were all respectful, professional, and honest with each other about our healthy low-carb lifestyle. What a thrill it was to see over 125,000 page views in just the first month and I'm so ecstatic about how many people have been positively impacted with the message of livin' la vida low-carb through that forum in the years since. And this includes all the Kim-kins refugees who followed my lead in turning away from that diet for good and landing in a safe place online where they could receive real support for their healthy low-carb lifestyle.

A very brave decision was made about a month after I left Kimkins by three extra special angels in God's eyes: Becky Winn, Christin Sherburne, and Deni Huttula. For those of you who are familiar with these awesome women and followed the Kimkins story, then you would probably recognize them as the primary faces of the Kimkins diet in the early days.

Becky was always providing thorough and direct posts on the Kimkins fo-rum to questions posted by members. Christin was the cover girl in *Woman's World* magazine in June 2007 and a big cheerleader on behalf of the Kimkins diet after losing over 100 pounds in five months. Finally, Deni was also in the *Woman's World* article for her weight loss and was a Spirit-filled spiritual leader for so many going through this journey.

But you'll notice I said "was." All three of them left Kimkins in September 2007. It started with Becky when she announced it was time for her to leave. Here's an excerpt of what she wrote at the Kimkins site:

"What led to my dawning awareness that it was time to go was more than irreconcilable differences of opinion, more than self-protective concern, and more than current controversy. What led to my regretful realization that I would have to leave is another story for another time."

Then, in a Labor Day surprise, both Christin and Deni wrote detailed blog posts announcing their sudden departure because of many of the same concerns I had about Heidi Diaz and the claims regarding her Kimkins diet. Christin admitted her hair started to fall out after four months on Kimkins and she didn't have a period for five months in her farewell post on the Kimkins forum. She began to wonder what price she was paying with her health by following a plan like Kimkins for long-term weight loss.

"So while I do agree and whole heartedly support that there is everything to be said for protein sources to be lean, and eating fresh vegetables, there is also something to the fact that God created things like whole grains and fruit for our bodies as well. However, I saw those things as a short term sacrifice for a long term gain. But sacrifice at what cost?"

For Deni, she believes God had her at Kimkins for a time and a purpose for a season and now it was time for her to move on to the next phase of her life according to His Will for her life. Her growing concerns about Kimkins led her to no other conclusion.

"I am leaving because I have learned some things that make me doubt the integrity of the founder, and because I have been used for purposes that go against my personality, my moral, and my conscience. I was deceived, and yet I still do not regret or doubt that the Lord called me to be there. I simply accept now, that my work there is done and that the plans HE had for me there have been completed."

Part of the reason why Christin and Deni decided to leave Kimkins was due to health problems they both started dealing with. For *Woman's World* cover girl Christin who lost 100 pounds in five months on the Kimkins diet, she began having severe chest pains, among other health issues. For Deni who lost 60 pounds in three months on Kimkins, she says there should have been a "warning label" about the Kimkins diet after she began experiencing some rather odd side effects such as extra periods, hair loss, dizzy spells, blurred vision, heart flutters, and intense cravings. Ironically, all of this came in the pursuit of weight loss so she could live a healthier life for her family.

Is it mere coincidence that two of the most prominent Kimkins weight loss success stories who were the poster children for the diet had to deal with these kinds of health concerns? Why is a web site like Kimkins even allowed to exist when real people like Christin and Deni have documented proof that they have been damaged as a result of this diet plan cooked up by an anonymous woman hiding behind a computer?

With the departure of such strong and faithful leaders as Becky, Christin, and Deni from Kimkins (and other members at Kimkins quickly followed their lead), I opened up my new forum to the Kimkins refugees looking for a place to call home where they could reconnect with one another in fellowship and community. So many of them came willingly to this new safe place on the Internet free from judgment and ridicule and switching to solid low-carb plans like Atkins, Protein Power, and more.

Then in September 2007, a web site operated by the husband of Catherine Mac-Donald named Martin posted some startling private investigator photos and video footage of the real Heidi Diaz that appeared on his Slamboard.com web site — and now the gig was up! After years of fooling people into believing she had lost 200 pounds although she had refused to come out in public, the truth was right there for everyone to see that she was a 300-pound woman who had never lost weight at all. Heidi Diaz had lied about her alleged triple-digit weight loss!

I was stunned while at the same time reassured. Seeing those photos of Heidi Diaz absolutely confirmed many of the exact reasons why I decided to apologize and completely sever ties with Kimkins just weeks prior to this and I expected there would be even more investigations into the business practices and ethics of Kimkins and those behind it. People started writing to the Better Business Bureau of California complaining about the Kimkins web site and they ended up grading her diet plan with an "F" after receiving numerous negative comments from people who had been duped by Heidi Diaz. This is when everything started to unravel for Heidi Diaz and the Kimkins diet.

Some of the most ardent former supporters of this diet began speaking out about how the Kimkins diet program had negatively impacted their health and it even got picked up by a local television station in Los Angeles (KTLA-TV) in October 2007. Then the Kimkins diet story was given a nationally-televised audience for the first time in November 2007 when it was featured on FOX-TV's "The Morning Show with Mike & Juliet" where Christin and Deni shared their concerns about Diaz and the ultra-low-calorie diet plan she was pushing on the members of Kimkins who joined as a result of the *Woman's World* story. They warned that this diet simply promoted "anorexia" and should be avoided.

The public spokesperson for the Kimkins diet at the time all this was happening was a woman named Jeannie Battinger who quickly severed ties with the organization following the airing of this show in response to her own concerns about the now-exposed Kimkins founder. Even as Battinger was trying to defend the indefensible during her appearance on "The Morning Show," you could tell she knew that something was awry. Her resignation took place less than a week after the show aired.

With all the media exposure of this dangerous diet plan, the most significant took place in early 2008 when *ABC News* was looking for people harmed by Kimkins and ran a story that was featured on "Good Morning America." The tidal wave of concern about Kimkins apparently grew to the point after that segment aired that *Woman's World* finally came to their senses and decided to post the following statement on their web site in February 2008:

A statement from Woman's World Magazine. Please accept our apology. We at Woman's World pride ourselves on finding inspiring diet successes to share with our readers every week. That's why we were so distressed to learn that Kim Drake, the founder of Kimkins.com, gave us inaccurate information about herself and her weight loss. Though the article appeared several months ago, in our June 12, 2007 issue, and nutritionists assure us the diet information we provided was accurate, we deeply regret having shared with you a story we can't stand behind. Your trust means everything to us, and we want to bring you the very best magazine we can, each and every week.

It was great to see Woman's World magazine acknowledge the cover story they did on the Kimkins diet contained some "inaccurate information" after literally thousands of concerned readers flooded them with letters and e-mails begging them to print a retraction of their June 2007 story featuring the Kimkins diet so prominently with two real people — Christin Sherburne and Deni Huttula — and a fake photograph and story about Heidi Diaz' falsified 200-pound weight loss. In fact, in keeping with her propensity to stretch the truth, Diaz was referred to in the magazine as Kim Drake.

Considering all the preponderance of the evidence that had previously come out in the eight months that happened between the story being published and this apology from *Woman's World*, it should not have taken this long for action to be taken. At least they took SOME kind of action to right this wrong that set in motion a flood of new Kimkins members to the web site to be sucked in by an opportunist who has continued to bilk members out of $80 long after all these revelations have come to light. As of September 2009, she's STILL in business and charging nearly $100 to be a member of her diet web site.

After all these revelations came out on television about Heidi Diaz including the fake before and after pictures of Russian brides she used on her web site, the lies about her own alleged weight loss success, and all the rest of what had become the Kimkins diet scandal, I decided to give Kimmer/Heidi Diaz a call for myself. I used the same number she gave me to call her for the podcast interview we had previously done, so I KNOW it was her number beyond any shadow of a doubt. I wanted to ask her why she was still claiming she lost nearly 200 pounds when the private investigator unveiled an entirely different story altogether. I also wanted to settle the question about her name being Heidi Diaz or not.

The resulting "conversation" was one of the strangest exchanges I have ever participated in. It was so beyond surreal, I can hardly describe it for you. You're just not gonna believe this really happened, but it is 100% true. I called and asked for Heidi and she attempted to portray the babysitter by taking a message for her. But I recognized her voice and noted that I wanted to talk to her and again Heidi acted like she didn't know who I was. Finally, at the end of the call, she said I must have dialed the wrong number and then she hung up on me.

Did Heidi Diaz think I wouldn't recognize her voice after conducting a nearly 90-minute interview with her just a few months prior? She even acted like she was watching kids and talking to them asking who Jimmy Moore is. What was really funny is she said Heidi was out and that she'd take a message, but then at the end she changed her story and said that I must have dialed the wrong number. How very odd.

I have interviewed several former prominent Kimkins members at my blog and podcast show about their experience being on the diet, including Jeannie Battinger, Amy Bryant, and Christin Sherburne to get the message out about the dangers of going on the Kimkins diet. At the beginning of 2009, Heidi Diaz was unfortunately still in the diet business...but that could be changing very soon for two reasons.

First, the Kimkins diet has been exposed and was named the Healthy Weight Network's "Worst Diet Product of 2008" in their 20th Annual Slim Chance Awards. Here's what they wrote about the dubious "winner":

It must have seemed an easy way to get rich quick. Founder Heidi "Kimmer" Diaz set up a website and charged members a fee to access the Kimkins diet, boasting they could lose up to 5 percent of their body weight in 10 days. "Better than gastric bypass," there was "no faster diet," and in fact she herself had lost 198 pounds in 11 months. Stunning "after" photos were displayed. In June 2007 Women's World ran it as a cover story, and that month alone PayPal records show the Kimkins site took in over $1.2 million. Then users began complaining of chest pains, hair loss, heart palpitations, irritability and menstrual irregularities. This was not surprising since Kimkins is essentially a starvation diet, down to 500 calories per day and deficient in many nutrients (shockingly, laxatives are advised to replace the missing fiber). In a lawsuit, 11 former members are uncovering a vast record of Diaz's alleged fraud. They found that the stunning "after" photos, including one of Kimmer herself, had been lifted from a Russian mail order bride site. According to a deposition reported by Los Angeles TV station KTLA, Diaz admitted using fake pictures, fake stories and fake IDs, and a judge has allowed the litigants to freeze some of her assets.

The other reason Heidi Diaz and her Kimpire is in big trouble is the class action lawsuit waged against her by former Kimkins members who were harmed by the diet. The plaintiff's motion for class certification action by Jeanessa Fenderson led by chief counsel for the plaintiffs John Tiedt (TiedtLaw.com) is on the court docket in Riverside Superior Court in California. To make matters worse, Diaz is having trouble finding an attorney willing to defend her dubious actions.

As a sign of desperation, Diaz even went so far as to file a cross-complaint lawsuit against the members of the class action suit as well as others, including myself, allegedly for inflicting economic damage, slander and libel, invasion of privacy, civil conspiracy, and inflicting intentional emotional distress — all worthy of "damages" totaling in excess of $1 million. Hilarious, isn't it? That frivolous lawsuit was summarily dismissed just weeks after it was filed.

Now she's sending out cease and desist orders to people who have written negatively about her or the Kimkins diet. This is one of the reasons why you have to be so careful about Internet opportunists like her who are lurking online. They seem to only be in this for the money and unfortunately that's what Heidi Diaz has done.

On Monday, January 12, 2009, Heidi K. Diaz submitted the paperwork to United States Bankruptcy Court in the Central District of California just two days before the class action lawsuit against her and her Kimkins diet program was set to be heard by a judge to determine certification to move forward with the case. An automatic stay in the *Fenderson v. Diaz* class action lawsuit was faxed to lead prosecuting attorney John Tiedt in the class action case to inform him what Diaz had done and that any action against her civilly would have to be put on hold or transferred to bankruptcy court. In other words, this was even more stall tactics to delay justice against this woman who has purportedly bilked well over $1 million out of unsuspecting dieters worldwide while leaving the weight and health of many Kimkins victims in disarray.

Lead attorney prosecuting the case against Diaz, John Tiedt said he was not surprised by this move by Diaz and has sought diligently to prosecute her to the fullest extent of the law spending thousands of hours and much of his own money building a case against her over the past few years.

"We will not be deterred. We will not stop until we have justice," Tiedt said. "We anticipated the possibility of bankruptcy. This is Ms. Diaz's third bankruptcy. We are now obtaining a bankruptcy litigator to join our team. Our attack on the bankruptcy will start immediately. I will never stop."

But, you know, fate had a way of working things out for the good against people like Heidi Diaz. You see, Riverside County Superior Court Judge Michael B. Donner never got the papers about Diaz' bankruptcy ploy, so he went ahead and heard the case for proceeding forward with the class action lawsuit by Tiedt on Wednesday, January 14, 2009 at 8:30am.

Jeanessa Fenderson finally got what she had been fighting for nearly a year to see — CLASS ACTION CERTIFICATION! This was HUGE because now anyone who had been harmed physically, monetarily, or otherwise by Heidi Diaz and the Kimkins diet could seek damages by joining this lawsuit. A formal order was prepared and served to Heidi Diaz who said she was going to represent herself in court. As of the writing of this book, the class action lawsuit against her is still ongoing and John Tiedt has vowed to continue fighting this until a judgment has been made against Diaz. It's only a matter of time now.

You'd think all this real-life drama in her life would make Heidi Diaz reflect and take a personal examination of the wrong she has done to others and back away from the Internet dieting business. Nope! Believe it or not, this woman not only has the kahunas to start up another web site venture, but another DIET WEB SITE!!! Oh yes, you're not gonna believe this one. The header of her new diet web site reads "Simple Choices: Weight Loss for Busy Lifestyles" and basically looks like Kimkins reincarnate. You go through a week-long "Detox" and then move on to a "low-glycemic Flash Start" program.

It's a low-carb, low-fat, low-calorie, portion control diet designed to help you "lose weight fast" for only $19.95 a month? Other than the price, which is a huge jump up from the flat rate "lifetime membership" she offered at Kimkins, this sounds a whole lot like another diet Heidi Diaz has put her fingerprints all over, doesn't it? The system sounds way too familiar to me. This has Kimkins written all over it because Heidi had these same things at her other site, too. What you can eat, support forums, diet tools — this is nothing new at all. And, of course, she's offering an affiliate program to entice people to sign up all their friends and blog readers. As someone who was fooled by this woman once before, don't fall for it!

Let this Kimkins example be a lesson that you need to do your own research for detailed information about anything like a diet plan. For so many of these opportunists out there like Heidi Diaz, this is nothing more than a ruthless money-making scheme that has been perpetrated on unsuspecting victims by someone who doesn't seem to care a bit in the world about the weight and health of the people she comes into contact with. Anyone who doubts this should get introspective and take a long, hard look at all that has transpired over the past few years with Kimkins and is still going on to this day. If you do that, then there's no other choice for you but to distance yourself as much as possible from people like her. It is for the best and you'll be so glad you did.

The moral of this story surrounding the Kimkins calamity is simple: be very careful about who and what you choose to associate yourself with. I learned my lesson as have many others who were sucked in by this. What began as merely a raw business deal has now turned into something much worse. It's without a doubt dangerous to the health of those who are on this low-fat/low-carb/low-calorie diet plan.

One of my fellow weight loss bloggers Muata Kamdibe from MrLowBodyFat. com interviewed me in 2008 and he asked me why people continue to support a "big fat fraud" like Kimkins. Here was my response:

I wish I knew why in light of all the evidence showing the Kimkins diet fraud which was created by a morbidly obese 300+ pound woman named Heidi Diaz who has been a well-known opportunist for years is still so attracted to this plan. It is basically a ZERO fat, ZERO carb, and protein-only diet that is causing some really dangerous health complications to happen in the desperate and unsuspecting dieters who try it. The calorie intake of the people following this plan as Diaz, who is neither a doctor nor a nutritionist, wrote it out is around 500 a day. Yikes! This diet is nothing more than a one-way ticket to anorexia and death due to malnutrition. I suppose people are so desperate for weight loss that they'll even try something this drastic to see if it will work for them. It's a sad day in our society when people are more concerned about weight loss than they are about improving their health. The latter is worth so much more to your body long-term which is why I emphasize that fact more and more in all that I do. National television exposure of the fraud as well as an ongoing class action lawsuit against Diaz will eventually come to a head and hopefully bring this diet imposter down for good. For the sake of the tens of thousands of people who got sucked in by this scheme, I can only hope that day will be sooner rather than later.

So let this serve as a warning...there are people just like Heidi Diaz out there right now waiting to pounce on your sincere desires to lose weight and get healthy. Be very cautious and careful about whomever you come across on the Internet to make sure they are legitimate. Here are five practical clues to help you find people you can trust about giving you solid diet advice online:

1. They are willing to share their real names and photos.
2. They do not require you to pay to access their columns.
3. They tend to put themselves out there on YouTube and podcasts.
4. They can be seen in public and confirmed as real people.
5. They aren't hiding behind a cloud of secrecy and deception.

As disappointing as it can be to have one put over on you like I was with the Kimkins diet ordeal, there are also some pretty amazing things that can happen in your life when you least expect it. Following my low-carb weight loss success, I have had the privilege of seeing once-in-a-lifetime experiences happen in my life that never would have happened had it not been for my healthy low-carb lifestyle. That's what I'll be sharing about in the next lesson!

LESSON #18
Sometimes when you least expect it,
amazing things will happen

"As Joseph Campbell said, when you're on the right path, you will receive help when you least expect it. Everyone told me the odds of finding distribution for an independent film made by first-time filmmaker were about a thousand to one. My reply was that if I don't give it a shot, the odds are zero. As Wayne Gretzky said, you miss every shot you don't take. I took the shot, and now I receive emails from people all over the world who've seen my movie Fat Head. A clear goal is like a magnet that attracts the right people, the people you need. Once I fully committed to making Fat Head, it was like the universe decided to play connect the dots. The composer, co-producer, music producer, sound engineer, animator, medical experts...they all just seemed to show up when I needed them "

— **Tom Naughton**, director and star of the low-carb documentary film project *Fat Head* (FatHead-Movie.com)

When average, ordinary people who happen to be carrying around quite a few extra pounds on their body set out to lose weight, I am convinced that most of them (myself included!) have no clue about how much their life will be changed following their weight loss success. Sure, you think about how good you'll look, how much healthier you'll be, and all of the predictable things that come with losing a significant amount of weight like I did in 2004. But the fringe benefits of losing triple digits worth of weight cannot be experienced until you actually do it.

Because of my low-carb weight loss success five years ago, I have had the privilege of appearing on television, radio, and in newspaper stories many times, publishing my first book in October 2005, quitting my job in customer service and working full-time spreading the message of healthy low-carb living since October 2006, launching a successful twice-weekly online radio show podcast that has been among the Top 20 best Nutrition & Fitness shows on iTunes since 2006, and becoming the owner of one of the most successful diet and health blogs on the Internet today read by hundreds of thousands of people each month. All of these have been some of the most outstanding opportunities ever since I started livin' la vida low-carb.

But sometimes, when you least expect it, some really amazing things will happen.

In December 2006, I had the privilege of doing something that some would consider "once in a lifetime." There was an open audition being held about 20 miles away from where I live in Greenville, South Carolina to appear in a Universal Pictures film featuring Academy Award-winning actor George Clooney, along with John Krasinski and Renee Zellweger called *Leatherheads*.

If you haven't seen the movie which came out in theaters in April 2008, it is a period film that takes place in the early days of the birth of football in America in the 1920's. Clooney was the director and star of the film as an aging football player named Jimmy "Dodge" Connelly who attempts to recruit an extremely talented young college football star named Carter Rutherford (portrayed by NBC-TV's "The Office" star Krasinski) to play in the newly-developed professional league to provide an incentive for fans to come out and support the football games. But a female reporter from the Chicago Tribune named Lexie Littleton (played by Zellweger) gets into a love triangle with Carter and Dodge that makes for good on-screen drama and comedy.

Because this was a "football" movie, the producers were looking for Caucasian males 20-35 years old, between 5'9" and 6'3" tall, and weighing 160-250 pounds to fit the prototype of the typical 1920's football players (African-Americans were not yet a major part of professional football at that time). While playing football in high school or college was not required, the applicant was required to be "athletic."

At the time of this audition, I was days away from turning 35, 6'3" tall, 220-something pounds, and played regular competitive volleyball and basketball along with working out at the gym. I felt I was qualified to at least put my name in the pool of applicants to be considered even though I was on the high end with my age and height. Besides, why would I pass up a chance to possibly appear in a Hollywood film?

I had heard about the tryouts for *Leatherheads* earlier in the week on the television news and then again on the local talk radio station. My initial reaction was "what a unique opportunity to be a part of something like this!" So, why not give it a shot? This was a neat chance to be a part of something that not that many people get to do. So I went for it!

The process was supposed to last from 9AM-3PM, but it was obvious when I arrived right at 9AM that this wasn't going to be the quick in-and-out ordeal like I had originally expected. The line of men who were waiting to be a part of this movie wrapped around the inside of the building with at least 750 people and then another 300-400 guys outside the door. And there were people of all shapes and sizes, too. Some were big and bulky, pushing that 250-pound weight limit to the max while others were weak and puny and probably didn't come anywhere close to reaching the required height and weight. But they didn't care because this was their chance to be a star. Or so they had hoped.

While waiting near the back of the line, I had a friendly conversation with a 32-year old financial advisor named Brian who said his wife urged him to come to the audition. He said he wanted to enjoy the experience of trying out to be in a major Hollywood movie and that it didn't really matter if he made it or not. We had plenty of time to talk, too, finally leaving the parking lot at around 11AM with a handful of "souvenirs" — the papers we were given as our reward for coming — three hours after standing outside in the cool breeze of that early winter morning.

Once inside the building and into the audition room, we were handed an instruction sheet and application which asked for your name, contact information, Social Security number, clothes sizes including shoes, and athletic experience. Then you stood in line to hand your application to someone who assigned you a number which was handwritten on a white sheet of paper — mine was #371 — that you then took to a photographer to snap your full-body photo holding your number. Finally, an assistant producer with the film did an on-the-spot informal interview with each applicant asking about their experience playing sports.

All in all, it was quite an adventurous Saturday morning and I was hopeful for a chance to be cast as an extra in *Leatherheads*. However, my lack of football experience in high school or college I thought would likely hamper my chances and disqualify me from being considered. Yet, considering my chances would have been exactly ZERO had I not lost 180 pounds by livin' la vida low-carb in 2004, I considered the tryout a BONUS in my life. That's something pretty amazing if you ask me.

Losing weight gave me what was an unbelievable shot to forever be a part of cinematic history. Okay, perhaps that's a bit hyperbolic, but I think you get the picture. To be in a film with one of this generation's biggest Hollywood actors — George Clooney — would be an honor indeed. The producers said they would choose 50 men to fill the three teams featured in the film and that I would hear back from them via telephone or e-mail by mid-January 2007. Filming would begin in February 2007 in North and South Carolina just a few miles from where I live in Spartanburg, South Carolina.

And so I waited...and waited...and waited...

December came and went as did January. I knew from the get-go it was going to be a very long shot that I would ever step foot on the set of *Leatherheads* since they could only choose 50 men total out of thousands who applied to make up the various football teams in the movie. I held out hope for the best, but was bracing to be rejected. To be honest, I never seriously expected the producers to call me since I didn't play football in high school or college. But you know what, good things can happen to people in the strangest ways sometimes.

When the end of January 2007 arrived with nary a word from anyone about the *Leatherheads* movie, I just assumed the opportunity had passed me by this time and honestly I had forgotten all about it. But, imagine my surprise when my cell phone rang around 5:00pm on the last Tuesday afternoon in February that year from what showed up as a "Private Call." I always wonder if I'm getting a telemarketer when that shows up on my caller ID, but this time I decided to take the call anyway. I'm so glad I did!

On the other end of the line, the very nice lady said, "Hi, I'm from the *Leatherheads* movie and we'd like to know if you are still interested in being an extra in the film?" After picking my jaw up off the floor, I thought to myself "Ummmm, let me think about it...YES, yeppers, yip-yip-yippee!" I think I said, "Yes ma'am, I sure would!" I couldn't believe I actually got the call two days shy of March because they had already started filming a couple of weeks prior. Even still, here was the call I had been waiting for but not really ever expecting. WOW!!!

The very nice lady on the other end of the call said I needed to come by the makeshift office building in Greer, South Carolina on that Thursday morning to get fitted for my costume. I was assuming I'd be outfitted with football gear, but grew suspicious when she asked me to bring some size 13 black-laced shoes to wear. Hmmmmm...

She also asked if I was available on that coming up Sunday for filming and I asked what time. "It will be all day long," she responded. Oh, okay...er, yeah! I'm there, baby! This is the movies, the "chance of a lifetime" that I wouldn't miss for the world. Yee haw! What an extraordinary opportunity to experience something I can tell my grandkids about someday. Although the funky looking football uniforms certainly would take some explaining.

Once I arrived at my costume fitting on that Thursday morning, I quickly realized I would not be appearing in *Leatherheads* as a "football-playing extra" as I suspected. Actually, it turned out they liked my height and broad shoulders, so I would be playing the part of the doorman in front of a hotel in the 1920s. Actually, this was even better because I ended up being the ONLY doorman in the movie which gave me a good shot at being in the final cut.

The filming of the scene where I played the doorman took place on that first Sunday in March 2007 in downtown Greenville, South Carolina. The costume was quite exquisite with three layers involved, including a white shirt, vest, and huge blue-green overcoat that looked very classy if you ask me with a black tie, black shoes, and white gloves. Lookin' sharp! I received instructions to call a special super-secret telephone number on that Saturday night prior to filming so I could find out what time they would need my character for the scene they were shooting.

There were three pages of detailed information explaining what was going to happen. The biggest theme they attempted to communicate was patience and focus on the day of the shoot. And more than anything else, the producers wrote in the instructions, try not to gawk at George Clooney when he walked on the set. I didn't think I'd be close enough to see him anyway, so it wasn't a big deal either way to me.

My appointed time to check in for the hotel scene was at 10:30AM on that Sunday morning. But since they had partitioned off two or three blocks around the area they were filming, I had some difficulty finding a place to park. I ended up parking in a bank parking lot that allows free parking on the weekends.

Sweeeeet! I remember walking briskly towards the hotel not really knowing where to go when I got there.

Cameras, lights, and crew were everywhere and as I get closer I could hear several women screaming, "George, George, look over here!" These were the Clooney groupies that would literally spend hours waiting on the outer edges of the set just to see their favorite movie star for a few brief seconds. It was kind of funny to watch, but that wasn't the end of it. Clooney-mania was in full force throughout the filming of *Leatherheads*.

After trying to figure out where I needed to be, finally I stopped and asked one of the crew members, "Where are the extras supposed to be?" He pointed me in the right direction and I ended up in the holding room to check in. "Are you Jimmy Moore, our doorman?" the beautiful young blonde woman asked. "Yes ma'am, that's me," I replied. She said she had just left me a message on my cell phone which I had turned to vibrate so I wouldn't forget and have it on during one of the scenes. That wouldn't be good in a 1920's period film now, would it?

After filling out some paperwork so I would get paid (can you believe they actually PAY people to do this?!), she told me to go get my costume and get dressed, get my hair styled, and then to makeup. Hoo boy, this was the real deal now! But there was only one problem — where the heck was the costume trailer? I walked around with all these men and women dressed in 1920's garments and I was still dressed in 2007 street clothes.

Finally, I went back to the registration and asked if they could have someone show me where to pick up my costume and one of the crew members took me to where I needed to be. Hallelujah! It turned out I needed to be about 2 blocks over from the hotel, so there's no way I would have ever found that on my own. After getting my costume, I rushed back to the men's dressing room which was filled with a bunch of guys changing out of their 21st century blue jeans and T-shirts and into the kind of clothes worn by the men in the 1920's — semi-formal dress pants with an overcoat and top hat. There were two guys who had a similar costume to me portraying bell hops, but mine was the only doorman costume.

I was able to put all of it on except for the collar and tie. I just couldn't figure it out on my own (and left wishing my wife Christine was with me to help), so I headed to the hairstylist and makeup room. Each line was full of 20-25 extras waiting to get primped and glamorized for the scene we would all be taping just a few hours later. It was all starting to sink in at that point that the time for our Hollywood movie experience was getting closer and the excitement was in the air.

Of course, for many of these extras, this was not their first time in *Leatherheads.* A lot of them said they had been in a previous scene on the football field on Friday and expressed how muddy it was out there since we had a nearly 3-inch downpour on that Thursday prior. They were happy it was sunny and dry for this particular day's shoot.

One of the explicit instructions we were given in our instructions sheet was this: "NO CAMERAS OR VIDEO EQUIPMENT IS ALLOWED. FAILURE TO COMPLY IS GROUNDS FOR REMOVAL FROM SET."

Yikes, I knew I wouldn't be caught dead with a camera then! I was not even going to risk it, so I left my digital camera at home. But imagine my surprise when I saw just about everybody click, click, clicking their cameras in seeming violation of this rule. When I inquired with one of the perpetrators of such blatant malfeasance about it, they told me the crew said they were fine with pictures being taken in the holding area, just not on the set. Gee, thanks a lot, I wish I had known that!

As I was waiting to get my makeup on, a woman asked me if I would come out to speak with her for a moment. It turns out she was a groupie and she was just fascinated that someone from the movie was actually talking to her. If she only knew how irrelevant my character was in the grand scheme of this movie, then she wouldn't have bothered with me. Actually, I convinced her to help me put my collar on and she enthusiastically agreed to help me. I thanked her and said I needed to get back in line for makeup.

That was just a little too weird for me, but it was also a little bit fun, too. People are strange when they get around other people they think are famous. I enjoyed it in a sadistic, self-absorbed kind of way. But this was probably my only chance of ever doing anything like this, so I was soaking it all in moment by moment.

Back to the holding area I went and all the extras waited there for about 30 minutes before one of the assistant directors came in to tell us to line up for wardrobe to fix us up perfectly since the scene we would be in was getting ready to be shot. EXCITING! It was a couple of minutes later as I was waiting in the back of the line that I heard the assistant director say, "Where's Jimmy Moore?" I raised my hand to identify myself and she said, "Come here." She then explained that I needed to move to the front of the line because I was gonna be in the main part of this scene with "George" — as in George Clooney! You're kidding me! Not only was I getting to be a part of this incredible atmosphere, but now I'd probably end up being in the movie in a scene with George Clooney himself. COOL!

After getting tugged on and fitted to make sure all of our costumes looked snazzy, we were led out to the filming site to wait and wait and wait...(did I mention we waited a while?)...for our next instructions. The crew was already in action setting up the cameras and lights for the shoot while the primary director for *Leatherheads* (besides Clooney) David Webb was walking the scene with his fellow assistants. I recall him walking right up to me and saying, "This is what I want you to do" while proceeding to demonstrate my part of the scene telling me to look straight ahead and stoic as George rides up on the motorcycle and then give him an incredulous look. "Can you do that?" he asked. "Yes sir!" I quickly answered.

Then we went through take after take after take rehearsing this 20-30 second scene. Everything was in motion and almost ready to begin shooting with cameras rolling. It was about this time that Clooney appeared on the set and started observing the scene while making his recommendations about how it should go. All the extras started mumbling to themselves that THE star had arrived. I'm not all goo-goo, ga-ga over the man, but I admit it was pretty neat seeing George Clooney in the flesh within eyeshot.

Tick-tock-tick-tock...before I knew it, the time was already 3:00PM and we had been doing this scene over and over for several hours. But it was getting close to Showtime when we'd be shooting the scene with George since he was there now. One of the sound guys came running straight at me as we were waiting and said, "George wants to mike you up for a possible line. Can you handle that?" I confidently replied, "Sure!"

So they hooked me up with a fancy wireless microphone and got me all ready to say something. Are you kidding me?! Not only am I in this movie and in a scene with George Clooney, but now I might have a line in it talking to him too? WOWSERS! This just keeps getting better and better. All I needed was five little words in a speaking role and I would have been given my Hollywood actor's guild card and paid MUCH more money than the typical extras pay.

The first take with Clooney was a bit surreal for me. I looked straight ahead and did my look as instructed by the director, but I was completely enamored by the amazing acting skills that George displayed. His character in *Leatherheads* was quite cocky and you could see that shine through in those few seconds he stood about one foot in front of me for that scene. What's amazing is we shot that scene about ten more times with Clooney before they decided it was as good as it was gonna get.

In my doorman scene, he spoke a line to me (although that line was ultimately cut from the final version of the film). In fact, I was the ONLY extra in that particular scene that he uttered a single word to. Awesome! Here's what he said to my character — "Keep it close, will ya?" I was fascinated by Clooney's acting abilities when on the various retakes he would ad lib an extra word in that line. One time he added, "Captain" on the end as in "Keep it close, will ya, Captain?" Another time, he said "Keep it close, will ya, fella?" I kept wondering if "dude" or "man" was coming next!

Although we weren't supposed to ask for autographs or engage in small talk with the actors, after about the sixth take when the director yelled "cut" I looked over at George Clooney standing a couple of feet away and uttered, "Hey George, I think I've got your line memorized by now." He looked back and smiled with a slight little chuckle as if to say "welcome to the grit work of Hollywood...Captain!"

As for my big speaking debut in a Hollywood movie — uhhhh, well, it never really materialized. Honestly, I think they forgot about it after putting that microphone on me, but that's okay. At least I was pretty sure at the end of taping that day that I'd end up in the movie with my doorman role in this scene. It was a load of fun to be a part of, but tiring. Even still, I think I could handle doing this kind of work every day of my life!

We broke for "lunch" which ended up being around 3:45pm and were fed a delicious spread of gourmet food prepared buffet-styled and yes I got to eat low-carb. I had green and WHITE asparagus (never heard of it before, but it was good!), salad greens, meatloaf, pulled pork, and honeydew for dessert. We weren't sure if we would be needed anymore after our meal, so we all filled up just in case we'd have a few more hours on set.

During the meal, I was able to tell the people at my table about my livin' la vida low-carb experience. They were amazed by my weight loss success story and seemed genuinely interested in what I was saying. Of course, all the while I was talking about ditching sugar from my diet, the other extras were eating chocolate chip cookies and banana splits for dessert. Oh well! Old habits are very hard to break.

It was kind of funny all the people who wondered if I was some professional actor from Hollywood since I got to be in the scene with Clooney and they miked me up for a possible speaking part. You could tell they all wished it was them who had that role of the doorman since the likelihood of their making it into the final cut of *Leatherheads* for more than a split second didn't look good. I responded that I was no different than them and just had the good fortune of being able to fit the doorman costume (like that famous episode of *The Brady Bunch* where Greg got the singing gig because he "fit the suit").

A little more than an hour after we ate lunch, we were beginning to wonder what we would be doing next when the assistant director came in and yelled, "Thank you very much, you can go home now!" WOO HOO! Getting out of my doorman costume was a lot easier and faster than getting into it was and I was so ready to wear blue jeans and tennis shoes again. But I was not complaining...this was a magical and memorable experience that I would not soon forget.

When I went to check out and get my paperwork for getting paid, they asked me if I would be available as an extra for several more dates at the end of the month. Really?! I get to do this again? Yes, please sign me up! I'd be back in a heartbeat and wouldn't miss it for the world. So that's how my first experience in a Hollywood movie went.

A few weeks later, I got another call from the casting office for *Leatherheads* asking me if I would like to do some more extra work. Uh, let me think about it... HOW MANY WAYS CAN YOU SAY YES?! They said filming would begin on that Thursday and last through Saturday if I could make it. You bet your sweet bippy me, myself, and I will all be there. And what a weekend it was!

The scenes were shot in a town about 45 minutes from my house called Travelers Rest, South Carolina and they were all about simulating a football game during the part of the movie where Clooney's team, where he is the quarterback, along with John Krasinski, who portrays the rising star of this new football league, are on their way to the big championship game. That's where some nearly 400 or so extras were strategically placed in certain sections of the stands and given instructions to cheer, react, and make the moviegoer believe we were responding to what was happening on the field even when no action was taking place. Through the magic of CGI and creative editing, they made us look like about 20,000 people in the final version of the movie. Neat stuff!

I don't think people have any idea how much time and energy goes into making a two-hour film happen, but I will tell you it is quite exhausting just being an extra. And I was only on the set for a few days — I can't imagine what it was like to be a member of the crew for the 5AM reporting time to be on set and then working until past 8PM most nights. You think I'm joking, but those are the grueling hours so they can try to squeeze in every last second of work into each day to make the film what it needs to be. But you won't hear me complaining about it, though, because this is Hollywood!

The hourly pay was only $7.00 for extras, but I would have done it for FREE just for a chance to be seen in a film expected to be watched by millions of people worldwide on the silver screen and then when it comes to DVD and cable television. Although my second experience on the set began on a Thursday, they actually began shooting these particular scenes in Travelers Rest on that prior Sunday when the co-star of *Leatherheads* Renee Zellweger was on the set. Oh dang, I hate I missed that and wish I'd been there! I never did get to see her on the set in any of the scenes I was in. Bummer.

The extras that were there on Sunday and then again on Wednesday told me I was lucky I didn't work those days because the heat was so unbearable. We had record-high temperatures in the Upstate of South Carolina with the temperatures reaching in the mid-to-upper 80's in the middle of March. That wouldn't be bad if this was a movie set on a beach or if the costumes were shorts and T-shirts. But they had everyone wrapped up in layers of wool coats, scarves, and top hats like they wore in the 1920's that got just a wee bit toasty under the baking sun.

Wearing a big wool coat, scarf, hat, dress pants, shirt and tie, and dress shoes is definitely not the attire of the 21st century, but that's exactly what the men wore day in and day out back then. So we had to dress the part whether it was 85 degrees outside or 45 degrees. It was like we stepped back in time seeing each other dressed like this and the women were all dolled up with their cute hats and bright makeup. I swear all the women looked exactly alike — gorgeous, of course.

When I arrived on the set that Thursday, there was a significant cooling trend that had come through and kept the highs only in the lower 60's. Ahhhh, much better. Even still, it was very windy, cloudy, and a fine mist of rain was coming down for a while during our filming — perfect football weather! In fact, at one point the rain began coming down hard enough that they sent us all back in-side to eat lunch while they waited for Mother Nature to cooperate. I suppose unpredictable weather is one of those things that filmmakers deal with and can't really control.

We ended up waiting in the extras holding area for about seven hours before a member of the casting crew came in and said, "Okay, you can go home for the day." Yep, that's how it goes. The natives were getting restless from being bored out of our minds doing nothing and we were hoping for more action to come the next day. And we weren't disappointed.

After another 5AM call time, we were on the set by 8AM and got in a lot of filming of various takes, retakes, retakes, and...(did I mention we had some retakes?) before lunch came at 2:00pm. There were several times when the camera passed right in front of where I was sitting, walking, or standing. It's all orchestrated to make the scene look as authentic as possible. Unlike my scene as the doorman where I was all but assured to be seen, these football "fan" scenes were hit or miss whether they'd actually show up in the final cut. We had to wait and see when the movie hit the big screen to find out.

One of the scenes I participated in at the Travelers Rest filming was with Cloo-ney doing the Statue of Liberty play where Krasinski was supposed to come behind him for the handoff. Unfortunately, these are actors and not athletes, so we saw a few fumblerooskis and dropped balls along the way. It was funny because all of the extras in the stands would start booing them. But it was all in good fun and they eventually pulled the scenes off to make them look be-lievable. Clooney threw a pretty good spiral, by the way!

Speaking of the aforementioned Mr. Krasinski, who I admittedly had never heard of before this movie (I don't get the comedy on "The Office"), he was a hoot on the set. We were about 100 feet away from him sitting in the stands, but you could hear him cracking jokes and keeping the football actors, extras, and crew loose on the set. They had him running the length of the field down the sideline for a big play his character makes in the scene and he did the take about 10 times. Instead of hopping on the camera cart, he simply turned around and sprinted back to his starting position. That's impressive for an actor although he did look a bit lanky running down the field. Through the magic of Hollywood, you knew he'd look like a pro in the final cut!

We were graced with a little bit of extra excitement during filming that day when one of the football-playing actors portraying the character of "Big Gus" (you'll know exactly who this is when you see the movie — he'll be hard to miss because of his weight) noticed a member of the paparazzi hiding in the woods ostensibly trying to take photos of Clooney for his newspaper or magazine. When "Big Gus" saw this guy, he suddenly started pointing and yelling to the top of his lungs, "Hey, hey, get out of here. I see you, you've been outed. Now get out of here."

Of course, everyone on the set looked in the direction "Big Gus" was pointing and saw an obviously embarrassed photographer scrambling and stumbling all over himself to get away fast enough. As the guy tripped several times while attempting to leave, all the extras started laughing at him and then cheered "Big Gus" for spotting this creep. A few days earlier, local police had actually snuck up behind another photographer and arrested him, according to the extras who were working that day. The officers found him covered in kudzu attempting to camouflage himself — it didn't work! Are these people that hard up for a photo of Clooney?

During some of our downtime in the extras holding area on Friday, they had a drawing for some *Leatherheads* knick-knacks. My name was pulled out of the jar and I won a banner from the film which is a nice reminder of my experience. But I'll also have many more memories in my head watching Clooney in his role as both actor and director. This man is very good at what he does and showed it quite often during the making of this movie. What an honor it was to be a part of his film.

As we were wrapping up work on the film for the weekend, all the extras got a signed letter from the Extras Casting Director for *Leatherheads* Tona B. Dahlquist thanking us for being a part of the movie. Ummmm, I think WE should be the ones thanking YOU for the opportunity to be a part of something like this — so, THANK YOU! I don't know how people do this for a living with all the hard work that goes into it, but it sure is exciting for those of us who live somewhat "normal" lives by comparison.

But my Hollywood experience wasn't over yet! They asked me after the Travelers Rest filming to travel a couple of hours north to Charlotte, North Carolina for more scenes as a football fan on the following Thursday, April 5, 2007. The wake-up call for the Charlotte scenes I was going to be in was really, really, REALLY early — 2:30am! EEEK! What's really bad is I didn't get to sleep until midnight that night, so I barely got any rest at all before making the drive up I-85. Why was I up so early? Extras were told to report to the check-in between 4-7AM. I wouldn't get home that night until nearly 8PM!

Yep, it was a long day for us, but we had to cram in a full day of filming which turned out to be the opening scene of *Leatherheads* where Krasinski's character Carter Rutherford is playing college football for Princeton against Penn. We moved around all over the stadium doing the same scene over and over again from different angles and in different positions. During filming, we got to see George Clooney and John Krasinski a LOT. In fact, Clooney was dressed in regular clothes for the scenes we shot in Charlotte since he was not on the field portraying his "Dodge" Connolly character that day. Nevertheless, since he was the director of *Leatherheads*, he had to be there to make sure the movie looked exactly like he wanted it to.

Of course, Clooney couldn't have directed *Leatherheads* all by himself, so he got ample help from his 1st Assistant Director David Webb. Man, what a pro this Webb guy was! From the first time I saw him on the set in Greenville, I could tell right away he knew exactly what he was doing and would keep the day flowing right along. He was the one who would say "Action" through that infamous bullhorn. Of course, all of us extras were also accustomed to hearing him say "Cut — back to 1" which meant we would be doing the scene over...AGAIN! But you knew when he said "That's a wrap" that they got the shot they were looking for.

At one point during the Charlotte shoot, Clooney climbed up into the stands smacking his gum and coming within just a few feet of us extras. We weren't supposed to talk to him, but a few extras got in some comments to him anyway. Constantly keeping us loose by giving acting instructions with a bit of his trademark dry humor, you could tell Clooney absolutely loved his role as both director and leading man in *Leatherheads*.

As for Krasinski, this guy was absolutely hilarious! Even still, when the cameras were rolling he was all business and did his job extremely well. Classy guy, too! It'll be interesting to see if he keeps that same good head if he ever becomes a superstar like Clooney someday. There was one memorable moment on set during that Charlotte scene at the beginning of the movie where Krasinski's character runs in the end zone for a touchdown and he is swarmed with people running up cheering for him. A group of guys lifted him up on their shoulders like a hero and he's pointing to the crowd. Anywho, they had to do that scene over about three or four times because the extras were inadvertently pushing John's head into the camera which doesn't make for very good filming. Their new instructions were to "Get excited, but not TOO excited." Hmmmm, how does that work?

As fun as it was being an extra on a Hollywood movie, it is certainly not a job I would necessarily want to try to support a family on — not by a long shot, no matter how thrilling it is to do it. I left the *Leatherheads* set for good after the Charlotte filming and it was indeed a fun ride. They kept filming in North Carolina for about another month afterwards and then it was in production where the fate of the scenes that all of us extras were in fell in the hands of the person with the scissors in the cutting room!

Would I do something like being an extra in a movie again? Heck yeah, in a heartbeat, baby! But I couldn't do this line of work every single day of my life for the money they pay. Give me blogging about the healthy low-carb lifestyle and a "normal" life thank you very much!

After we finally had the opportunity to see the trailer during the Super Bowl in January 2008, the big moment arrived on April 4, 2008 — the day *Leather-heads* premiered in movie theaters across the United States. After anxiously and excitedly waiting for over a year to see if my once-in-a-lifetime experience working on the set of a Hollywood movie actually resulted in face time in the movie, I was thrilled and honored to see that I was indeed in the final cut as the doorman.

Christine and I couldn't wait to visit our local movie theater in Spartanburg, South Carolina just after noon for the first showing of *Leatherheads* to see if my scene as The Doorman opposite Clooney himself ended up in the final version. I was pretty confident that it would since this was the only thing we worked on for an entire Sunday filming about 20-30 seconds worth of a scene. I was looking for it and within 15 or so minutes of watching the flick on the silver screen, there it was!

I'm the big tall guy standing there looking down with a condescending face at Clooney's character coming off of his motorcycle! In all, this scene was about

15-20 seconds long total and I was on screen with Clooney for about 5 seconds. It wasn't much screen time when you think about a two-hour movie, but I felt extremely fortunate to have gotten that much. Many of the hundreds of other extras either got a flash-in-the-pan blip on the screen or nothing at all. I was indeed lucky and appreciated the opportunity to be a part of something so special and memorable.

Now, Christine on the other hand was as giddy as a little schoolgirl when she saw me on the screen and couldn't keep quiet in the sporadically-filled matinee showing. As soon as she realized that was me standing at attention next to George Clooney on that spittin'-and-sputterin' motorcycle in front of the hotel, I thought they were gonna throw her out of the theater for causing such a ruckus. She started whoopin' and hollerin' pointing her finger up at the screen saying, "Oh my God, there you are, oh my God, there you are!" I tried to get her to put her hand down and lower her voice as people were starting to stare at us. She was proud and happy to see her man in a real live movie. What a neat moment I'll always treasure for the rest of my life.

Just a couple of hours after the early showing of *Leatherheads* we enjoyed at our local theater, Christine and I got all dressed up in formal attire and headed down the road a few miles to Greenville, South Carolina where a group of several hundred extras got together for an official premier viewing of the movie to watch and reminisce about our time on the set. It was neat meeting up with many of the extras who I shared hours upon hours of waiting and waiting and waiting with the previous year just so we could make it to this moment of glory. Everyone was grateful this time had come and we even got the royal treatment from the local press, too.

They rolled out the Red Carpet for us and we had local television personality Jack Roper from the CBS-TV affiliate in Greenville/Spartanburg, South Carolina WSPA News channel 7 on hand to announce our names as people gathered along both sides of the carpet cheering for us and taking our pictures as we entered the movie theater. When Jack introduced me and Christine, he said, "Next up we have Jimmy Moore and his friend." Uh, yeah, she's my friend known as my WIFE, Jack! I quickly corrected him to stay out of the doghouse. Okay, now that was weird! But I liked it and ate every bit of it up! How often do you get a chance to do something that this?

As the movie was getting close to the end, I leaned over to Christine and said that we should leave early (since we had already seen the film once that day) to beat the crowd over to the BMW Zentrum where the extras after-party would be taking place. She agreed and we headed out the door. Three seconds after walking out of the front door of the theater we heard a loud explosion as a bright light filled the stormy sky — a transformer had blown from the major thunderstorm that was moving through the area and the entire block immediately went black. Boy, what great timing! It turns out the movie had just ended and the closing credits were showing, so nobody missed any of the movie itself.

At the earlier showing, we stayed all the way through the ending credits to see if my name would be there as "The Doorman." It wasn't. I guess they only put your name in there if you had a speaking part and I did not have one — although it was very close to happening. Interestingly, even if I did end up having that speaking role in the scene I was in, it looks like it would have been cut. They chopped off the last 5 seconds of that scene where the line was scheduled to happen and went right to the next scene where Clooney's character clashes with Zellweger's character inside the hotel. Oh well!

All in all, this romantic comedy set in the 1920s about the birth of professional football is a fun movie to watch (although it didn't do very well commercially at the box office) and I was humbled to be able to play even a teeny tiny little role in it. I've had people in my church and blog readers tell me they recognized my doorman character in the film. And it was odd seeing it playing on HBO in the summer 2009 over and over again — yet another reminder of the good things that can happen to you when you least expect it. I'm thankful for the memories that I have from this experience and if given another chance to be an extra in a Hollywood film, I'm there!

At the after-party, I was interviewed by a reporter from *The Greenville News* and they quoted me first in their story. It was an unbelievable experience that will give me something to talk about besides livin' la vida low-carb for the rest of my life. If you haven't seen *Leatherheads* yet, then do yourself a favor and GO SEE IT! It's a cute film that just about everyone will love and enjoy. And about 15 minutes into the movie, you'll get to see someone you actually know.

See, sometimes when you least expect it, amazing things will happen! Switching gears back to low-carb again in the next lesson, we'll take on many of the negative studies about low-carb and explain why this kind of sloppy research is misleading people about the incredible health benefits of carbohydrate restriction.

LESSON #19
You can't always trust or believe the negative studies on low-carb

"It is unfortunate that sensationalist headlines replace the positive results of carefully controlled objective research results for very low-carbohydrate diets. In research there are numerous studies that provide reasons why low-carbohydrate diets are linked to poor weight maintenance and negative health consequences; none of these negative results are based on objective carefully controlled data and all too often they are skewed by various limitations and other factors that affect the outcome of the study. A low-carbohydrate diet can be safe and effective and it is a healthy way to eat for a lifetime."

— **Valerie Berkowitz**, MS, RD, CDN, CDE, co-author of *The Stubborn Fat Fix*, blogger at "Valerie's Voice: For the Health of It" (ValerieBerkowitz. wordpress.com)

You've seen me highlight lots and lots of studies supporting the idea of carbohydrate restriction for weight loss and health in this book. But I know what you're thinking — what about all the research that contends high-carb diets are good for you and that low-carb is just a bunch of hooey? What do you say to that Mr. Livin' La Vida Low-Carb Man? You know, I'm glad you asked because that's precisely what I want to share about in this chapter because you can't always trust or believe the negative studies that come out about low-carb. Let's take a look at a few of the most prominent ones to come out over the past few years.

Eating Sugar Is Good For Mental Health?

A so-called scientific research study presented at the annual meeting of the Society for Neuroscience in Washington, D.C. in November 2005 claimed that lab rats that were fed sugar water twice a day became less agitated and reduced stress levels when put in a stressful situation than the control group of lab rats that were not fed the sugar water.

Lead researcher Yvonne Ulrich-Lai, psychiatry fellow from the University of Cincinnati, took blood samples from the rats and found the stress hormone glucocorticoids were lower in the hypothalamus region of the brain where stress originates than the control group that was fed either saccharin water or just plain water.

"We actually found that sugar snacks, not artificially sweetened snacks, are better self-medications for the two most common types of stress—psychological and physical," Ulrich-Lai explained.

Excessive presence of glucocorticoids weakens the immune system and causes fat to store in the abdomen, the researchers added. They concluded that people who consume sugar to deal with stress are actually helping themselves deal with it in a positive manner.

"I think this research is giving us insight into something that many people may be doing already without realizing it," Ulrich-Lai says. "A lot of people when they are stressed will say that they like to eat food that tastes good."

Comfort foods like cookies, cakes, pies, candy bars, chocolate, sugar, sugar, and more sugar — where will it stop? When do you draw the line between what is good and healthy for your body versus the innate desire to be mentally happy?

The study notes that increased sugar consumption causes weight gain, but that the rats were able to self-monitor their calories enough to lower their intake sufficiently to keep their weight under control. Well good for the rats, but what about humans? How many of us have the gumption or know-how to "balance out" our caloric intake when we consume more sugar? Sounds complicated if you ask me and not something that many will be able to easily implement in their lives.

When I started livin' la vida low-carb on January 1, 2004, I gave up eating sugar in large quantities for good. It was very hard at first to overcome my sugar addiction as I detailed in my first book, but it has been the best thing I could have ever done to help myself lose weight and improve my physical and mental health. Just the thought of eating sugar today is repulsive. With my blood sugar under control, my emotions and mental health are excellent and I don't need sugar to de-stress me.

But I have a sure-fire way to help people lower their stress and increase their energy. It's called EXERCISE!!! Just 30 minutes at the gym or playing your favorite sport a few times a week will do wonders for your body and release all the natural endorphins that make your body relax and tingle (in a good way!) all over. Leave the granular white stuff alone and try the basketball court or swimming pool instead.

Ulrich-Lai admits that fruits and vegetables, many of which are acceptable on a healthy low-carb lifestyle, may have the same effect on the brain in reducing glucocorticoids as sugar.

"I think the key is eating something you enjoy eating," Ulrich-Lai concludes.

I do. They're called low-carb foods and I wouldn't trade them for all the sugar in the world! Give up sugar for good because it is poison for your body. You don't need it and you will survive. Again, I'm living proof of that!

The lead investigator of this particular study named Dr. James P. Herman contacted me in an regarding my comments on his research regarding the relationship between sugar and its effect on stress levels:

I am writing in response to your blog concerning the press reports on our work on sugar and stress. I am the principal investigator on the project. I want to note that, as is often the case, the press reports missed the point of our study. Our work indicates that eating sweets may be a form of 'self-medication' against stress; we feel that this is a physiologically maladaptive response to stress that is a likely contributor to our current 'obesity epidemic'.

Our next step is to understand how food reward blocks stress, and evaluate alternatives to food as stress preventatives. Indeed, you are right on about exercise; there is some evidence to suggest that exercise has similar stress-reducing effects in similar animal models.

In no way do we advocate carbs, sweets, etc. as a therapy for stress. I hope this clarifies the issue you raised.

Sincerely,
James P. Herman, PhD

Absolutely it clarifies the issue, Dr. Herman. THANK YOU for writing and I apologize if my concerns about your study reflected poorly on your organization in any way. I have a major problem with the way the media twists solid and clear research into the story they want to tell. It's a shame to see your outstanding work warped by them like that and I for one will not stop shining the light on it when I see it happening. Again, thanks for making your work available to the public and for working on ways to reduce stress and obesity in America.

You know, I've noticed a trend since I started blogging about livin' la vida low-carb in April 2005. While there are negative articles against the Atkins diet and other low-carb programs here and there throughout the year, it seems the media and the current health experts like to orchestrate a huge negative splash against low-carb every six months in an attempt to discredit this wonderfully healthy and effective way of eating.

In August 2005 after the Atkins Nutritionals bankruptcy announcement, the press had a field day firing away at low-carb with every barrel they could find to lock, load, and unleash. They declared it was the end of low-carb and urged readers to just move on. There was just one problem: People were still losing weight and getting healthy on low-carb!

Then six months later in March 2006, the media were at it once again with all-too-eager health "experts" to provide them with a quote or two expressing their great concern over the safety of the Atkins diet. This time around it was about a case study of one person who went on the Atkins diet and allegedly experienced health complications. This "study" got tons of press, but as you will see it was much ado about nothing.

Atkins Diet Case Study "Proves" Low-Carb Isn't Safe?

Dr. Klaus-Dieter Lessnau, a clinical assistant professor of medicine at New York University Medical School points to one case study of a 40-year-old obese woman who allegedly experienced health complications in 2004 during her experience on the Atkins diet.

Of the millions upon millions of people who have gone on a low-carb diet at some point in their life, they found one person who had trouble with it. It comes out to about 0.000000000000000000001 percent of the entire pool of people who have ever been on a low-carb diet! So why in the world were there huge headlines claiming "Atkins Diet Safety Questioned," "Atkins Diet Not Safe," "Low-Carb Unhealthy," and much more all over one person claiming it caused her trouble? Am I the only one who finds this just a wee bit suspicious?

Now, I'm not so naive to think there aren't other cases of people who may have experienced similar health problems while being on the Atkins diet (although it is unclear even in this case study whether the low-carb diet is what caused the problems or not). But to make a blanket statement about everyone who is on the low-carb lifestyle based on this one case study is preposterous.

Using that logic, I suppose we can say that all journalists are guilty of plagiarism and just make up the news. What do I base this on? Well if you use former *New York Times* journalist Jayson Blair as your case study, there's no other conclusion to draw. Since Blair was found to be deceitful and manipulative with the facts in his newspaper stories, then I suppose every single reporter in the entire world must be the same way, right?

What's the difference between what I just did to journalists and what these journalists criticizing the Atkins diet are doing with low-carb? The answer is nothing! And therein lies the problem that people like me and other low-carb supporters have with the irresponsible journalism in reporting about livin' la vida low-carb.

This research from Lessnau appeared in the March 18, 2006 issue of the medical journal *The Lancet*.

According to Dr. Lessnau, this patient he studied had ketones build up in her blood as is commonplace when you restrict your carbohydrate intake. The process of ketosis, which causes the body to emit ketone bodies, is what makes the body burn fat and help people lose weight on a low-carb diet. Apparently for this patient, though, she experienced something not even remotely the same as ketosis called ketoacidosis and was hospitalized for it because it caused her to have breathing problems. This condition is serious, but entirely treatable.

Concluding that this problem is much more commonplace that people think, Dr. Lessnau said it must be "not well-diagnosed or may be underreported."

"The Atkins diet is not a safe diet in everybody," Dr. Lessnau said. "It can cause potentially life-threatening problems."

With all due respect, Dr. Lessnau, the Atkins diet is completely safe for the majority of people who try it. Nobody with any sensibility about them will deny this very clear fact. I will grant you leverage that there are some people who may not do well on the Atkins diet for a variety of reasons, but that doesn't mean we should throw the baby out with the bath water and discourage everyone to avoid low-carb! Most people respond very well to low-carb by losing a whole lot of weight and restoring their health.

Had it not been for the low-carb lifestyle, I would probably be a dead man today lying in an extra extra extra extra extra large casket six feet beneath the ground! Just a few short years ago I was walking around as a 410-pound ticking time bomb just waiting to explode. I had tried and failed on diet after diet, but that Atkins diet you are claiming can cause potentially life-threatening problems saved my life. Today, I'm healthier than I've ever been in my entire life and I wouldn't think of any other way to eat than low-carb.

Unfortunately, a lot of people are listening to these scare tactics from researchers and thinking they need to move on to another weight loss plan instead of low-carb. All I can say is don't let fear-mongering cause you to wander around in the diet wilderness indefinitely for years on end trying to find a way to get your weight problem under control when the answer is sitting there right under your nose just waiting for you to try it. Low-carb works and I'm living proof.

Dr. Lessnau had some of his health colleagues join him in this anti-Atkins bash party, too. Temple University's Gary D. Foster said any weight loss program should be slow and methodical under a doctor's care.

"Losing weight quickly brings its own set of problems," he said. "We have known for a long time that losing weight quickly is a bad idea medically."

Is 180 pounds in one year considered "quickly?" Perhaps, but it was necessary for my dire situation.

University of Minnesota assistant professor Dr. Lyn Steffen had a few more choice words for livin' la vida low-carb.

Low-carb is *"not a diet for life,"* Dr. Steffen asserted.

Dr. Steffen is of the opinion that any diet that people choose to lose weight should be "sensible" and "healthy" as part of an active lifestyle. I agree, which is why I chose the low-carb life.

"My recommendation is to develop healthy eating habits for life," Steffen said. "The low-carbohydrate diet is not a diet for life."

I have personally been eating this way for over five years and my health has never been better. I know people who have been low-carbing for over a decade and yet their health is as strong as ever. In fact, one senior citizen friend I know who lost well over 100 pounds on low-carb quite a few years back was recently told by his doctor that he's got the heart of a young person. Does he just have good genetics or could the Atkins diet have something to do with that?

Dr. Steffen wasn't the only one hurling stones at the Atkins diet, though. Check out the comments from Yale Medical School professor Dr. David L. Katz, who wrote *The Flavor Point Diet*.

"The Atkins diet is at odds with a strong foundation of knowledge about the fundamentals of healthful eating and sustainable weight loss," Dr. Katz asserts. "But the burden of proof has always been the other way around: diets at odds with conventional dietary wisdom must prove themselves healthful. In my opinion, the Atkins diet never did, and never will, meet this test."

I am living proof. My photos show it, my medical history shows it. As a morbidly obese man I dealt with high cholesterol, high blood pressure, and serious breathing problems. Now I don't worry about any of those conditions as a result of being on a low-carb diet.

What we have here is a red herring. These self-proclaimed health "experts" along with their willing accomplices in the media want you to think low-carb diets such as Atkins are unhealthy so the focus can be taken away from the legitimate failure of the low-fat diet as evidenced by strong published research which I've highlighted earlier in this book. People are wising up and educating themselves about all the alternatives that are available to them.

If you are one of those seekers, then let me welcome you to the best thing you could ever do to improve your health. Putting up with negative headlines and information about livin' la vida low-carb is something us low-carbers have grown accustomed to. We don't let those things get us down because we have seen the success for ourselves. Let the naysayers do and say what they want, but they will never convince me that the low-carb lifestyle is anything but the healthy, delicious and nutritious approach to losing weight, keeping it off forever, and making me a vibrant and athletic man. That's what makes me proud to say I support the Atkins/low-carb diet 100%!

You know what's funny is Dr. Lessnau can't possibly expect us to believe all this hoopla he stirred up in the media was over just ONE patient? Can you imagine what would have happened in the media if he had, say, 100 patients who had problems while following the Atkins diet? THEN, he might have had a leg to stand on. Instead, he's just another "expert" trying to gang up on the Atkins diet!

I contacted Dr. Lessnau regarding my concerns about his study and I actually heard back from him with his comments on my criticisms of his research. He posted his comments at my blog and claimed that he stands by his study's conclusion that his patient got sick after meticulously adhering to the Atkins' diet.

What does that mean? Did the patient read *Dr. Atkins New Diet Revolution* and follow it exactly as prescribed? Or did she merely cut back on her carbs and only eat steak, bacon and eggs all day as the media would have us believe represents the Atkins di°et? I think it is extremely important to distinguish between the two. Urging me to shell out the big bucks to read his ridiculous case study report in its entirety at *The Lancet*, Dr. Lessnau said his patient was forced to be admitted into intensive care because of the Atkins diet.

"Generally speaking, you do not want to start a diet and end up in the intensive care unit," Dr. Lessnau exclaimed.

Who's to say it was the Atkins diet that caused your patient to end up in ICU, Dr. Lessnau?

Dr. Lessnau said he is now looking for "any alternative explanation of this severe metabolic acidosis" that his patient had to deal with.

"I would be happy to know if there is any other cause that could explain such a severe disease," Dr. Lessnau inquired. "We could not explain it by any other disease."

I'm uncertain why this woman's disease has been attributed to the Atkins diet, but it appears that this singular account has convinced Dr. Lessnau that this is often what happens with people who try low-carb. Why not ask more of us about our low-carb diet and results? I'd be happy to share mine.

"Please let me know if you have a better idea how to explain this severe metabolic acidosis," Dr. Lessnau pleaded.

There were plenty of researchers and physicians who stepped up and offered reasons why this could happen and none of them came to the same conclusion that it was because of the Atkins diet. But I had an assignment for Dr. Lessnau, too. Since he claimed this problem was so prevalent, I asked him to find me 100 more cases of people who by following the Atkins diet were hospitalized for "severe metabolic acidosis." Since he made the assumption that this is such a widespread problem, I wanted some hard evidence. If the prevalence of this condition was so normal then I didn't think he would have any problem getting those examples to me rather quickly.

But he couldn't find even one more case at all which all but proved to me his theory was badly mistaken.

The great low-carb researcher from the University of California-Davis Dr. Stephen Phinney weighed in at my blog about this with his explanation of what happened to Dr. Lessnau's patient.

For starters, I applaud Dr. Lessnau for bringing this interesting case up for discussion. That said, however, Dr. Lessnau seems a bit too eager to blame carbohydrate restriction for his patient's metabolic acidosis. With apologies for my rather formal style, here's why I think he shot from the hip.

In the Lancet case report, Chen and Lessnau (see ref 1 below) suggest that a carbohydrate-restricted diet can induce ketoacidosis in a non-diabetic patient, but the data presented do not support this conclusion.

First: the reported anion gap of 26 represents a 12 mM anion excess above the upper limit of normal. The serum beta-hydroxybutyrate (the dominant circulating ketone moiety in humans), reported at 390 ug/mL, translates to a concentration of 3.7 mM. That is, the ketones in this case (both beta-hydroxybutyrate and acetoacetate) account for only about a third of the apparent anion excess. Thus the ketonemia in this case represents only a minor fraction of the anion excess, and thus is not the primary factor in the reported metabolic acidosis.

Second: the normal physiologic state of nutritional ketosis, also called starvation ketosis, is associated with serum ketones in the 1-5 mM range (as in this case), and this is not normally associated with metabolic acidosis (see refs 2,3,4). So given that nutritional ketosis does not cause acidosis despite up to 5 millimolar ketones, how is it credible to blame 4 millimoles of ketones for a 12 millimolar of excess anions in this case?

Third: in their case report, Dr. Lessnau states that they provided the patient with dextrose at the rate of only 38 g/d (5% dextrose at 30 ml/hr). This is not enough carbohydrate to reverse nutritional ketosis, and yet the patient improved. If the ketogenic state was the cause of her problem, why did it improve on a homeopathic dose of glucose?

Fourth: Yes, a barcarbonate of 8 and an anion gap of 26 are worrisome, and any ER doc would admit this patient for evaluation and rehydration. However most of us would save the term "severe acidosis" for anion gaps greater than 30 and blood pH values under 7.1. Calling an arterial blood pH of 7.19 "severe acidosis" is a bit of hyperbole.

Fifth: patients with pancreatitis can have an elevate lipase but normal serum amylase (see ref 5). Given her elevated lipase, white blood cell count of 13×10. ninth, and gastrointestinal symptoms, why was this not just a case of mild pancreatitis? We all know that CT scans of the abdomen in someone with a BMI of 41 are notoriously difficult to interpret for soft-tissue injury.

Sixth: I agree with questioning the frequency of events such as this case during low-carbohydrate dieting. As an academic physician with 30 years of experience in adult weight management, I have not seen a similar case in over

3000 patients followed closely during a very low calorie ketogenic diet. Given this experience, I think that it is likely that the current case represents as-sociation without causality. Not having this experience, it is unfortunate that Dr. Lessnau chose to conclude causality rather than raising it as a hypothesis.

Stephen D. Phinney, MD, PhD
Professor emeritus, UC Davis
Elk Grove, CA, USA

References
1. Chen TY, Smith W, Rosenstock JL, Lessnau KD. A life-threatening compli-cation of Atkins diet. The Lancet 2006;367:958.
2. Cahill GF. Starvation in man. N Engl J Med 1970; 282:668-675.
3. Phinney SD, Horton ES, Sims EAH, Hanson JS, Danforth E, LaGrange BM. Capacity of moderate exercise in obese subjects after adaptation to a hypoca-loric, ketogenic diet. J Clin Invest. 1980;66:1152-1161.
4. Phinney SD, Bistrian BR, Wolfe RR, Blackburn GL. The human metabolic response to chronic ketosis without caloric restriction: physical and biochemi-cal adaptation. Metabolism 1983; 32:757—768.
5. Sharma P, Lim S, James D, Orchard RT, Horne M, Seymour CA. Pancrea-titis may occur with a normal amylase concentration in hypertriglyceridaemia BMJ 1996;313:1265.

One high-saturated fat meal will clog your arteries, damage heart

Another very small study funded by Pfizer, maker of the statin drug Lipitor, a top-selling cholesterol lowering medicine came out in August 2006 where lead researcher Dr. Stephen Nicholls, a cardiologist and Associate Director of the Intravascular Ultrasound Core Laboratory at the Cleveland Clinic, along with his colleagues at The Heart Research Institute in Sydney, Australia, observed 14 men between the ages of 18 and 40 (average age: 29.5) who ate two meals exactly one month apart consisting of a piece of carrot cake and a milkshake.

The two meals had one primary difference between them — the kind of fat used in them. The first meal consisted of coconut oil which is high in saturated fat while the second meal used safflower oil which is high in polyunsaturated fat. Dr. Nicholls conducted his study under the archaic assumption that satu-rated fat leads to the buildup of fat in the arteries causing them to get clogged and lead to heart attacks and strokes. Newer research in recent years has proven these long-held beliefs are inaccurate, but medical researchers and doctors still adhere to these older beliefs.

Three hours after the saturated fat meal was consumed, Dr. Nicholls said he looked at the lining of the arteries and noticed they were unable to expand to increase blood flow in those study participants. After six hours, he said the anti-inflammatory qualities of the HDL cholesterol were actually reduced. On the other hand, the polyunsaturated meal resulted in improvements in the anti-inflammatory qualities with less visible inflammatory markers present in the arteries following the meal than before the meal.

This study appeared in the August 15, 2006 issue of *Journal of the American College of Cardiology.*

I'm certain supporters of low-fat diets loved this study but unfortunately this research was so narrowly-focused and contradictory of previous research on saturated fat that it was all for naught. In fact, another study of healthy and successful individuals on weight loss who had lost at least 30 pounds and kept it off for over one year found that their consumption of saturated fat rose from 12.3g daily to 154.0g daily, an unbelievable increase of 1,250 percent!!!

As shocking as it may sound to people like Dr. Nicholls and the countless others in the medical profession like him who promote low-fat as the dietary answer to every ailment, the truth of the matter is that saturated fat can be good for you!

The head of preventative cardiology from the New Orleans, LA-based Ochsner Clinic Foundation Dr. Richard Milani was quoted in response to this study as being impressed by it because it is so "simple" and "very straightforward."

"Given a choice between something with polyunsaturated fat and saturated fat, please avoid the saturated fat," Dr. Milani said.

When I asked Anthony Colpo, author of a fabulous book entitled *The Great Cholesterol Con*, to respond to Dr. Milani's comment about avoiding saturated fat, here is what he said.

"My advice would be to avoid this man's highly misguided advice like a putrid smell," Colpo stated. "The researchers allegedly showed negative

arterial changes and increases in inflammatory agents from ONE SINGLE meal...Whoopee!!" Colpo exclaimed.

Citing previous randomized, controlled clinical trials showing people on high polyunsaturated diets for the long-term actually show higher levels of inflammatory agents and free radical activity than those on high-saturated diets, Colpo said there is no evidence that reducing saturated fat intake actually leads to improved cardiovascular or overall mortality rates.

"In fact, a number of these trials observed worse outcomes in the high-polyunsaturate group," Colpo noted.

That's the problem with studies like this, not enough research over the long-term. Fourteen people were in this study and everyone is excited about how much this proves saturated fat is bad.

Despite how small his study was, Dr. Nicholls said he was proud of the results of his study and boldly proclaimed it has a great "take-home, public-health message."

"It's further evidence to support the need to aggressively reduce the amount of saturated fat consumed in the diet," he concluded.

It truly does not suggest this. Perhaps the cake and shake meal may have had too many carbohydrates and sugar in it to do a person any good. Saturated fat is not the great nutritional enemy that you want people to believe it is, Dr. Nicholls. The body needs the fat that comes from consuming grass-fed and organic sources of beef, pork, lard, poultry fat, butter, cheeses, coconut oil, and cocoa butter, among other foods. Plus, these generaly taste so much better than those fake soy and vegetable oil versions that are actually bad for your health.

Colpo was so fired up about this so-called study that he wrote an entire column in response to it that was too good not to share in this book:

"One High-Saturated Fat Meal Harms Your Arteries? Rubbish!"
by Anthony Colpo

For over five decades, the health and medical establishment has been telling us that saturated fat and cholesterol cause heart disease. My recently published book, The Great Cholesterol Con, explains clearly and concisely why this theory is utter rubbish. For most laymen, that sounds like an outrageous claim, but I readily challenge ANYONE to refute the arguments I have presented in my book.

The medical orthodoxy has successfully perpetuated the highly lucrative lipid hypothesis simply by ignoring contradictory evidence and promoting the living daylights out of 'supportive' evidence (health authorities also have no qualms about taking unsupportive evidence and 'reinterpreting" it so that it appears supportive—my book gives numerous examples of this very phenomenon).

A textbook perfect example of the establishment practice of ignoring contradictory evidence but relentlessly hyping 'supportive' evidence occurred this last week, with the publication of a study comparing the effects of a single high-saturated fat meal with a single high-polyunsaturated fat meal. According to the study, the saturated fat-enriched meal produced harmful increases in inflammatory factors and negative changes in arterial function. Headlines in the ever-compliant media immediately trumpeted the study as further proof that saturated fat was public health enemy number one. In robot-like fashion, media outlets all around the world mindlessly parroted the Associated Press headline "One High-Saturated Fat Meal Can Be Bad."

The study that caused all the kerfuffle was performed in Sydney, Australia. On two occasions one month apart, fourteen healthy subjects consumed a high-fat meal comprising a slice of carrot cake and a milkshake. The fat source in one of these meals was safflower, while the other contained highly saturated coconut oil. The researchers collected blood samples from the subjects before the meals, and 3 and 6 hours after. They extracted HDL from these samples, placed it into a solution containing human umbilical vein endothelial cells, and then observed the effect of the HDL on the endothelial cells expression of intercellular adhesion molecule-1 (ICAM-1) and vascular cell adhesion molecule-1 (VCAM-1). For those of you not familiar with scientific gobbledegook, adhesion molecules adhesion molecules play vital roles in numerous cellular processes. They are believed to play an important role in the atherosclerotic process by facilitating the components of atherosclerotic plaque to proliferate at the site/s of arterial damage.

So let's be clear: The researchers were not observing actual plaque formation in human arteries; this objective would be impossible in such a study. They were instead observing the effects of HDL extracted from humans after eating the test meals on the amount of ICAM-1 and VCAM-1 expressed by umbilical vein endothelial cells in a petri dish.

The other reported outcome was forearm blood flow. To listen to the mainstream media reports, one gets the impression that the subjects' arteries were struggling to cope with blood flow after eating the saturate-enriched meal. A look at the data helps put the results into better perspective. Both meals caused decreases in arterial flow mediated dilation by a "whopping" — wait for it — 0.9 and 2.2% in the polyunsaturated and saturated groups respectively. With these piddling changes, we're not exactly talking life-threatening arterial spasm! Furthermore, looking at the data, one sees that the baseline flow mediated dilation was higher when the subjects ate the highly saturated test meal; was the greater reduction in FMD due to saturated fat, or simply a reversion-to-the-mean effect? Who knows, and who cares, because the difference was not even statistically significant! To quote the researchers themselves:

"Flow-mediated dilation (FMD) decreased at 3 h following consumption of the saturated meal (p _0.05 compared with pre-meal) but not 3 h after the polyunsaturated meal (p _ NS compared with the fasting state), although the difference in post-prandial change in FMD between the meals just failed to meet the conventional criteria for statistical significance. The FMD at 6 h after both meals did not significantly differ compared with the fasted state..., There was no significant change in the vessel size, estimated flow within the brachial artery, and glyceryl trinitrate response following both meals."

Please note the section I have highlighted: "the difference in post-prandial change in FMD between the meals just failed to meet the conventional criteria for statistical significance."

Translation: "As much as we really want to dump on saturated fat, the differences were not statistically significant, damn it!"

And what about the changes in ICAM-1 and V-CAM-1? Both ICAM-1 and V-CAM-1 were higher at 6 hours after consumption of the saturate-rich meal, but lower after consumption of the polyunsaturated-rich meal. It's anyone's guess as to the long-term relevance of acute reactions observed in a petri dish to plaque formation in human arteries. To claim that these reactions demonstrate that saturated fat is indeed atherosclerotic is to make a massive leap of faith. But that's just what the researchers and many of their peers did.

Stephen Nicholls, the head researcher, had no qualms about making the great leap when he stated: "the take-home, public-health message is this: It's further evidence to support the need to aggressively reduce the amount of saturated fat consumed in the diet." According to Dr. James O'Keefe, a cardiologist at the Mid America Heart Institute in Kansas City, the study showed "a really important concept - when you eat the wrong types of food, inflammation and damage to the vessels happens immediately afterward." Also jumping with unbridled anti-saturate abandon was Dr. Richard Milani, head of preventive cardiology at Ochsner Clinic Foundation in New Orleans, who advised: "...given a choice between something with polyunsaturated fat and saturated fat, please avoid the saturated fat."

Let's now find out why you should avoid Milani's advice like a putrid smell. When I ride my bike up a steep hill, or perform a weight training session, my blood pressure temporarily rises to very high levels. In fact, when high-intensity exercises like squats or deadlifts are performed with heavy weights, blood pressure often rises to astronomical levels. Does that mean I should stop lifting weights or riding my bike? If we applied the mentality of the researchers conducting the single-meal study, the answer would be yes. But if we use common-sense and reason, the answer is a resounding "NO!"

Why?

Because the increases in blood pressure evident during physical exertion are not permanent, but transient. When I'm out of the gym or off my bike, my blood pressure is a perfectly healthy 110/70, which is actually lower than average. All that riding and pumping iron is actually stimulating my heart and arteries to become more efficient! The short-term blood pressure elevations I experience whilst exercising in no way reflect the long-term decrease in blood pressure that I have enjoyed.

The take home message is that it is the long term effects of diet and exercise that matter. Atherosclerotic heart disease is a process that takes many years to develop, which is why the majority of heart attacks occur in those over 65 years of age. Heart disease is not caused or prevented by a single meal.

So if it's the long-term effects of diet or exercise that matter, then that is exactly what should be tested. This may sound like commonsense to many of you, but commonsense is a quality sadly lacking among a large proportion of those conducting research and dispensing health advice today.

There have been numerous randomized controlled CHD prevention trials conducted since the 1960s, in which people have been given either high-polyunsaturate diets or high-saturate diets as the sole intervention. In these trials, extending up to eight years, no cardiovascular or overall mortality advantage has ever been observed that can be attributed to saturated fat restriction. In fact, a number of these trials observed poorer mortality outcomes in the high-polyunsaturate group (these trials are all discussed at length in The Great Cholesterol Con).

Healthy subjects placed on high polyunsaturated diets for 4 week periods have exhibited higher levels of free radical activity and blood clotting markers than those on high-saturated diets. In animal studies, polyunsaturated vegetable oils consistently promote cancer growth; an eight-year trial with real live humans that observed significantly higher cancer incidence in the polyunsaturated group suggests this phenomenon is not merely confined to lab rats. This same study, by the way, showed little difference in extent of atherosclerosis among autopsied subjects from the high-saturate and high-polyunsaturate diets. If anything, the aortas of those eating the polyunsaturated-enhanced diet tended to show more plaque build-up.

So when clueless health 'experts' tell you to opt for polyunsaturated fat instead of saturated fat, ignore the living daylights out of them. Doing so could well save your life. The study discussed in this article was supported by a Pfizer Cardiovascular Lipid award. Pfizer makes over ten billion dollars per year from sales of Lipitor, the world's best-selling cholesterol-lowering drug.

Dr. Nicholls is supported by a postgraduate research scholarship from the National Heart Foundation of Australia. Co-author Dr. Rye is a National Heart Foundation of Australia Principal Research Fellow. The National Heart Foundation of Australia operates a program in which it charges a fee so that food manufacturers can display the "Heart Foundation Tick". Polyunsaturated vegetable oils and margarines contribute a significant portion of certified products.

Another co-author of the study, Dr. Lundman is supported by postdoctoral scholarships from the Swedish Heart and Lung Foundation, which counts among its sponsors Unilever, the food giant that manufactures numerous vegetable oil and margarine products.

References
Milicia J. One High-Saturated Fat Meal Can Be Bad. Associated Press, Monday, August 7, 2006.
Nicholls SJ, et al. Consumption of saturated fat impairs the anti-inflammatory properties of high-density lipoproteins and endothelial function. Journal of the American College of Cardiology, 2006; 48: 715—720.
Dayton S, et al. A controlled clinical trial of a diet high in unsaturated fat in preventing complications of atherosclerosis. Circulation, 1969; XL: II-1-63.

You gotta love the way Colpo explains things and he blew that saturated fat study completely out of the water! But there are always more studies waiting in the shadows attempting to put livin' la vida low-carb in a bad light.

Three-day study of 15 people claims Atkins is unhealthy

Lead researcher Dr. Chin Moi Chow, senior lecturer in the School of Exercise and Sport Science of The University of Sydney in Australia, claimed that after she observed 15 people on the Atkins diet over a THREE-DAY period she noticed that the study participants experienced more mood swings, fatigue and even extreme dreams allegedly as a result of being on a low-carb diet. Dr. Chow said more of the Atkins dieters were able to sleep deeply (18 percent) than the control group on a normal diet (14 percent) because the higher fat intake supposedly stimulated the release of a hormone called cholecystokinin that made them tired. But she was quick to point out the trade-off for this deep sleep included vivid dreams and frequent waking up in the middle of the night as the body "struggled to break down hard-to-digest foods," apparently referring to the additional fat and/or protein consumed by low-carb dieters.

While only 20 percent of the study participants on a normal diet remembered their dreams, 53 percent of Atkins dieters recalled how "unpleasant" their dreams were.

"Some people didn't remember much about their dreams but they definitely remembered that they were unpleasant," Dr. Chow stated. "Others reported being chased or experiencing nasty stresses related to their daily lives."

The negative impact of this manifested itself during the daytime for the Atkins dieters who were tired, moody, irritable, lacked concentration, and could not focus. In fact, Dr. Chow made the following grim conclusions about people who go on the Atkins diet.

"It might make you lose weight and sleep more deeply but the side effects are so bad that they seriously affect your life," Dr. Chow exclaimed. *"So that's not good on your work situation or social situation, and if you have a lapse of concentration while you're driving that could be fatal."*

She added that the Atkins dieters in her study were also suffering from low blood sugar levels and ketosis which she describes as "chronic starvation." Who would ever want to put themselves through something like this?! Dr. Chow presented her findings at the Australasian Sleep Association Conference in Perth, Australia on October 7, 2006.

Does this sound like a weight loss plan YOU would want to do after reading a study like this? Heck, if I hadn't already lost triple-digit weight on the Atkins diet already, then I'm not so sure I'd want to do it with the way Dr. Chow blasted it in her study.

I'm the first to admit there are some rather unpleasant temporary side effects to beginning a low-carb program affectionately known as Induction flu because most people are addicted to carbohydrates — severely addicted! I know I was. I personally wanted to kill myself on the first day of my Atkins diet experience because I felt so unbelievably weak, drained of any energy whatsoever, had a massive headache from Hell...I think you get the picture. My wife Christine will tell you that she has never seen me get as sick as I did on January 1, 2004 when I embarked on this journey to lose weight on the Atkins diet.

But is this a reason to not start a low-carb plan? Heck no! It's very natural to make your body go through the sugar and refined carb withdrawals in those early days because it is a necessary step to getting to the best part of livin' la vida low-carb — weight loss and health improvements. Had I given up after just three days, Dr. Chow, then I would have never tasted the thrill of an enormous weight loss and vastly improved health. My life was RADICALLY changed for the better because of the Atkins diet.

Plus if this was a study about the Atkins diet, then why was it done for only three days? That's not even close to being the Atkins diet. It doesn't even take you through one-fifth of the first phase of the Atkins diet. If you are going to accurately look at the Atkins diet that was created by the late great Dr. Robert C. Atkins, then you need to go at least two weeks to get through the Induction phase and then another 8-24 weeks to see how the dieter progresses during ongoing weight loss (OWL) from being controlled by carbs to taking back control of their eating habits again.

Sure, it can be rough in the early days of Atkins and nobody in the low-carb community is denying that. But that's like leaving a movie theater five minutes after the movie starts because a character you liked was killed off. Does this mean the movie was going to be bad because of this? Of course not! And neither does any pain or struggles that come early on in a low-carb plan.

Although Dr. Chow admitted these Atkins diet side effects had not been evaluated over longer periods of time, she still insisted on making this three-day experiment indicative of ALL low-carb dieters at any point on the diet.

Have you heard of the American marathon runner named Roy Pirrung? At the age of 32, he was tired of being overweight and was ready to quit smoking. So what did he do? He started running like Forrest Gump. Run, Roy, run and he hasn't stopped running since. He is now a renowned world athlete having competed in races both at home and abroad. He is an American record-holder and a member of the USA Track and Field Masters Hall of Fame. All of these accomplishments are worthy of sincere accolades for a job well done.

Unfortunately, Pirrung wrote a guest column about diet and health that was published in *The Sheboygan Press* in 2006 where he had some decidedly poor interpretations of what the Atkins diet is all about. This all-American athlete had little good to say about this way of eating at all.

In his column entitled "Fewer calories, not carbs, important to weight loss," Pirrung said he blames Dr. Robert C. Atkins and Atkins Nutritionals, Inc. for fooling people into believing that removing carbohydrates from their diet will result in weight loss. He believes the Atkins diet is only good "for a time."

"Most diet plans that are promoted through books, TV ads and the like are usually effective for a short period," Pirrung stated in his column.

While that is true because the hype behind most of those highly-promoted diet plans are based on faulty science, the Atkins diet is built on very sound scientific research that proves it is quite effective as a permanent lifestyle change that people can do for the rest of their lives for the sake of their weight and health. Even Pirrung admits the Atkins diet is good for "dramatic weight loss," but he contends that it doesn't last.

"What is wrong now, is that some people still follow this plan, or at the very least, believe carbohydrates are to be avoided," he lamented.

Consider me among those who still follow this plan and substantially reduce my intake of such junk carbs as sugar, white flour, starchy vegetables, and processed foods. Your body just doesn't need these kinds of carbohydrates and you are better off without them. My weight loss and health have never been better and it can be a good long-term way of eating for people who wish to maintain their weight and live healthier than they ever have before.

Pirrung goes on to quote a study, but doesn't say who conducted the study, which university or organization funded the study, when it took place, how long the study lasted, or what scientific journal or conference published it.

Here are the details about the "study" that Pirrung quoted:

A study of about 50,000 women with an average age in their lower 60s were placed on a low-fat, high-carb diet to see what impact the addition of carbohydrates in place of fats would have on weight stability and general health. The study participants were fed foods like fruits, vegetables and whole grains in place of the fats in their diet. The low-fat diet participants ate 53 percent of their total caloric intake as carbohydrates while the control group averaged 45 percent carbs. The low-fat dieters ate 120 fewer calories than the control group. After a year had elapsed in the study, the low-fat dieters had not experienced a significant weight loss or gain and the researchers concluded that a low-fat, high-carbohydrate diet was not a contributing factor in weight gain and eventual obesity.

Pirrung said this study proves the veracity of low-fat, high-carb diets as a healthy way to eat while low-carb makes you eat too much fat and calories. But wait a minute. This study didn't even look at what most of us would consider a low-carb diet since the control group ate 45 percent of their calories from carbs. The results are flawed because 45% carbohydrates is not low-carb; in order to be low-carb the carb counts should be closer to single digits.

He contended this study (again, where did it come from?) proved that "the weight loss [on low-carb] was short-term and not an effective plan for long-term weight loss." How does it prove that? Even if I do believe this study you cite in your column without any references to back it up, it just doesn't add up. Put a 54 percent carb diet against a 10-20 percent carb diet head-to-head any day of the week and even drop the calories of the low-fat, high-carb diet to 500 calories below the low-carb, high-fat diet to create a calorie deficit and you will see something remarkable — incredible sustained weight loss that continues on as long as the low-carb diet is followed. It's only short-term if the person stops eating that way.

Pirrung described the Atkins diet as contradictory and says the high-fat intake is why it is so unhealthy compared to low-fat high-carb diets which are allegedly beneficial in reducing breast cancer, colon cancer and heart disease. He also contends weight management is about watching your calories along with regular exercise, not carb-counting.

"The authors of these studies have stressed the importance of a diet plan that includes cutting back on calories, not necessarily one of the food groups, and exercising on a consistent basis," Pirrung contended. "They also were adamant that the study has proven, to people who still swear by the Atkins plan, that they have nothing to fear by eating foods containing carbohydrates, only more calories."

There is no talk about the quality of these calories. Science is proving that it is healthier to eat sugar-free, low-carb, high-fat (and delicious, I might add) foods, and that's for me. I'm livin' la vida low-carb until the day the good Lord decides to take me home. And that won't be for a very long, long time.

Lean pork weight loss study disregards positive role of dietary fat

It seems like we are seeing lots of research coming out all the time regarding the health and weight benefits of eating meat because of the healthy levels of fat and protein it provides. These exciting new scientific foundations for protein consumption are revealing what many of us who are livin' la vida low-carb have already discovered — protein and fat in animal-based foods are playing a major role in keeping hunger satisfied while aiding in permanent weight loss. It's about time, right?

Lead researcher Dr. Wayne W. Campbell, associate professor of Foods and Nutrition in Purdue University's Laboratory for Integrative Research in Nutrition, Fitness and Aging, and his fellow researchers observed 46 overweight and obese women between the ages of 28 to 80 with a BMI of 26-37 over a period of 12 weeks. What they wanted to know was the impact of dietary protein on weight loss, appetite, mood, as well as cardiovascular and kidney health.

Each of the study participants were placed on one of two specific low-calorie diets:

NORMAL-PROTEIN (NP) GROUP — A 750-calorie diet with 18% protein
HIGH-PROTEIN (HP) GROUP — A 750-calorie diet with 30% protein

Both of these groups were also split into pre-obese and obese subcategories according to their BMI. The HP group was provided with 6 ounces of lean pork on average daily as part of their high-protein consumption. At the end of the study, all of the participants involved had lost weight, fat mass and lean body mass. But the lean body mass losses were less in the HP group than the NP group. In fact, the pre-obese HP group lost less lean body mass (3.3 pounds) than the obese NP group (6.2 pounds).

Nothing is said about the carbohydrate or fat content of the diet Dr. Campbell put these study participants on, but we can infer from the lean pork that it was lower in fat and higher in carbs. Additionally, the HP group experienced greater satiety than the NP group, thus the perceived pleasure of the diet was increased with the HP group and decreased with the NP group. Finally, blood pressure and cholesterol levels improved for all groups while kidney function had no significant change, regardless of the protein consumption. These findings were important since people who oppose high-protein diets worry about damage to the kidneys and heart.

The results of this study were published in the February 2007 issue of *Obesity*.

Dr. Campbell said the presence of protein from the lean pork consumed by the HP group made the difference in weight loss and lean muscle mass preservation.

"After 12 weeks, our study found that the group of women who followed a reduced-calorie eating plan while consuming a higher level of protein was more

effective in maintaining lean body mass during weight loss compared to those who consumed the same amount of calories with less protein," he said.

Maintaining muscle mass helps burn more calories which is crucial in bringing about faster weight loss and eventual weight control, Dr. Campbell added. Plus, hunger was a non-factor among the study participants who ate higher amounts of protein which led that group to feel more confident and energized as they went through their diet.

"The women on the higher protein diet rated themselves more positively in terms of overall mood and feelings of pleasure during dieting which could help dieters stay true to their weight loss plans longer," the researchers contended.

Interestingly, this was the first such study on high-protein diets for weight loss where pork was the primary source of the protein. While that is significant primarily as a marketing tool for the National Pork Board, who commissioned and funded this study, I believe they missed an excellent opportunity to educate and discuss the health benefits of consuming the fatty cuts of pork as part of a healthy diet, too.

We already know fat is important for so many aspects of health, including the heart. But why must we obsess over finding the "lean" portions of pork? The researchers could have very easily placed the HP group on a high-fat, moderately-high-protein, and low-carb diet and seen even better results. A fat/protein/carbohydrate ratio of 60/30/10 would have been VERY easy to implement and produce even better results with weight loss and health improvements.

But that's not what they did with their study which is a real shame. Trying to appease the low-fat crowd for whatever reason, the marketing people representing the pork industry highlighted the six cuts of pork that fall within the USDA's definition of the word "lean" for having less than 10g fat. Why hide and be ashamed of your fattiest cuts of meat? That's just selling yourself short and doing a great disservice to the public about the amazingly healthy products you have to offer them.

I'd love for Dr. Campbell and his researchers to do this exact same study again except this time make the HP group a high-fat and low-carb diet group as well. I would bet they would see a MUCH more pronounced difference in weight loss and lean muscle mass preservation among this group than any other diet comparison. I'd love for my theory to be tested.

High-protein, low-carb diets lead to higher mortality rates?

Oh no! I guess all of us low-carbers need to make sure our will is written because it looks like we're all headed for a one-way ticket to the cemetery because of our low-carb lifestyle. Well, that's what some are claiming after reading a May 2007 *European Journal of Clinical Nutrition* study about mortality rates of people on a high-protein, low-carb diet.

Lead researcher Antonia Trichopoulou from the Department of Hygiene and Epidemiology in the School of Medicine at the University of Athens in Athens, Greece wanted to examine the mortality rates of people who stay on a high-protein, low-carb diet over the long-term. Using the Greek population to comprise her pool of study participants, Trichopoulou observed the diet of 22,944 healthy adults and assessed their diet by way of a questionnaire. The researchers paid especially close attention to the protein and carbohydrate levels of the people in the study and more specifically their relationship to the rate of death among specific categories of people.

What she found was that 455 deaths happened over the 10-year period which Trichopoulou contributed to "high values of the additive low-carbohydrate-high protein" diet. She also added that the study participants who ate such a diet saw more cardiovascular and cancer deaths than those who ate a high-carb diet. What was Trichopoulou's grim conclusion? *"Prolonged consumption of diets low in carbohydrates and high in protein is associated with an increase in total mortality."*

While it is certainly an interesting study to look at, I'm not buying it. Whenever you leave the study data in the hands of the participants as they did in this research, you are opening yourself up for suspicious results. But, despite my doubts about the veracity of the study results, my readers and I were publicly challenged by a board certified dietitian named Dr. Steven Acocella to refute the findings under the assumption that this was a legitimate study. Before I share with you his challenge, I think you need to know a little more about this gentleman first.

This man is no fan of the late great Dr. Robert C. Atkins and his low-carb nutritional approach. As a fellow colleague of low-fat vegetarian diet advocate Dr. Joel Furhman, we can presume he too believes meat should not be a major part of a healthy diet. Thus, a study like this one from Greece seems to further his position.

So, here was his challenge to people who are livin' la vida low-carb:

Dear Jimmy and blog members:

I know that the low-carb approach focuses caloric intake on high-fat but we all agree by default this diet style is also low-carb and high in protein, as fatty foods are often derived from high-protein foods. I know I'm in the lion's den here but Jimmy often posts opposing view and allows hearty debate. My post will hopefully inspire such discourse.

I will not editorialize on the study, but simply listen to you and your reader's comments. I will say that there's no reason that we need to dispute the efficacy of the study itself. Let's go from the position that the study is not flawed. Let's discuss the science and findings.

The conclusions of the authors are reproducible and consistent. What do you all think? If you do post this study I applaud your willingness to explore the science and not ignore nor dismiss it.

I am keen on hearing the comments.

Dr. Steven Acocella
Board Certified Dietitian
Doctor of Chiropractic Medicine
Master of Science Human Nutrition
Fellow - American College of Lifestyle Medicine
Diplomate - American Clinical Board of Nutrition

One fatty meal will send your blood pressure through the roof?

In April 2007, I'm sure you saw all the news stories out of Calgary, Alberta Canada about a study showing how dangerous eating one high-fat meal supposedly is to your blood vessels. Lead researcher Dr. Tavis S. Campbell, assistant professor of psychology at the University of Calgary, along with his fellow researchers observed 30 healthy adults who fasted the night before consuming one of two predetermined meals:

A HIGH-FAT FAST FOOD BREAKFAST or
A LOW-FAT CONTINENTAL BREAKFAST

Take a good hard look at the "high-fat" breakfast: A McDonald's meal with a sausage McMuffin, an egg McMuffin, and two hash brown patties. The "low-fat" breakfast was dry cereal with skim milk, a cereal fruit bar, fat-free yogurt, and a glass of orange juice.

Both of these meals had about 800 calories, but the "high-fat" meal consisted of 42g fat while the "low-fat" meal only had 1g fat. The researchers also added a sodium supplement to balance the salt differential between the two meals. A couple of hours after the meal, the study participants were put through some stress tests to see how their bodies would react to both mental and physical stress. For example, they were asked to perform public speaking about a sensitive and personal subject as well as dipping one of their hands in ice water.

The researchers measured their cardiovascular response, including blood pressure, heart rate, and resistance within blood vessels. What they found was the "high-fat" study participants experienced higher blood pressure than those who ate the "low-fat" diet. They conducted the experiment twice to confirm the results. Therefore, Dr. Campbell concluded that eating just one "high-fat" meal can induce stress which is a precursor to cardiovascular disease. In other words, the researchers believe it's the fat that may bring on a heart attack or stroke.

But they would be wrong. Why? Just take a look at the macronutrient breakdown of the "high-fat" meal again. Yes, it is indeed high in fat, but it is also high in something else. Carbohydrates! Is it possible that the combination of a high-fat and high-carb diet brought about the "exaggerated cardiovascular reactivity" and not solely the saturated fat content of that meal? I'd love to know what Campbell and his researchers would have found in their study if the participants had thrown away the English muffins and replaced the hash browns with a salad and full-fat Ranch dressing (thus making it a low-carb meal).

There's no doubt in my mind the results would have been MUCH better compared with the high-carb, sugar-loaded, low-fat meal. It's amazing how researchers like to look past the high-sugar, high-carb content of these "high-fat" foods in their experiment and just automatically assume it's the fat that is the culprit.

This study was published in the April 2007 issue of *Journal of Nutrition.*

Dr. Campbell expressed grave concern about the findings of his study.

"It's been well documented that a high-fat diet leads to atherosclerosis [hardening of the arteries] and high blood pressure, and that exaggerated and prolonged cardiovascular responses to stress are associated with high blood pressure in the future," Dr. Campbell contended. "So when we learn that even a single, high-fat meal can make you more reactive to stress, it's cause for concern because it suggests a new and damaging way that a high-fat diet affects cardiovascular function."

It would be wise for researchers to read up on some of the latest studies about how protective fat consumption is when it is combined with a reduced carbohydrate intake conducted by such respected researchers such as Dr. Jeff Volek, Dr. Eric Westman, Dr. Stephen Phinney, Dr. Jay Wortman, Dr. Richard Feinman, and Dr. Mary Vernon. There are many many more as well.

With such misinformation about a high-fat diet like this, it is more important now than ever before that we distinguish that it is the carb consumption and not the dietary fat that leads to heart disease. One of these days that truth will finally get through.

High-fat Atkins diet damages your blood vessels?

Despite being called out by Gary Taubes in his book *Good Calories, Bad Calories*, the use of sensationalism and colorful innuendo by the active players in modern health research and journalism hasn't changed one iota! Want another perfect example of this? Just look at this November 2007 headline from Reuters to see what I mean:

"High-fat Atkins diet damages blood vessels: study"

Lead researcher Dr. Michael Miller, director of preventive cardiology at the Baltimore, MD-based University of Maryland Medical Center, and his colleagues wanted to see what effect a maintenance diet has on blood fat levels, cholesterol, and other markers for inflammation. They observed 18 people over a ONE-MONTH period following one of three diets:

ATKINS — 50 percent of calories from fat
SOUTH BEACH — 30 percent of calories from fat
ORNISH — 10 percent of calories from fat

The researchers made sure that NONE of the study participants lost weight so the results would not be skewed by weight improvements since it was about weight control and not weight loss. Each of them had their blood tested for all of the health markers checked out for the study.

What was the result?

The ATKINS group allegedly saw an increase in their cholesterol levels and inflammation which the researchers concluded would cause "long-term damage to blood vessels" and could very likely lead to heart and arterial disease. On the other hand, the SOUTH BEACH and ORNISH groups saw their cholesterol levels come down and artery function was improved. Using an ultrasound machine to measure flexibility and dilation of the blood vessels as well as proteins in the blood, the researchers found major inflammation in the ATKINS group.

"Some markers of inflammation were increased by as much as 30 to 40 percent during the Atkins phase, whereas during the South Beach and Ornish phases, the markers either were stable or went down, some by as much as 15 to 20 percent," Dr. Miller remarked.

I've been livin' la vida low-carb for MUCH longer than one month (over five years and counting!) and I have not been harmed by my high-fat, low-carb Atkins diet. What's most interesting about the conclusion that the Atkins diet is dangerous is that it is based on the results of six people.

So, was this study published in some prestigious medical or science journal? No. It was presented as a paper at the Scientific Sessions of the American Heart Association held in Orlando, Florida in November 2007. No peer review. No long-term observations. The lack of substance in this study along with some rather suspicious and shady implications about what the Atkins diet is should have made anyone with a brain at this AHA conference stand up and question the validity of such research.

Did it happen? Not a chance.

Was anyone else struck by the almost-exclusive focus on the dietary fat content of these diets? What was the ratio of the other two macronutrients — protein and carbohydrate? If that "Atkins" diet with 50 percent fat was matched up with say 30-40 percent carbs, then it is not the Atkins diet. If that's the case, then no wonder their LDL cholesterol went up. Fat consumption is only healthy when carbohydrate intake is kept to a minimum.

Most of us who are following the Atkins plan as outlined in *Dr. Atkins' New Diet Revolution* (the only Atkins diet plan that really counts since it is by the book!) know that even in maintenance people are consuming no more than 20 percent of calories in the form of carbohydrates. And yet Dr. Miller expressed his concerns about the Atkins diet because of his study results.

"It really is the Atkins diet that is the worst," he told Reuters. "The Atkins diet caused the LDL levels to go up by about 7 percent, whereas in the Ornish and South Beach diets...they went down 7 to 10 percent."

What about the HDL "good" cholesterol, the triglycerides and particle size in LDL cholesterol in the Atkins group? We don't have any of this pertinent information about the study participants in this research. Needless to say, it seems this study was flawed and inconclusive at the very least.

While the diets used in this study were supposed to simulate what would happen when you begin a maintenance plan on the various plans, there is something to be said for those of us who actually DID lose weight on these methods and then continued to follow them long-term after the weight has come off. When I weighed 410 pounds in 2004, my weight was bad, but my health was getting much worse. Without the Atkins diet, I never would have regained my health and become the energetic man I am today.

And my lipid profile did improve and has continued to do so five years later. But Dr. Miller believes any positive impact of livin' la vida low-carb will only reach a certain level before your health begins declining again.

"When you lose weight everything looks good but after a while you plateau and you hit a maintenance stage," Dr. Miller contended.

That's what happens on virtually any nutritional lifestyle change when you begin as an overweight or obese person and do something about it. Whether you choose low-fat, moderate-fat, or low-carb, the end result is still the same when you stick with it — lasting and permanent weight and health control. If one option doesn't work, then another one should be tried. That has always been my motto in trying to help people in their own journey to better health. Low-carb is definitely one of those permanent weight loss solution options that people should consider and do proudly if it works for them.

"We don't recommend the Atkins diet," Dr. Miller concluded. "Why not start out with a diet that will be healthier for you in the long run after weight loss?"

We all know what kind of diet this implies, but a one-size-fits-all plan will never work for all people. Drawing broad-based conclusions about a healthy nutritional approach like the Atkins diet, and looking at a very short-term study with a small sample size and attempting to extrapolate long-term consequences from such limited data is irresponsible. The very point of research is to help people better understand what may happen to their health in a given circumstance.

What we need are researchers who can get back to doing what they were meant to do. And that's looking at problems objectively, following research protocol precisely, and then letting the results show what they show. It's the right thing to do.

The Atkins low-carb diet is absolutely sound nutrition, pure and simple. For the past three decades, we have seen excellent independent research validating every single point that the late great Dr. Robert C. Atkins wrote about in his books as well as in real people like me who lost triple-digit body weight and have now kept it off for over five years. This is a long-term personal experiment for each of us and since there are so many of us, we feel it warrants a true study that mirrors our efforts.

A high-carb, protein-packed breakfast good for weight loss?

Have you heard about that study presented at The Endocrine Society's 90th Annual Meeting in San Francisco, California in June 2008? A researcher claimed to have found a way to overcome the problem with cravings on a diet which eventually leads to dieters regaining their weight. It's a big top-secret bit of nutritional advice that they've unleashed on the world.

Wanna know what it is? Eat a huge high-carb, high-protein breakfast and then eat low-calorie, low-carb meals for the rest of the day. That's it! If you eat this "big breakfast," then you are guaranteed not just to lose weight, but to keep the weight off long-term, according to the author of the study Dr. Daniela Jakubowicz from the Hospital de Clinicas, Caracas, Venezuela.

I'm sorry, Dr. Jakubowicz, but with all due respect to your research my body does not need to be inundated with carbohydrates early in the day in order for me to feel satisfied and free from cravings the rest of the day. It can be argued that eating those carbs in the morning even with a high-protein intake will result in a severe spike in blood sugar leading to a quick mid-morning crash and hunger like you wouldn't believe. That's why I started livin' la vida low-carb so I wouldn't have to deal with that rollercoaster ride anymore.

Of course, if you are gonna consume a large amount of carbs, then it is better for it to be earlier in the day so you have time to burn them off as part of your daily activities. But this does not abdicate the body's natural response to them over the course of the day which can have health implications if this high-carb breakfast strategy is implemented long-term. You know, when I first heard about this it kind of sounded like a reverse of Drs. Richard and Rachael Heller's ill-advised *Carbohydrate Addict's Diet* if you ask me.

The study itself was conducted in conjunction with researchers from Virginia Commonwealth University in Richmond, Virginia and Dr. Jakubowicz wanted to see what the long-term impact of satiety (the feeling of being "full") and cravings using a strict low-fat, low-calorie, low-carb diet and one that included the "big breakfast" on 94 obese inactive women.

Well, there's your first problem. A truly effective low-carb diet cannot be calorie-restricted or fat-limited. Fat is the fuel for your body when you remove the carbohydrates, so limiting your calories from this macronutrient while cutting your portions down to minimize your caloric intake is setting your diet up for disaster from the beginning. I've said it many times before, but I'll say it again: Don't mix low-fat and low-carb together! It will only lead to a miserable weight loss experience.

There were a total of 46 women placed on the very low-carb diet with the following macronutrient and caloric breakdown:

FAT — 78g
PROTEIN — 51g
CARBOHYDRATE — 17g
TOTAL CALORIES — 1,085

This is a miniscule amount of food! While the ratio of fat/protein/carbs is excellent at around 79/14/7, the calories are way too low. I even added up the numbers and I only came up with 974 calories — over 100 calories less than the researchers claimed. If you multiply 78 X 9 calories for each gram of fat, that gives you 702 fat calories. Add that to the 51 X 4 calories each for the protein to give you a total of 204 protein calories and 17 X 4 calories each for the carbohydrate to give you a total of 68 carb calories. Adding up these three numbers, you only get 974. Do I need to tell you how deficient this is for a healthy low-carb diet? The percentages are fine, but the portions are inadequate.

Their breakfast was the smallest meal of the day at just 290 calories and they could use up to 7g of carbs in the form of bread, fruit, cereal and milk and only 12 grams of protein coming from meat and eggs, for example. The researchers were trying hard to keep this control group from having a "big breakfast" with too much protein.

Who follows a low-carb lifestyle and has bread, fruit, cereal and milk for breakfast? Anyone? I've never heard of someone who is livin' la vida low-carb eating such foods because they are NOT permitted during Induction as this group was supposed to represent. The Induction phase doesn't include any of those things. Instead, it's all about consuming healthy amounts of fat and adequate protein to keep your hunger at bay to help you get through the day. That's what Dr. Atkins advocated, NOT this made-up version of low-carb these researchers were promoting.

Conversely, there were 48 women placed on the "big-breakfast diet" with the following macronutrient breakdown:

FAT — 46g
PROTEIN — 93g
CARBOHYDRATE — 97g

TOTAL CALORIES — 1,240

The ratio of fat/protein/carbs is about evenly balanced coming it at around 36/31/33, which isn't exactly low-carb by any real stretch of the imagination. And once again the calories don't seem to add up only totaling 1174 — 66 calories less than what the researchers stated. If you multiply 46 X 9 calories for each gram of fat, that gives you 414 fat calories. Add that to the 93 X 4 calories each for the protein to give you a total of 372 protein calories and 97 X 4 calories each for the carbohydrate to give you a total of 388 carb calories.

Regardless, it's quite easy to see that the huge high-carb "big breakfast" meal at the beginning of the day for the dieters in this group greatly skews their macronutrient totals for the day making this an odd "low-carb" diet. They consumed a 610-calorie breakfast with 58 grams of carbohydrate, 47 grams of protein, and 22 grams of fat. Their lunch was 395 calories of another high-carb, low-fat meal followed by supper being a 235-calorie meal that's very low-carb, high-fat. I can only imagine what the bodies of these poor women were thinking on this diet. What in the world are you doing to me?

So, what were the results of this suspicious eight-month study? Four months focused on weight loss followed by another four months of weight maintenance. The strict low-carb, low-calorie group lost an average of 28 pounds compared with the "big breakfast" group who only lost 23 pounds. Statistically, this is not a big difference, according to the researchers.

But the "ah ha" part of this study Dr. Jakubowicz wanted people to remember about it is what happened at the end of the eight months — after four months of maintenance. The low-carb, low-calorie dieters regained an average of 18 pounds for a net weight loss of 10 pounds — just 4.5 percent of their body weight. Meanwhile, the "big breakfast" group lost an additional 16.5 pounds for a total weight loss of 39.5 pounds — an amazing 21 percent of their body weight. Dr. Jakubowicz reminds people that the women who had the "big breakfast" said they weren't as hungry before lunch and lacked the cravings for carbohydrates that the low-carb, low-calorie dieters did.

"Most weight loss studies have determined that a very low-carbohydrate diet is not a good method to reduce weight," Dr. Jakubowicz concluded. "It exacerbates the craving for carbohydrates and slows metabolism. As a result, after a short period of weight loss, there is a quick return to obesity."

My experience has been that eating a truly low-carb diet (not one that starts off your day with cereal or bread!) keeps the cravings away and consuming plenty of fat and moderate amounts of protein as every good low-carb diet does will rev up your metabolism into a fat-burning machine while you enjoy delicious foods that will keep your energy levels up all day.

The major flaw in this study was the restriction on calories it placed on the low-carb dieters in the control group. Have them get rid of the fruit, milk and bread for breakfast and let them eat all the eggs and sausage they need to satisfy their hunger. Then at lunch, have them eat a hamburger patty or two with some cheese on top and a little mayo with a side salad and Ranch dressing. For supper, let them cook up a nice fatty steak and serve a little steamed broccoli or cauliflower with butter on the side. Snacks in between those meals can include almonds, macadamia nuts, sugar-free chocolates, string cheese, pepperoni slices, and other snackable low-carb foods.

If your control group was allowed to truly eat a healthy low-carb lifestyle as outlined above, then they would have lost more than 28 pounds in four months and they most certainly would not have gained anything back. Speaking of that, how did they gain the weight back? Did they add back more calories in the form of carbohydrates to go along with the fat they were eating? Anyone with a brain knows that a high-fat, high-carb diet is unhealthy, so why should it be surprising they'd gain the weight back? This just seems so strange to me that they're pointing the finger of blame at the low-carb diet itself.

Low-carb works only when you work it. If you stop doing it, then you are no longer following a low-carb diet. Dr. Jakubowicz says only 5% of low-carb dieters are still at it two years later, but I know many people who have been eating this way for quite a few years and they've done just fine sticking with it.

Dr. Jakubowicz also says that low-carb living does not address addictive eating impulses, but I could not disagree more. When you eat this way, you bring so much balance back into your health and eating habits by getting off of those blood sugar swings that are causing insulin to spike inside of your body and setting off a whole string of adverse health consequences.

I heard back from the researcher's son Dr. Salomon Jakubowicz after posting my commentary about this study at my blog and he said that the media distorted what his mom's research was all about. Here's what he wrote on my blog:

"Regarding my mother Daniela Jakubowicz's study she tried to make a low-carb diet including breakfast for both subjects and controls but the journalists increased the importance of the carbs during breakfast incorrectly calling it a 'High-Carb And High-Protein Breakfast.' She does know that protein's satiety power is bigger than carbs or fats. Your review is challenging although not very respectful for a health researcher."

Well, #1 I'm not a health researcher. I'm a guy who lost weight and got healthy on a truly low-carb diet. That notwithstanding, I think it is incumbent upon your mother to set the record straight since the headlines completely skewed what her study intended. I invited Dr. Salomon to ask his mother if she would like to appear on my podcast show to clear the air about how her study was misinterpreted. She never responded to my request.

Low-carb diets make you forget?

A study from a group of psychologists out of Tufts University claimed that people on a carbohydrate-restricted diet performed poorly on memory-based exercises compared to those on a high-carb, calorie-restricted diet. A total of 19 women were voluntary placed on a low-carb or low-calorie, macronutrient balanced diet. Nine women went on the low-carb diet and 10 chose the low-calorie one. Here's yet another study on low-carb diets with an extremely small amount of people in it.

Five cognitive memory tests were given to the study participants, including before they began the diets, two during the first week, and then two more in the second and third week of the diet which, ironically, included the low-carb group adding back in carbohydrates to their diet?! What the heck?

The low-carb dieters allegedly experienced a decrease in their memory-related tasks compared with the low-calorie dieters. Reaction time was slower, but short-term attention span was better for the low-carb group. Hunger wasn't an issue for either group and the low-calorie participants experienced some confusion in the middle of the study (maybe they were REALLY hungry and were trying to fight it off).

Answering the question about why the low-carb diet group started adding the carbs back in, it was to return the cognition to normal, according to the researchers led by Holly A. Taylor.

"The popular low-carb, no-carb diets have the strongest potential for negative impact on thinking and cognition," she explained. "Although this study only tracked dieting participants for three weeks, the data suggest that diets can affect more than just weight. The brain needs glucose for energy and diets low in carbohydrates can be detrimental to learning, memory and thinking."

Well, what about other research studies that have showed there is no difference as it relates to cognitive and psychological function between low-carb and high-carb diets? Noted neurosurgeon Dr. Larry McCleary, author of *The Brain Trust Program*, said in my blog interview with him in 2008 that "if you want to age your brain just eat the typical [high-carb] diet most Americans consume. That will lead to memory, attention and mood difficulties and will hasten the path to Alzheimer's." It's not low-carb diets that are the culprit in memory loss...it appears it is the high-carb, junk-based diets that dominate American culture nowadays.

Taylor contended the brain uses glucose as the primary fuel source but cannot store it in the body. That's why your body needs carbohydrates so it can turn those carbs into glucose which is then delivered to the brain by the blood to be used as energy. Therefore, in her reasoning, reducing the carb intake takes away from giving your brain the energy it needs, right? Not exactly. This line of thinking is dead wrong because it forgets that the brain functions BEST on ketone bodies. Again, I turn to my blog interview with Dr. McCleary as he explains how this process works.

"[There is] an alternative energy source the body developed millions of years ago for times when the brain couldn't depend upon glucose. This alternative fuel is ketone bodies which are merely partially burned fats. They are burned differently than sugars and the brain loves them. They have been shown to help a multitude of brain afflictions from memory loss to migraine headaches to hot flashes. An easy way to produce ketone bodies is simply by restricting carbohydrate intake."

So, as you can see, carbohydrate intake for the sole purpose of making glucose for your brain's energy needs as Taylor suggests is invalid. The brain prefers ketone bodies for energy just as the Eskimos, Inuit, and Paleolithic man (just to name a few!) all survived consuming a low-carb diet. And their memory did just fine! This study entitled "Low-carbohydrate weight-loss diets. Effects on cognition and mood" appeared in the February 2009 edition of the scientific journal *Appetite*.

Weight loss is all about the calories and nothing more?

It's all about the calories you put in your mouth. Whether it's low-fat, low-carb, high-protein or whatever, in the end the only thing that makes a difference when it comes to losing weight is calories. That's the conclusion of a study published in the February 26, 2009 issue of *New England Journal of Medicine* paid for by the National Heart, Lung, and Blood Institute of the National Institutes of Health that you undoubtedly saw plastered all across the media at the time. Unfortunately, though, the researchers failed to include a genuine Atkins-styled low-carb diet in the comparison!

Lead researcher Dr. Frank Sacks, a professor of Cardiovascular Disease Prevention in the Department of Nutrition at Harvard University, and his researchers observed 811 overweight or obese older adults and put them on one of four diet plans with the following fat/protein/carbohydrate ratios over a period of two years:

DIET #1: 20/15/65 (low-fat, low-protein, high-carb)
DIET #2: 20/25/55 (low-fat, moderate-protein, high-carb)
DIET #3: 40/15/45 (moderate-fat, low-protein, moderate-carb)
DIET #4: 40/25/35 (moderate-fat, moderate-protein, moderate-carb)

Not a single one of those diets even comes close to any reputable low-carb diet plans like Atkins. Only DIET #4 approaches the lower-carb plan created by Dr. Barry Sears' called *The Zone Diet* which has a 40/30/30 ratio. A genuine low-carb diet would look something like 60/20/20 at the highest level of carbs and most likely 75/20/5 for people who have read *Dr. Atkins' New Diet Revolution*. It's a very high-fat, moderate-protein, low-carb diet during the weight loss phase. More on why this was omitted from the Sacks study in a moment.

Each of the diet plans used in this study were forced to comply with the "heart healthy" guidelines that restricted saturated fat calorie intake to less than 8 percent of total calories, generous portions of fruits, vegetables and whole grains, and a minimum of 20g of fiber daily. The template for the diets was the infamous DASH (Dietary Approaches to Stop Hypertension) diet rather than any of the more popular diet books over the past decade, including Atkins and Dr. Arthur Agatston's *South Beach Diet.*

The study participants were asked to attend weight loss meetings and keep a journal of their food intake on the Internet. Each individual was provided a calorie goal which was approximately 750 calories below their daily needs to allegedly create a "calorie deficit" to induce weight loss. However, none of them were allowed to dip below 1,200 calories a day. As for exercise, they only had to engage in some kind of moderate physical activity for 90 minutes a week so it would not be a major factor in the weight loss. Dr. Sacks wanted the diet composition to be the driving force in the study above everything. So, what were the results?

After six months on each of the diets, all of the study participants lost an average of 13 pounds regardless of the diet they were required to follow. By the end of the two-year study, they had kept off an average of 9 pounds and shed 1 to 3 inches off their waist — again, it didn't matter which diet they were on, it produced the same results. Likewise, increases in HDL cholesterol, drops in LDL cholesterol and triglycerides were all ditto at six months and two years. The study participants all said they experienced satisfaction, fullness, and hunger control on their particular plans.

While this study seemed somewhat interesting to the researchers, it really doesn't mean anything regarding the differences in weight loss and health benefits of any significant macronutrient ratio comparisons. Why wouldn't you want a 10/20/70 low-fat diet like Dr. Dean Ornish would prescribe for producing weight loss and health improvements as well as a 70/20/10 low-carb diet closer to the one Dr. Robert C. Atkins dedicated his life to? Dr. Sacks had his reasons for purposely omitting a truly low-carb diet.

"People don't stick with low-carbohydrate intake and we didn't want to try anything unrealistic," he said. "We tried a big range but a reasonable range of fats, protein and carbohydrates."

With all due respect, how did you come to the conclusion that people who eat a carbohydrate-restricted diet don't stick with it? Since you're a researcher, wouldn't you want the evidence to guide you rather than coming into an important research study with some pre-disposed ideas about what the truth is? I've been eating a high-fat, low-carb diet for over five years as have hundreds of thousands more who visit my blog — what exactly is "unrealistic" about this way of eating?

Dr. Sacks said his study promotes *"a very simple message that cuts through all the hype: To lose weight, it comes down to how much you put in your mouth — it's not a question of eating a particular type of diet."* When you leave out one of the most popular diet plans over the past decade from this comparison study, I can see how you would think all diets work the same — or should I say how they all don't work the same way. A 9 pound loss in two years for overweight and obese people is hardly progress.   And adherence to the chosen weight loss plan was poor to the point that virtually all four diets were virtually identical — so it stands to reason the results would be similar. The researchers say their study will "give people lots of flexibility" to choose the plan that's right for them.

"Weight loss is very simplistically just reducing the amount of calories that you take in, and any kind of healthy diet that allows you to do that is the best," they concluded.

We'll never know based on this study if a high-saturated fat, ketogenic low-carb diet which may allow more calories than any of the four diets in this study would produce even better health and weight loss results. Losing weight is about so much more than just watching out for your calories...it's about making the right choices of food for YOU. A Type 2 diabetic, for example, needs to eat a very low-carb, high-fat diet to stabilize insulin levels so that weight loss and blood sugar control can ensue.

I asked a few of my low-carb expert friends to weigh in on this study with their thoughts.

Dana Carpender, noted low-carb cookbook author who wrote the foreword to this book, said that *"the researchers commented that they tried to make their diets 'heart healthy,' low in cholesterol and low in saturated fats. This tells me that they're working with a paradigm I consider to be thoroughly disproven."*

Dr. Scott Olson, author of the book *Sugarettes*, said *"If they had really wanted to test a low-carbohydrate diet, they would have tried an Atkins diet, or the sugar-free diet I suggest. Those diets keep your blood sugar low and, therefore, keep you from adding weight. Calories mean nothing when you are talking about weight loss."*

Jackie Eberstein from Controlled Carbohydrate Nutrition (ControlCarb.com) responded to this study by describing it as *"an unfortunate waste of money. It was flawed from the beginning."*

"It's clear that the intent was to do a lower carb diet than the typical Western diet but to avoid using the proven very low-carb diet. If they used a very low-carb diet such as Atkins, the results would have been better and it would be harder to sustain the calories in-calories out theory. By designing the study this way they made sure that didn't happen.

Why not use Atkins? Because those involved with the study seem to have a strong anti-low-carb bias. The designers of this study made sure that on the most carb restricted version the amount of carbs was well above the amount one would eat on Atkins. When carbs are too high, as in this study, the positive metabolic advantages, such as significant fat burning, that occurs with low-carb are lost and it simply becomes another calorie-controlled diet.

The bias of one of the researchers was clearly demonstrated with the statement that an Atkins diet wasn't used because people don't stick with a low-carb intake. Tell that to the millions of people who do every day—in the process they get thinner, healthier, improve their quality of life and reduce or eliminate medications."

Well said, Jackie! Let's see what the always entertaining and on-point Brooklyn, NY-based SUNY Downstate biochemistry professor **Dr. Richard Feinman** from The Metabolism Society (NMSociety.org) had to say about this Sacks study.

"I suspect that it is part of a new paradigm on the part of the nutritional establishment which is a kind of 'scorched earth policy.' In other words, having clearly failed at low-fat, they are now trying to say that no diet is good. The technique is NINO — nothing in, nothing out. That is, make minimal changes and then show that nothing happened."

Finally, **Dr. Jay Wortman** from the *My Big Fat Diet* documentary film (MyBigFatDiet.net) chimed in with his own feedback about the study.

"Both Sacks and his co-investigator, George Bray, are on record as being very opposed to the idea of a low-carb diet. For them to say that a low-carb diet is as good as a low-fat diet is progress of a sort, I suppose.

I attended a lecture by Sacks a couple of years ago at a big conference where he was promoting the idea of high protein. When I pointed out that to achieve an increase in protein he reduced carbohydrate and that the benefits may have been attributable to the lowered carb, he launched into an angry diatribe about how low-carb had no scientific merit.

The other thing about this study is that the diets were 'goals' and the fact is that most people didn't stick to the assigned diet. A final observation — 35% carb is not low enough for people who have developed insulin resistance. For these people, a very low-carb diet almost magically reverses their health problems. You would not expect to get this kind of metabolic benefit from a diet of 35% carbs or greater.

Bottom-line: this study adds nothing to our understanding of diet and is being used to shore up the untenable position that macronutrient content is irrelevant, that only calories count. There is a growing scientific literature telling us quite clearly that this is not true. These guys are on the wrong side of a major paradigm shift."

And I couldn't have summarized this study any better than that. Do you believe the researchers purposely left out the inclusion of a ketogenic low-carb diet to skew their results? It certainly appears that way.

Whenever a new study or health research is released to the public, we are always greeted by many of the same people over and over again to interpret the findings and tell us what the take-home message is. And these people are usually deeply rooted in conventional wisdom regarding a "healthy" diet — namely, strong advocates of a low-fat, high-carb, and vegetarian-styled diet. Although Dr. Dean Ornish gets his fair share of media ink on his opinions about diet studies, another name has become almost as popular — Dr. David Katz.

He's does all that he can to get his name published in any article related to diet, nutrition, weight loss, and fitness. He commented on the Atkins diet when Atkins Nutritionals filed for bankruptcy in 2005 by stating his disdain for the Atkins diet:

"The Atkins diet is at odds with a strong foundation of knowledge about the fundamentals of healthful eating and sustainable weight loss," Dr. Katz asserted at the time. "But the burden of proof has always been the other way

around: diets at odds with conventional dietary wisdom must prove them-selves healthful. In my opinion, the Atkins diet never did, and never will, meet this test."

His own bias against low-carb diets such as Atkins even led him to personally come after me as an amateur who does not have a right to share educated opinions on the subject of health.

"The fact that you've lost weight does not make you a nutrition expert," he wrote to me in 2006. "I have driven over suspension bridges — doesn't make me an engineer."

One of my regular blog readers and nutritional science blogger David Brown (NutritionScienceAnalyst.blogspot.com) responded to comments made by Dr. David Katz about this study with the cold hard facts. He e-mailed Dr. Katz directly about the statements he made in an Associated Press story about the Sacks study that weren't exactly backed up by the science. Here's what David wrote to Dr. Katz:

Dear Dr. Katz,

Apparently, you consider saturated fat to be atherogenic. In the column "Low-carb? Low-fat? Study finds calories count more," this is what was attributed to you.

Dr. David Katz of the Yale Prevention Research Center and author of several weight control books, said the results should not be viewed as an endorse-ment of fad diets that promote one nutrient over another.

The study compared high quality, heart healthy diets and "not the gimmicky popular versions," said Katz, who had no role in the study. Some popular low-carb diets tend to be low in fiber and have a relatively high intake of saturated fat, he said.

Both experimental and observational evidence I'm familiar with do not seem to link clogged arteries to saturated fat intake when adequate supportive nu-trition is included in the diet and excessive refined carbohydrate is not con-sumed. In fact, fructose research by Peter J. Havel, Richard J. Johnson, and several others suggests that excessive fructose consumption may be driving the obesity/heart disease/diabetes/metabolic syndrome epidemic. You may want to examine their findings.

Below is a comment at the close of the Chang article.

Other experts were bothered that the dieters couldn't keep the weight off even with close monitoring and a support system.

"Even these highly motivated, intelligent participants who were coached by expert professionals could not achieve the weight losses needed to reverse the obesity epidemic," Martijn Katan of Amsterdam's Free University wrote in an accompanying editorial.

It's likely that if the researchers (in the Sacks study) had not limited experimental parameters to a "heart healthy" diet (35% carbohydrate is not low-carb and 40% fat is not high-fat) and if they had included foods with high saturated fat content, they likely would have observed what carbohydrate restriction can accomplish.

I'm not suggesting that carbohydrate restriction is the only way to control weight. The Kitava Study hints that carbohydrates derived from grains have a different effect from carbohydrates derived from root crops and vegetables (Note that Kativans have high triglycerides and low HDL cholesterol but experience no strokes or heart attacks). I suggest you familiarize yourself with current lipids research furnished by the Nutrition & Metabolism Society.

Finally, I urge you to read some of the comments submitted to the 2010 Dietary Guidelines Advisory Committee in January, 2009.

Regards,
David Brown

Well done, David! It probably won't change Dr. Katz' mind about anything, but at least he knows that people like you and me are out here watching what he is saying.

Dr. Feinman added a few more comments about the Sacks study with his own brand of skepticism and scorn.

"In any other science, the fact that [Sacks] wanted people to take in 15% protein vs. 25% and they did not do it would be considered that the experiment failed and they would not have published it," he wrote in an e-mail to me. "In fact, when he looked at the actual behavior of people in the experiment, protein did correlate with weight loss, just the opposite of what he said."

I say kudos to Dr. Feinman for adding his voice to the growing list of people who are exposing bad science when they see it. I appreciate the incredible yeoman's work he is doing at the Metabolism Society (NMSociety.org) sharing genuine research that will benefit both doctors and patients with quality information to help them treat conditions like obesity, diabetes, metabolic syndrome, and other health conditions. We need more people like him in the low-carb research world willing to expose fraudulent studies like this one when they arise.

Plant-based "Eco-Atkins" diet better than traditional low-carb?

As if the original Atkins high-fat, low-carb diet wasn't good enough already, researchers attempted to make it better by using a plant-based low-carb, low-calorie diet instead in a study published in the June 8, 2009 issue of *Archives of Internal Medicine*. The theory was to see if similar weight loss results from previous studies could be replicated while simultaneously seeing drastic reductions in LDL cholesterol.

This so-called "Eco-Atkins" was designed to create a vegetarian Atkins diet which sounds like an oxymoron if you ask me. The researchers observed 44 overweight men and women with high LDL cholesterol and put half of them on a diet high in vegetable proteins from gluten, soy, nuts, fruits, vegetables, cereals and vegetable oils or on a high-carb, low-fat diet including low-fat dairy and whole grain products for a period of four weeks. Both groups only consumed about 60 percent of their caloric needs to produce an alleged "calorie deficit" and they lost close to exactly the same amount of weight (almost 9 pounds). However, the "Eco-Atkins" study participants saw their LDL cholesterol and blood pressure decrease more than those on the high-carb, low-fat diet.

All I can say about this study is big whoopdi-freakin'-doo! We already know from many other previous research studies on the low-carb diet that this way of eating produces weight loss and reductions in blood pressure and that the traditionally meat-based Atkins diet kept LDL cholesterol levels stable while significantly raising HDL and lowering triglycerides — both key indicators in cardiovascular health. Why wasn't HDL and triglycerides measured in this "Eco-Atkins" study?

What was also missing from this study was the kind of LDL they were measuring. As you know from my earlier chapter on cholesterol, all LDL cholesterol is not the same. You have the small, dense LDL particles that are the dangerous kind that can lead to atherosclerosis (hardening of the arteries) and heart disease. And then you have the large, fluffy LDL particles that are virtually harmless to your health.

Arbitrarily lowering LDL just to be lowering it is useless which is why taking a statin drug to accomplish this is just about as stupid as it comes. Eat a high-fat (and it can even come from animal sources), low-carbohydrate nutritional plan to make these healthier LDL particles, increase your HDL, and lower your triglycerides. You don't need to turn to an "Eco-Atkins" because the REAL Atkins diet works just fine for producing amazing changes in your weight and health.

Eating red meat will kill you — OH NO!

Another day, another study about how red meat is supposed to kill you! I'm sure you heard all about the March 2009 study that claimed consuming red meat will put you on your death bed. If not, then check out just a few of the thousands of health headline stories that were blaring from coast to coast about this:

Study: Too much red meat shortens life
Live longer by reducing red meat intake
Are You Eating Too Much Meat?
The Growing Case Against Red Meat
Red meat increases risk of death from cancer
Too much red meat will kill you — study
Eating Red Meat May Boost Death Risk

And my favorite one of all...

Death link to too much red meat (won't we ALL die of something someday?)

As with most studies about health that are released to the public, the average Joe or Jane on the street will simply look at these headlines, hear it talked about on *Good Morning America*, *The View*, Oprah, and their local news, rationalize in their minds that it makes sense, and decide to cut down on their red meat consumption — even if it is only temporary. Our pop culture society doesn't demand much more investigation into supposedly scientific claims that are made like this and a lot of people are gullible enough to believe the reporting of these studies without doing their due diligence in checking them out for themselves.

This purposeful veganization (that's my new term for the radical vegetarians and vegans who would like nothing more than to have everyone in the entire world eat the way they do) that has been going on for the past few decades is so easy to see through that you'd have to have your mind shut down to miss it. And yet how many of us low-carbers will see friends and family and hear them talk about this so-called "study" that warns about eating red meat and share their concerns about our health? You know it's gonna happen if it hasn't already.

While they'll be well-meaning in their comments, these people are utterly clueless about what a "healthy" meat-based low-carb diet like Atkins is really all about because of the anti-meat tenor of most health news coverage. However, this could be an excellent opportunity to educate them about the truth of livin' la vida low-carb, too. Never be ashamed to share the truth with others about what has happened to your weight and health eating this way.

So what about this study published in the March 23, 2009 issue of *Archives of Internal Medicine*? Lead researcher Dr. Rashmi Sinha from the NIH-based government group called the National Cancer Institute and her fellow researchers conducted a prospective study of 500,000 people who were a part of the NIH—AARP Diet and Health Study. These study participants ranged in age from 50-71 when the study began in 1995. Dr. Sinha states that this study is very likely the largest one conducted to date examining the dietary consumption of red and processed meats with cancer, heart disease, and death. Their premise was that a high intake of red or processed meat may increase the risk of mortality and the researchers wanted to see if there was a relationship between meat-eating and death.

A detailed survey questionnaire was distributed to the study participants to determine their food intake and the researchers kept tabs on them for a decade by tapping into the Social Security Administration database to see any deaths that took place. After ten years, a total of 47,976 men and 23,276 women had died. They divided up the participants into various categories according to the frequency of their red meat consumption. Red meat in this study was defined as beef, pork, bacon, ham, hamburger, hot dogs, liver, pork sausage, steak, and meats in foods such as pizza, stews, and lasagna. Processed meat included white or red meat that was cured, dried, or smoked, like bacon, chicken sausage, lunch meats, and cold cuts.

To establish a clear definition of what was considered "high" versus "low" consumption, Dr. Sinha said the group with the highest intake of red meat ate an average of just 4.5 ounces daily. Conversely, the group with the lowest intake of red meat ate on average about a half-ounce per day. As for the processed meats, the heavy consumers consumed 1.5 ounces daily while the lightest eaters ate a minuscule one-tenth of an ounce.

What did the researchers conclude about the connection between meat consumption and deaths as a result of the data they gathered? The biggest red meat and processed meat eaters were at a higher overall risk of dying during the study period with a specific increase in risk from cancer and heart disease deaths. Statistically speaking, the risk of dying was nearly one-third (31 percent) higher among the meat-eaters compared to those who ate the lowest amount of red meat. And for women it was worse — the biggest red meat eating females experienced a 50 percent greater risk of death from heart disease.

Dr. Sinha added that 11 percent of all deaths in men and 16 percent of deaths in women would have been prevented if the heavy red meat eaters would have adopted the habits of their fellow participants who ate less red meat. She contended that heart disease fatalities would have dipped by 11 percent in men and 21 percent in women had they backed off on the red meat. And the cancer risk was about 20 percent higher in those who ate the most red meat as well as 10 percent higher in those who ate the most processed meats. The researchers said white meats like chicken and turkey, generally lower in fat, were the most "protective" against deaths, including those associated with cancer.

My initial reaction to this study is that it doesn't prove anything. Many of the people in the study were already old when the study began and some of them very likely would have been in their 80's by the end of the study period. Can we not extrapolate that a good many of those deaths that occurred just happened because it was Grandma or Grandpa's time to go? Plus, who knows what their health was like apart from their diet prior to this study beginning?

You can't necessarily attribute causality between their meat-eating and their eventual death.

It would be the same as saying this — all of the people in the study who died breathed oxygen when they were alive, so surely it had to be the air they sucked in their lungs that killed them! Or, even more absurd, how about that survey all of the study participants filled out? Did you ever stop to think THAT could have been the reason for their deaths? It's just as ridiculous to blame the air and that questionnaire on the deaths as the red meat like the researchers did in this study.

But while we're attaching blame to the foods consumed by those involve in the study, isn't there also a possibility that the people who were eating the most red meat were also consuming a diet high in carbohydrates? You cannot overlook the negative impact that sugar/carbs very likely played on the cancer, heart disease, and death statistics found in this study. Would the results have been the same had the people consuming the red meat kicked the carbs while eating even more red meat? Who knows because Dr. Sinha doesn't tell us. Again, that's what makes this study so irrelevant.

Although Dr. Sinha feigns innocence and claims only to be interested in the science, she and her researchers have given more fuel to the fire of the vegetarian and vegan interest groups out there. I for one will not be giving up my delicious and healthy red meat consumption which is a whole lot more than 4.5 ounces a day! In fact, I have been known to eat a 13-ounce T-bone steak in one MEAL. That's three times the amount that allegedly killed these study participants, so is my risk of dying in the next ten years three times quicker?

When asked to elaborate on why she thinks it was the red meat consumption that led to these increases in cancer, heart disease and death, Dr. Sinha theorized the following:

- Meats produced carcinogens when they are cooked
- Cells are damaged from excessive iron intake
- Saturated fat leads to heart disease and cancer

There's no evidence to substantiate any of these claims and plenty of it to discredit the notion that meat in and of itself leads to any health complications.

Just face the facts — meat is an extremely important aspect of a healthy life-style when you keep your carbohydrate intake to a minimum. This point is irre-futable and backed by plenty of science already. Nevertheless, Dr. Sinha rec-ommends that people consume no more than 18 ounces of red meat weekly by limiting their consumption to no more than two days a week while giving up all processed meat entirely. She says people should become almost-vegetar-ians for the sake of improving their mortality rates.

With all due respect to Dr. Sinha, and her research, this changes nothing about how I choose to live a healthy lifestyle because red meat saved my life. When I weighed over 400 pounds in 2004 and decided to start on the Atkins diet to do something about it, red meat became a major part of my life. Whereas I used to eat a big bun and French fries with my hamburgers or a baked potato and dinner roll with my steak, now I forgo those wasted carbs and just stick with the healthy parts of those cuts of meat — the fat and protein! Today I am a new man as a result of consuming delicious and hearty cuts of red meat. And I'm not about to let you or anyone else rob me of the joy that has come from this incredible journey to better health.

12-week study on mice eating low-carb means atherosclerosis in humans?

In a study entitled "Vascular effects of a low-carbohydrate high-protein diet," lead researcher Dr. Anthony Rosenweig, Director of Cardiovascular Re-search in Beth Israel Deaconess Medical Center's Cardiovascular Institute and Professor of Medicine at Harvard Medical School, and his research team observed over a 12-week period an ApoE mouse model of atherosclerosis (plaque accumulation in the arteries leading to the heart — a precursor for a heart attack or stroke) and fed them one of three isocaloric diets with various fat/protein/carbohydrate ratios:

GROUP 1 — standard mouse "chow" diet (15/20/65)
GROUP 2 — a typical "Western diet" (42/15/43)
GROUP 3 — low-carb, high-protein diet (43/45/12)

Before we even get into what Dr. Rosenzweig found in this study, let's take a look at the diet they are using for this "low-carb" group. While it is indeed low in carbohydrate comprising just 12 percent of the total caloric intake, what's up with the astronomically high protein content? Most of the reputable low-carb plans out there such as Atkins, Protein Power, and the like are decidedly much higher in FAT (upwards of 70 percent of total calories coming from fat) with only moderate or adequate amounts of protein. A 45 percent protein low-carb diet is nothing at all like what so many of us who are livin' la vida low-carb would be consuming following a typical low-carb diet.

With that one caveat aside for now, let's take a closer look at what the researchers did with these mice. They examined them at the six-week and twelve-week mark to see what impact had been made on the various study groups. Weight gain in mice is expected, but GROUP 3 gained 28 percent LESS weight than GROUP 2 — not a surprising result since most scientists acknowledge previous research showing the effectiveness of low-carb diets for weight loss. But when they looked at the blood vessels of the GROUP 3 mice, the researchers found that plaque build-up was nearly double (15.3%) than what GROUP 2 experienced (8.8%). GROUP 1 showed little evidence of atherosclerosis by comparison.

The researchers expressed concern that humans consuming a high-protein, low-carb diet like the one consumed by these mice would lead to an inability to get the proper blood flow to the heart which could result in a cardiovascular event. Interestingly, the study found that the lipid profile of the GROUP 3 mice remained unchanged despite the supposed damage done to the blood vessels. This study was published in the August 24, 2009 online version of *Proceedings of the National Academy of Sciences*.

While mice can certainly be used in certain laboratory experiments to see what would happen to people in similar situations, I am not seeing the connection between a mouse and a human in this study. In fact, *Nutrition & Metabolism* (NutritionAndMetabolism.com) Founder and Editor Dr. Richard Feinman responded to this discrepancy by noting *"the scientifically correct title of this study should be 'Vascular effects of a low-carbohydrate high-protein diet in ApoE-/- mice' because that is what it is about."*

Dr. Feinman explained to me regarding ApoE that it is short for apolipoprotein E and is one of the protein components of the cholesterol and fat-carrying particles known as lipoproteins (LP) that circulate in the blood. It is required for efficient clearance of some of these particles. ApoE knockout mice (ones that have been genetically engineered to have no ApoE) are naturally prone to atherosclerosis because of the poor clearance of the LP particles.

Not surprisingly, the mice used in this study were ApoE-KO mice (genetically referred to as ApoE-/-) which have to be used to study atherosclerosis because normal mice don't generally develop atherosclerosis possibly because of the very high HDL cholesterol in their bodies. It is rare for humans to be deficient in ApoE but even those people who are and happen to have high cholesterol are not particularly susceptible to atherosclerosis.

Noted Milwaukee, WI-based cardiologist Dr. William Davis added another wrinkle to this study by sharing that *"there are three forms of ApoE mice (2,3,4), each of which responds differently to different diets. For example, ApoE2 people (and mice) respond to low-fat diets differently than ApoE4 people."* Now this is getting really interesting. So which mice did Dr. Rosenzweig need to use to extrapolate the best human application? It's anyone's guess!

Good Calories, Bad Calories author Gary Taubes explained that this study using mice actually contradicts a great preponderance of the evidence that we've already seen in human studies, including how an Atkins low-carb diet improves cholesterol panels, reduces inflammation, lowers blood pressure and more. So why are mice a better model for the development of atherosclerosis in humans than humans? Excellent question!

Although Dr. Rosenzweig admits it is "very difficult" to know how a diet is truly impacting cardiovascular health even in clinical studies, he insists that using mice fills in the gaps and answers the most pressing questions.

"We, therefore, tend to rely on easily measured serum markers [such as cholesterol], which have been surprisingly reassuring in individuals on low-carbohydrate/high-protein diets, who do typically lose weight," he stated. *"But our research suggests that, at least in animals, these diets could be having adverse cardiovascular effects that are not reflected in simple serum markers."*

Okay, let me get this straight to make sure I understand you correctly, Dr. Rosenzweig. Are you saying the improvements low-carb dieters in human studies have seen time and time again in their cholesterol, including increases in HDL "good" cholesterol, significant decreases in triglycerides, and an increase in the size of the LDL particles to the large, fluffy, and protective kind, are actually irrelevant as a true indicator of heart health because your mice happened to show negative cardiovascular effects even with all these improved markers? In other words, are we just supposed to chunk all that previous human data that shows otherwise and simply believe the mice in your study hold the key to truly understanding what a low-carb nutritional approach is doing in humans?

I'm gonna offer up a human case study that demonstrates how low-carb does NOT lead to plaque build-up in the arteries leading to the heart and it in fact does just the opposite.

A 37-year old male who has been eating a high-fat, moderate-protein, low-carb diet for 68 months had a CT scan of his chest conducted in August 2009 to see if there were any calcium deposits in the arteries leading to his heart. This heart scan would show any calcification of the plaque that has taken place as a result of his diet and assign a number to indicate the overall risk to cardiovascular problems. When the test results came back from this long-term low-carb eater, they showed his heart scan calcium score was zero. Despite eating a low-carb diet just as these mice did in this study, there was no calcified plaque at all.

By the way, the man featured in this case study is me, Jimmy Moore. WOO HOO!

Dr. Rosenzweig is probably not impressed by my phenomenal heart scan results attributed to low-carb living since he seems to be hedging all of his bets on mice. But the anti-low-carb bias is not just limited to him — another one of the researchers on this study named Dr. Shi Yin Foo, a cardiologist at Rosenzweig's lab, claimed that she wanted to do this study when several of her heart attack patients alleged to be livin' la vida low-carb. In fact, Dr. Rosenzweig was also eating low-carb at the time which came as a shock to Dr. Foo.

"Over lunch, I'd ask [Dr. Rosenzweig] how he could eat that [low-carb] food and would tell him about the last low-carb patient I'd admitted to the hospital," Dr. Foo exclaimed. *"[Dr. Rosenzweig] would counter by noting that there were no controls for my observations."*

That was one of the reasons why they decided to concoct this mouse experiment "so that we could know what happens in the blood vessels and so that I could eat in peace," Dr. Rosenzweig said.

Dr. Foo believes the diet composition they came up with most closely matches "a typical low-carb diet."

"In order to keep the calorie count the same in all three diets, we had to substitute a nutrient to replace the carbohydrates. We decided to substitute protein because that is what people typically do when they are on these diets," he explained.

No it isn't, Dr. Foo! Most people who have read just about any reputable book on low-carb dieting know that when you remove the carbohydrate you replace it with an increase in the percentage of fat in the diet. Generally it's not a significant increase in the amount of dietary fat consumed since combined with a reduction in carbs and an adequate amount of protein this way of eating is quite satiating.

But knowledgeable low-carbers are abundantly aware of the excessive glucose that comes from eating too much protein (there's that gluconeogenesis thing again!). And 45 percent of calories from protein are way too much by as much as double! I regularly get only about 20-25 percent of my calories from protein and my fat intake is a whole lot higher than 43 percent.

University of Connecticut researcher Dr. Jeff Volek, who has conducted numerous studies on low-carbohydrate diets, explained that *"no reasonable person would replace carbs with protein to the level these mice consumed."* He added that *"mice are horrible models of lipoprotein metabolism and atherosclerosis…because regular mice are resistant to atherosclerosis."*

The researchers expressed shock that all of the typical markers for cardiovascular disease such as cholesterol, triglycerides, oxidative stress, insulin and glucose all came back normal for the low-carb GROUP 3 mice.

"In each case, there was either no difference in measurements compared with the mice on the Western Diet [which contains the same amount of fat and cholesterol] or the numbers slightly favored the low-carb cohort," Dr. Foo added. *"None of these results explained why the animals' blood had more atherosclerotic blockages and looked so bad."*

To me it appears this study is being set up purposely to respond to low-carbers who have outstanding cholesterol, triglycerides, blood sugar and insulin levels as if to say, "Sure, your blood works comes back clean, but we really know what is happening to your arteries!"

Well, for Dr. Rosenzweig, the results of this study were enough to have him cease with his healthy low-carb way of eating.

"Examinations of the animals' bone marrow and peripheral blood showed that the measures of EPC cells dropped fully 40 percent among the mice on the low-carb diet — after only two weeks," he remarked. *"Although the precise nature and role of these cells is still being worked out — and caution is always warranted in extrapolating from effects in mice to a clinical situation — these results succeeded in getting me off the low-carb diet."*

Dr. Volek notes that a better animal model for conducting a study like this would have been guinea pigs which he says would *"have shown low-carbohydrate diets decrease cholesterol accumulation and inflammation in the aorta."* And he added that his own research of low-carb diets in humans has shown *"in the same 12 week period…that humans consuming low-carbohydrate diets have increased vascular function."*

Dr. Davis also chimed in that this study doesn't jive with what he's seen in his patients.

"I cannot reconcile what this study says with what I see in clinical practice: Low-carb diets yield not only extravagant weight loss, but also marked reductions in triglycerides, small LDL, blood pressure, blood sugar, reversal of pre-diabetic patterns and even diabetes, and is associated with reductions in CT heart scan scores," he noted.

When I asked Kansas low-carb diet practitioner Dr. Mary C. Vernon about this study, she quickly concurred with Dr. Davis in her trademark matter-of-fact way of saying things.

"This study just doesn't fit with what I have seen in patients. I have had patients with pre-existing coronary disease who should have had worsening of their artery blockage have no advancement of their disease when they had repeat cardiac catherization," she explained. *"To have no advancement of disease is unheard of in patients treated the standard way in the United States. I have seen patients with high levels of protein leaking from their kidneys return their kidney function to normal. And here is a twist — the diet people are taught to eat after bariatric surgery ends up being a low-carb one. So where is all the accelerated atherosclerosis in those patients?"*

What is the take-home message the researchers wanted to leave with people?

"For now, it appears that a moderate and balanced diet, coupled with regular exercise, is probably best for most people," they concluded.

This little study is absolutely irrelevant because it fails to acknowledge all the previous human studies that come to the exact opposite results. If you had a choice between believing a study of mice or a study of humans regarding your heart health, then which one would be more convincing to you? Obviously it's the human one. And there are plenty of human studies out there that could have been cited by these researchers — but they didn't do it! As Dr. Feinman said, *"For them not to cite papers that contradict their findings is dishonest."*

One of my readers shared with me regarding this study the fact that mice are herbivores and, as he put it so succinctly, *"may lack the physiological mechanisms to transport and utilize proteins and fatty acids as an energy alternative to glucose"* compared with humans. In other words, the diet fed to these mice is very likely unnatural *"if the creatures were forced to eat something they cannot metabolize, or metabolize poorly."*

This is something Dr. Vernon expressed concern about as well.

"Someone with more mouse knowledge than I have needs to address the mouse chow composition," she retorted. "What chow requirements are needed to produce nutritional ketosis in mice? Mice just don't generally eat this way. How do the researchers know that the change in the mice is from the decrease in carbohydrate? Maybe the mice don't tolerate the increase in protein in the study diet."

Dr. Vernon added that it is a great leap of faith to extrapolate human comparisons with these irregular mice diet models — human study participants are necessary to confirm or reject the findings in the animals.

"I would never plan my diet around what makes a mouse healthy — rodents just aren't very good models for humans. Of course, they reproduce rapidly and they make inexpensive research subjects, so a lot of research is done on mice. But follow-up studies using animals more like humans or humans themselves is needed before conclusions are reached," she expressed.

My reader went on to give the example of a carnivore like a tiger whose primary diet is fat and protein and imagined what would happen if the animal were to be fed a higher percentage of carbohydrate than normal. Would he be "healthier" than his fellow tigers? Not likely! But isn't this exactly what the researchers from Beth Israel have done with these mice? It's a fascinating thing to think about and pokes holes in what is unfortunately being promoted as a reputable study.

Dr. Vernon says she welcomes more research on this, but she will always be more apt to respond to the improvements she has been seeing in her patients over the years.

"I monitor my patients closely, because I know that each individual is unique and may demonstrate a response that I have not seen before. In that case, I would see advancing vascular disease. I haven't seen it yet, but I will continue to look for it," she said. "This is why I think doctors need to be involved in nutrition — because this nutritional intervention is as potent as many of the drugs we use and it treats the problem at the source rather than symptom without addressing the cause of the problem."

Dr. Volek summarized this so-called study in a pithy, yet thorough response.

"Let's put this paper into context — it used an unsuitable animal model to study the effects of a diet no one would consume and showed results opposite to that seen in a more suitable animal model and humans," he stated.

Is there anything else left to say after that? Releasing research like this and extrapolating human application is both irresponsible and unethical if you ask me. Researchers like Dr. Rosenzweig and Dr. Foo should know better.

Hopefully by now you can see why you can't always trust or believe the negative studies you read about low-carb living. While they will continue to throw everything they can at Atkins and low-carb diets to try to discredit them, the fact is much of the research is mere propaganda by those who despise this way of eating. We'll find out coming up in the next lesson why livin' la vida low-carb is so vitally important for helping to eradicate the skyrocketing childhood obesity rates which are running rampant in the United States and around the world.

LESSON #20
Childhood obesity could be eradicated
with low-carb living

"The inability to think differently on a subject even in the face of scientific evidence (think Galileo) is commonly referred to as a 'paradigm paralysis.' The longer we remain paralyzed on the issue of adolescent obesity, the longer our children will suffer. Allowing children to needlessly suffer is criminal at best and at its worst - I honestly have no word for it. Children today, thanks to the low-fat approach to dieting supported by the ADA, AMA, RDA and other health organizations have shifted caloric intake towards more (a lot more) carbohydrate. Children are taught to fear bacon and eggs and opt instead for a bowl of breakfast cereal with skim milk, toast and a banana. This breakfast will spill over 70 times the amount of sugar a child needs to keeps his blood sugar normal. Bear in mind this is just breakfast. And we wonder why our children are becoming obese at an alarming rate? If we really care about our children - if we really love them - we will snap out of our paralysis and instead embrace what research and basic biochemistry have been screaming at us for years - eat less carbohydrates and engage in exercises that build lean tissue, not burn calories. Anything else is insanity."

— **Fred Hahn**, personal trainer, founder of Serious Strength (SeriousStrength.com), author of *The Slow Burn Fitness Revolution: The Slow Motion Exercise That Will Change Your Body In 30 Minutes A Week* and *Strong Kids Healthy Kids: The Revolutionary Program For Increasing Your Child's Fitness In 30 Minutes A Week,* and popular blogger at SlowBurn.typepad.com

Just a little more than a couple of decades ago, the concept of childhood obesity was so rare you never even heard about it. Now the rates of severe childhood obesity have tripled in just the past quarter-century which considerably raises the risk for developing such preventable diseases as diabetes and heart disease according to National Institutes of Health (NIH)-funded research published in the September 2009 issue of *Academic Pediatrics*.

Lead researcher Dr. Joseph Skelton from Brenner Children's Hospital which is part of Wake Forest University Baptist Medical Center says the incidence of obesity in kids is not just a matter of them gaining a few pounds — they're gained a significant amount of weight rapidly which requires immediate medical supervision to help bring it under control before it develops into health complications down the road into adulthood.

"Children are not only becoming obese, but becoming severely obese, which impacts their overall health," he said. "These findings reinforce the fact that medically-based programs to treat obesity are needed throughout the United States and insurance companies should be encouraged to cover this care."

Dr. Skelton and his researchers observed information from the National Health and Nutrition Examination Survey (NHANES) to look at a representative study population of 12,384 U.S. children between the ages of 2 and 19 years old. An expert committee promoted using the classification of "severely obese" beginning in 2007 to those children whose body mass index (BMI) was in the 99th percentile for their age and gender. Although I believe BMI is questionable for measuring the ideal weight for both children and adults, those who fall in the 99th percentile are certainly putting their health at the greatest risk for being damaged.

This study was the first such research that demonstrated just how significant the problem of severe childhood obesity actually is in America. According to the most current statistics from 1999-2004, 2.7 million children in the United States are considered "severely obese" with the highest rates among African-Americans, Mexican-Americans and the poor. Dr. Skelton found that one-third of these severely obese children have metabolic syndrome, which includes anything that increases the risk of diabetes, stroke and heart disease, such as obesity, high triglycerides, low HDL "good" cholesterol, high blood sugar, hypertension and insulin resistance. This urgency of this point was not lost on the researchers.

"These findings demonstrate the significant health risks facing this morbidly obese group," they wrote in the report. "This places demands on health care and community services, especially because the highest rates are among children who are frequently underserved by the health care system."

And while the rates of childhood obesity continue to rise at astronomical rates, the overall obesity numbers for both children and adults is expected to reach the entire population by the middle of the 21st Century according to the findings of University of Missouri-Columbia researchers Dr. Frank Booth and Dr. Simon Lees. They said at the American College of Sports Medicine's 52nd Annual Conference in Nashville, Tennessee in 2005 that they expect childhood obesity rates to be at 100 percent by the year 2044 and adult obesity rates to reach that level by 2058.

Whoa! Is this really the inevitable fate of America? Well, if current indicators are any measure of what's to come, then the answer to that question is yes! In a way, I am pleased that two medical researchers have created a sense of urgency about the problem of obesity because we have not given it the lofty importance that it needs to find a viable solution. While I do not agree with much of what the government has been doing to try to deal with obesity, especially childhood obesity, I am convinced that people need to start taking this issue a lot more seriously than they are.

Part of that includes being open to the possibility that the traditional recommendation of a low-fat/low-calorie/portion-controlled approach to losing weight just doesn't work for everyone. This one-size-fits-all mentality has led us down a path of failure for so many years that you wonder why they even bother recommending it time and time again. If obesity reduction were a business, then it would have gone belly up a long time ago for being an utter failure.

The fatalistic prediction of Dr. Booth and Dr. Lees is based on the fact that Americans are not eating as they should and the fact that they are forgoing exercise as an ingredient in restoring their health to where it should be. It's like how the humans portrayed in the Disney/Pixar film *Wall-E* acted by just continuing to get bigger and bigger because of all the modern technological luxuries. I understand this dynamic personally because I used to be one of those who ate like there was no tomorrow and exercise wasn't even in my vocabulary. But when I decided I needed to do something to overcome my obesity problem, I turned to the low-carb lifestyle and exercise to get me there. Now, I have never felt this good in my entire life! It really can happen for people if they make up their minds to do this for themselves.

Do Americans care enough to "get off the ball and do something now" as Dr. Booth put it in an interview about his study? Otherwise, the research concludes that there will be an increase in early deaths, rampant spread of Type 2 diabetes (with the rates of that disease expected to triple by 2050), and the development of various forms of cancer. Interestingly, Dr. Booth puts the burden of doing something about this on doctors by asking them to inquire with their patients about their personal habits, including whether or not they exercise, what they eat, if they drink alcoholic beverages and if they are smokers.

If the American Civil Liberties Union doesn't get upset, then I'm sure there will be a lot of patients who will balk at their doctors pointing the finger at their problems so openly and honestly. But that's exactly what we need to have happen if obesity trends are going to be reversed. People need to suck up their own pride and get out of denial. It's time to wake up, America! We've sat back on our rears basking in the glory of our plentifulness for far too long that we are destroying ourselves from the inside. The fight against obesity is one that we all must take full responsibility for and do something about.

I know it may seem hard, but it must be done — for the sake of our children. While I am not a parent yet, I know that children are the future of this great country we live in. They are growing up in a world where childhood obesity is the norm, but we can change that for them. Take it from someone who's been through the struggle himself, it is entirely worth it. There are so many things I can do now that I could not do before I started livin' la vida low-carb. Simple things like standing up out of bed without having to jerk myself forward and roll out. Or even walking from the parking lot to the front entrance of Wal-mart without gasping for every breath of air. These little things and more are the rewards of restoring your health and regaining your life.

"The public also needs to start taking responsibility for childhood inactivity," Dr. Booth exclaimed. *"Children are not mature enough to make informed decisions about their eating habits and activity without instruction from adults."*

Dr. Booth is exactly right. If obesity is ever going to be reduced considerably in this country, then we adults are going to have to set the example for the next generation in both our eating and exercise habits. What are we doing to show them the importance of doing what is right in regards to their health?

I saw a group of children at my church recently who were eating sugary dough-nuts and I told the kids that eating foods like that wasn't very healthy for them. Their response to me was that they weren't worried about that because it's not hurting them today. And that's the main problem I see with fixing this issue. We wonder why Americans have gotten overweight and obese, but we don't look at what we are doing to contribute to the problem at an early age. Obesity will not go away on its own. Immediate action to correct this very real issue is needed to prevent the inevitable from happening in just a few short decades from now.

One of the things standing in the way of turning this childhood obesity crisis around is the government. A report released in 2005 about the current state of health of American children presented a conflicting picture of the reality of this problem. The Federal Interagency Forum on Child and Family Statistics, which is comprised of 20 different government agencies designed to research issues involving children and families, submitted their annual "America's Chil-dren: Key National Indicators of Well-Being" report for 2005 and revealed vari-ous health indicators led them to believe the health of children in the United States is doing pretty well. WHAT?! Even more egregiously, there were no warnings in this report about the rising obesity rates in children and only a scant mention of weight issues at all.

In the Health section of the report, it stated: *"The proportion of children ages 6—18 who were overweight increased from 6 percent in 1976—1980 to 16 percent in 1999—2002. Racial, ethnic, and gender disparities exist, such that in 1999—2002, Black-alone, non-Hispanic girls and Mexican American boys were at particularly high risk of being overweight (23 percent and 27 percent, respectively)."*

That was it regarding childhood obesity in this government report on adoles-cent health! There was nothing in this report about kids over-consuming sugar and getting fatter and fatter by the day. With warnings from overseas about the possible causes of childhood obesity, the United States needs to be lead-ing the way on this issue and not standing idly by hoping it will miraculously just go away on its own. It won't!

The fact of the matter is that kids are drinking way too many sugary sodas and eating large amounts of candy that are causing them to get fat. In addi-tion, they are not getting enough exercise to burn off all those extra carbs and calories they are consuming on a daily basis. In looking on the ChildStats.com contact page, it appears that nobody is assigned as the obesity contact under the Health heading. What is wrong with this picture?! Do we even care that our children are growing up to be overweight and obese, will carry that into their adult lives, and quite possibly have their own children someday who will go through the same vicious cycle? If you ask me, this is as disgusting as it gets and the government just turns a blind eye to it all.

This web site with the children's health report is run jointly by the U.S. Department of Education and The National Center for Education Statistics. Needless to say, they need to get serious about children's health by educating our kids about healthy eating choices that do not include sugar and excessive carbohydrates so that obesity rates will fall and the overall health of children will improve.

When the government does get involved in trying to do something about the childhood obesity rates in the U.S., they sure do come up with some ridiculous things like a Food Pyramid for kids! Sponsored by the U.S. Department of Agriculture in 2005 (and I'm sure they're working on one for the 2010 Dietary Guidelines update, too!), this kid-friendly version of the government-recommended Food Pyramid is aimed at reaching children between the ages of 6-11 by enticing them with a rocket ship-based computer game and cartoon graphics. They're trying to make it cool for the kids so they'll get excited about health, nutrition and fitness.

According to former *Washington Post* health columnist Sally Squires, this kid's Food Pyramid introduced in 2005 has some familiar themes you'll recognize regarding nutrition and fitness.

"It urges kids to fill up on fruit and vegetables, grab whole grains instead of more processed cereals, bread and pasta and to 'get your calcium-rich foods,' such as milk," she wrote. "Youngsters are advised to pick up protein — not the greasy fast food burgers, fatty hot dogs and deep-fried chicken nuggets that are often a staple of children's diets — but rather beans, nuts and sunflower seeds as well as lean meat, poultry without the skin and seafood."

That's not totally bad advice, especially regarding eating more of certain kinds of fruits and vegetables, staying away from processed and junk foods, consuming more protein that comes from all kinds of meats, and snacking on nuts and seeds. But I still think children could stand to stay away from high-carb staples such as bread, pasta, and milk. There are plenty of low-carb versions of these that would satisfy the nutritional needs kids have. The younger we can start kids on a healthy low-carb lifestyle, the greater chance obesity can be nipped early to prevent the onset of weight-related health problems.

In regards to dietary fat, Squires said the kids Food Pyramid promotes the good fats found in fish, nuts and olive oil which can help boost the physical and mental capacities of a growing child. And when it comes to exercise, the recommendation is to have an hour a day minimum, something Squires states "few children now meet." Part of the problem is that physical education and recess are all but obsolete in grade school now and nonexistent in middle and high school. A few years ago, I was a substitute teacher in my local school district and worked with a variety of students ranging from 4-year-old kindergarten all the way up to seniors in high school. Whenever I filled in on the elementary level, I was amazed the kids only got about 20 minutes at the most for recess usually just a couple of days per week. That's it!

I remember when I was growing up in the 1980's, we stayed out on the playground for about an hour playing all sorts of games like kickball, dodgeball, and more. They ran us ragged and I'm sure our moms and dads were grateful for it when we slept like babies at night. But those days are long gone in this world of video games, the Internet, and all the other technological distractions we now live with. Is it any wonder why obesity rates in children have jumped so dramatically in recent years?

Complaints about this Food Pyramid for kids being on the computer are centered around the fact that parents and children will have to seek out the information on the Internet to learn more about it. Although there was a lot of publicity about it when it came out with news stories popping up all across the media, what has happened in the years since? Did you even know there was a children's version of the Food Pyramid? Not likely.

The adult version of the Food Pyramid that released in 2005 was viewed by most adults as something negative (42 percent) compared with the people who saw it as a positive thing (37 percent) according to a BuzzMetrics survey of consumers who surf health web sites. The other 21 percent were unsure what they thought of it. An analyst for Buzzmetrics said the Food Pyramid "is barely a blip on the public conscience."

So why create a kid's version of it if the adult one has fallen so flat on its face? Do you expect to breed success out of such dismal failure?

As for the interactive computer game that involves a rocket ship, Squires continued in her column about it saying it "serves as a visual reminder of how well kids are doing for the day."

"When healthy food and more activity are recorded the rocket ship gets fueled. Put in enough of the right kind of fuel and it can take off. But put in food and drinks high in fat or added sugar such as sodas and the rocket ship could sputter on the launch pad, spewing black smoke," she wrote.

That's cute and all, but does anybody else see the irony in this? Here is a new health and fitness program designed to get kids to become more active and eat right and what is it encouraging them to do — sit in front of a computer screen and play this silly little game all day! "But mommy, I don't want to go outside and play, I want to sit here and stay fat while I play this computer game!" Was anybody thinking when they came up with this idea?

They began marketing this kid-friendly Food Pyramid in public schools, but to what end? What difference ultimately will this campaign and emphasis on a child version of the Food Pyramid make on the childhood obesity epidemic? If you ask me, it was one big waste of time, energy, and tax dollars. It's back to the drawing board because there's got to be a better way.

But we're missing the bigger question that needs to be asked. Until parents take a more pro-active role in getting their own weight problem under control, how can we expect their children to do any differently? Mothers and fathers who are the examples for their children to follow need to show their kids what good nutrition and fitness is all about by doing it themselves. We cannot and should not expect the government to play this role for us.

Whatever it takes to make it happen for you, do it. I've been in a situation where I allowed myself to become morbidly obese. I know the pain and the agony of trying and failing on diet after diet thinking nothing would ever work and wondering what was wrong with me. But there is something out there that will work for you. For me it was livin' la vida low-carb and it has helped me lose weight and keep it off now for over five years just when I was on my way to an early grave. Do it for your kids and they'll thank you for it when they become adults.

Some people may have concerns, though, about putting their children on a low-carb diet. Is it safe and effective for the little munchkins to eat a carbohydrate-restricted nutritional approach for the sake of managing their weight and health? A Gloucester, Massachusetts-based pediatrician named Dr. Brian Orr shared his opinion of livin' la vida low-carb for kids on the Fact-Monster.com web site:

"No diet is good for kids. You may have heard about some fad diets such as the Atkins Diet or the South Beach Diet. Adults follow these diets to lose weight. Most diets work at the beginning, but it's hard for adults to keep the weight off over a long period of time. As for kids, no diet is as effective as eating sensibly. You also need to exercise each day to keep you healthy and trim. So turn off the TV, get up and be active and eat your fruits and vegetables. Do I sound like your mother?"

Here's yet another current health expert attempting to explain away the incredible results of being on a low-carb lifestyle. Dr. Orr claims that "no diet is good for kids" and yet we have this growing and growing (literally!) childhood obesity problem that for some odd reason isn't going away. Why do you think that is, Dr. Orr? Could it be that the low-fat/low-calorie/portion control mantra that you and others have been pushing and promoting for the past few decades isn't working?

Describing the Atkins Diet or even the South Beach Diet as "fad diets" does nothing to diminish their effectiveness for people like me and the millions of others who have found success on them. Fad or not, there are a whole lot of people still losing tons of weight and restoring their health on low-carb. That fact is undeniable. Additionally, they are keeping that weight off over the long term when they continue to make low-carb their permanent lifestyle change. That's what I did and most of the weight has stayed off. There's no reason at all why people, young or old, cannot "keep the weight off over a long period of time."

Regarding the health habits of children, I agree that they need to be active and exercise to supplement good nutritional intake. Eating low-sugar fruits and non-starchy vegetables fits well within a healthy low-carb lifestyle as do good portions of protein and fats to give them energy to get through the day. Take the sugar and junk food out of their hands and soon the phrase "childhood obesity" will be eradicated from our dictionary!

Is low-carb healthy for children? You better believe it is! With childhood obesity getting worse no thanks to our government and the current health experts who are advising them, we can and must do something about it for the sake of the health of our children. After all, they are the leaders of tomorrow and we must protect that investment by whatever means necessary.

In December 2005, a position paper was released by the Institute of Medicine declaring childhood obesity and diabetes had grown significantly as a result of junk food advertising on television. The report entitled "Food Marketing to Children and Youth: Threat or Opportunity?" in essence blamed the junk food industry for enticing children with food and beverage products that are high in calories, sugar, salt, fat and carbohydrates with little if any nutritional benefits. As part of their recommendations to the U.S. Congress, they concluded in their report that food and beverage companies need to begin creating healthier products for consumers and to shift their advertising dollars to promote these better choices to young influential consumers.

So what is going to happen if they don't?

The authors of the report believe Congress should force companies to change their advertising practices to prevent junk food from being so heavily advertised and that incentives such as tax breaks should be given to companies who adhere to their goal of providing and promoting healthy products. Can you believe this is actually being proposed in the United States of America? While I am a strong supporter of individuals reducing the amount of junk food they consume to help them lose weight and get healthy, I am not at all in favor of the government telling a business what it can and cannot do. That's what natural market forces are for.

If there is enough of a public backlash on these companies to stop advertising their snack cakes, sodas and candies then the consumer will decide to move their dollars elsewhere. However, if the buying public does not see a problem with these products being advertised on television, then why should these companies adjust their marketing strategy? The bottom line is they shouldn't, no matter how revolting I may think their products are.

Rather than pointing fingers at advertisers of junk food for making their products so appealing to kids (isn't that the point of ANY good and effective business marketing campaign?), why don't we hold parents accountable for their role in this? The last time I checked, most kids don't hold down jobs and make money like their mom and dad does. Aren't parents acting irresponsibly with the nutritional choices of their children when they purchase them junk foods? Why are parents being let off the hook on this one?

The report notes that "early life environment is an important determinant of obesity later in life." I could not agree more. But that is further evidence that parents need to step it up as the leaders in their household and make healthy eating a priority by serving as an example for their children to follow. If Dad is sitting on the couch eating a whole bag of Doritos and mom is scarfing down chocolate chip cookie dough ice cream, then why should Junior act any differently? Try replacing that junk food with healthier sugar-free, low-carb whole food options and then go on a bike ride together as a family. Parents should begin cultivating a healthier lifestyle and you'll be surprised how quickly that will filter down to the children.

The sense of urgency about this issue comes at a time when childhood obesity has grown three-fold since 1965 and Type 2 diabetes has doubled since 1995. According to the Institute of Medicine report, there have been a series of "dietary patterns" which put our children's "health at risk," including poor eating choices being actively promoted in mainstream marketing. To reverse this trend, the report notes that there will need to be aggressive and sustained leadership from the government, parents, schools and the food and beverage industries.

Somebody tell me again why any of this is the government's business? Why is this the school's business? Why is this the food and beverage industries' business? The last time I checked, none of these entities were involved in the birth of the child that was conceived between his parents. They didn't wipe the nose when he caught a cold. They weren't the ones who offered a simple kiss on a boo-boo to make it feel better. No, it was the parents who did that!

Parents, listen to me. Take control of your own family and refuse to allow anyone to parent for you. If your child is overweight or obese, then take a pro-active stance in that situation by helping him overcome it. By modeling what your little one should be doing to keep his weight and health under control, you are teaching your child an invaluable lesson that he can pass down to his kids someday. We can end this cycle of obesity by educating our kids now about healthy and nutritional choices.

A panel of 16 of the best "experts" in the field of nutrition, advertising, marketing, childhood development and entertainment participated in the report. They based their findings on more than 120 studies on marketing, primarily television ads. They criticized the use of popular characters such as SpongeBob SquarePants and Spiderman to promote junk food and said these characters should only promote healthy foods for kids. What right do they have to require this to happen? Again, I agree with the premise, but why not let the businesses make those decisions?

Let's get one thing straight: Childhood obesity is not caused by junk food ads as this report suggests. No, if you want to know why this problem has gotten so out of hand, look no further than the parents of these obese children who have gotten bigger and bigger with little to no regard for what has happened to their child. Perhaps the adults could try modeling the low-carb lifestyle for their children to follow to help them lose weight and get healthy.

Of course, rather than stop junk food companies from marketing their products, there could be an adventurous and bold ad campaign educating parents about the harmful effects of sugar and high fructose corn syrup which is in virtually everything kids are eating these days. This is far more effective than mandating "healthy" advertising from food companies.

Ideas for dealing with childhood obesity are plentiful like what I found in a study presented at the Centers for Disease Control International Congress on Physical Activity and Public Health in April 2006 that concluded young overweight and obese children who play with toys that weigh heavier than normal helps contribute to more calories being burned and gives them extra exercise they wouldn't ordinarily experience. As crazy as it sounds, this is not a joke!

Lead researcher John C. Ozmun, acting associate dean of the College of Health and Human Performance and professor of Physical Education at Indiana State University in Terre Haute, Indiana, observed 10 children between the ages of 6-8 years old to see what effect adding more weight to their toys would have on their health. For the study, Ozmun replaced the normal, everyday block toys that are usually lighter in weight with ones that looked the same, but weighed three pounds each. What he and his graduate student researcher found was the children playing with the heavier blocks experienced a more rapid heartbeat and breathed deeper than they did with the lighter toys.

Can I interject some common sense into this for just a moment? I'm all for trying to help kids who are dealing with excess weight find a way to shed the pounds, but has anybody thought about how dangerous a 3-pound block would be with a group of children who may have the propensity for throwing their toys? Besides hitting another child with one of these "weighted" toys, what about when it hits a window and the glass shatters near other children? Then how bright will this idea be?

Ozmun admits "this is not going to solve the obesity problem," but he believes "it has a potential to make a positive contribution."

Perhaps. But the unintended negative consequences from weighing down toys to make them heavier may far outweigh any health benefits that would come from kids playing with them. There's a reason most toys are light — less dangerous! Plus, kids can burn a lot more calories during cardiovascular exercise they would get running around on the playground during P.E. or recess (that is, if they haven't abandoned this yet in your local public school!). Making toys heavier accomplishes very little towards fighting obesity IMHO! If childhood obesity is the big problem that everyone agrees that it is, then what can we do to help with that without causing potential harm to children?

Restricting advertisements on junk food is not necessarily the answer and neither is creating a children's version of the Food Pyramid! No, what we need is to take a serious look at what is causing all of this weight gain in children to begin with: sugary sodas, candy, snack cakes, cookies, crackers, juice, fast food, and millions of other high-carb food products their little bodies couldn't possibly burn off fast enough! For overweight or obese children, perhaps a long hard look at livin' la vida low-carb isn't such a bad idea after all. Are we just expecting this problem to go away all by itself?

Parents: STOP feeding your kids junk!
Teachers: DEMAND physical education at schools again!
Doctors: ADVISE young patients responsibly on good health habits!
Citizens: URGE even better nutritional education in schools!
Children: EXPECT more from those who lead you! MUCH MORE!

Ozmun said his study with the heavier toys is simply the beginning and that more studies would be needed to see if kids would keep playing with these toys or not over the long term. Even still, he is pushing for 3-pound stuffed animals to be required for physical therapy involving children.

"Having a 3-pound teddy bear may not only help with strength, but with balance and coordination," Ozmun said.

I still think that's way too dangerous for children. With all these warnings placed on children's toys these days, can you see the ones they put on these weighted teddy bears? "WARNING: This chunky-sized teddy may break bones, lead to deep bruising, or even death if thrown at another child or near glass." I wouldn't be surprised to see some kind of wording to that effect once the lawyers of the toy company that ends up manufacturing these sees the potential problems that will arise.

When I first heard about this story, I thought the teddy bears were going to literally be larger so the overweight and obese children will have a toy they could relate to. But that is an entirely different discussion altogether.

We already know that childhood obesity is a precursor to the development of a variety of health problems as an adult. But now a very large Harvard study says children who are still overweight by the time they reach adulthood have a proportionally higher risk of premature death due to their poor lifestyle choices and the subsequent obesity-related health complications that follow.

Study co-author Dr. Frank Hu, Associate Professor of Nutrition and Epidemiology in the Department of Nutrition at the Harvard School of Public Health, and his fellow researchers looked at 102,400 mostly Caucasian cancer-free at baseline female nurses ages 22-44 years old and found these women who were either overweight or obese when they turned 18 were much more likely when they were teenagers to drink alcoholic beverages, smoke cigarettes, and not exercise.

Actually, the study showed that even the women who never smoked at all were STILL more likely to die sooner if they were overweight when they turned 18. As a result, Dr. Hu found that the women who fell into the category of overweight or obese at 18 were most likely to die sometime between the ages of 36 to 56 years old. Yikes! In fact, the higher a woman weighs at the age of 18, the greater her chances of dying young will be, according to the researchers. The higher their weight, the higher the mortality rates — double yikes! Shockingly, the moderately overweight women at the age of 18 were 50 percent more likely to die before they reached the age of 30(!) while the obese women at 18 years old were more than double risk for a premature death than their normal weight peers.

Doesn't all of this just take your breath away to hear? This is an epidemic that is killing off people long before they can ever worry about getting old. I mean, come on, the research has found obesity is causing death to come before the age of 30 for those whose weight problem is most severe! Doesn't this scream at us that we need to do something about childhood obesity ASAP? Where are the bold headlines on this?! Why do we pay so little attention to a problem that has only been perpetuated by our own poor lifestyle choices? It's all been swept under the rug like it's not happening, but that dust is now beginning to pile up to the point that it can no longer be ignored.

Reading this study just breaks my heart and the saddest part about it is that this is all preventable! Note I didn't say it was easy, but the fact is losing weight can and should happen for these children who are overweight or obese so that by the time they become an adult they will have good habits in place ready to take them forward in life. No, don't expect the government to lose weight for you either.

Unfortunately, so many of us pick up the bad habits we learned as children and carry those over into adulthood. I know I did. How else can you explain someone who weighed 250 pounds when he graduated high school at seventeen, 300 pounds when he graduated college at twenty, 350 pounds when he got married at twenty-three, and kept growing and growing his weight until it reached 410 pounds at the age of 32?

Thankfully for me, the low-carb lifestyle came at just the right moment in January 2004 to save me from the certain devastation that would have befallen me had I not stopped the constantly rising weight gain when I did. I praise God and celebrate the gift of my weight loss experience every single day for helping me overcome my obesity problem and take back control of my weight and health once and for all.

Of the women who experienced death in this study, 258 of them died of cancer, 55 from heart disease or stroke and 61 committed suicides. That latter group of women are likely the ones who couldn't take the ridicule and scorn of their weight any longer and just decided to give up on life altogether. My heart aches for those hurting young people now which is why I do what I do today to educate, encourage and inspire others with my blog and books as a beacon of hope for anyone who believes they'll be stuck being fat forever. Oh no you won't!

Dr. Hu said his study results should be a wake-up call for parents to do everything they can to make sure their children are living a healthy lifestyle as they are growing up to prevent premature death from happening.

"This paper underscores the importance of efforts to prevent excessive weight gain in children, not only to prevent obesity but also to prevent moderate over-weight (people)," he said.

I'm gonna step on some toes here (so what else is new?), but any parent who allows their child to become overweight or obese and doesn't try to actively help them lose the weight is guilty of child abuse. That's right, child abuse! I know that sounds harsh, but I believe it with all of my heart. Any parent who thinks it is okay for their children to walk around 25, 50 or 100 pounds more than what they should weigh and just turns a blind eye to the problem like nothing is wrong should be locked up in jail for neglect and should never be allowed to be a parent again!

While I realize there are many reasons for weight gain in children that aren't always tied to their diet, most overweight and obese children got that way because they loaded up on junk food, fast food, and high-carb convenience foods their parents freely bought for them while all but rejecting any form of physical activity in favor of television, video games, and computer stuff. Parents can create a healthier environment to help their children eat better and engage in fun exercise routines to bring their weight under control. It is possible!

If you have a chunky kid, then now is the time to do something about it. And parents, YOU will need to be the ones who need to take the lead on this by becoming an excellent example for your kids to follow. Don't demand your child live healthier while you plop down in front of that television munching on whole bags of Cheetos and boxes of Twinkies right in front of them! How hypocritical! The fact is they'll eat better and get active when they see you doing the same thing. This will also help keep you accountable in managing your own health, which probably needs some work as well. Can I get an amen to that? Doesn't this seem like a win-win proposition? You betcha!

Dr. Hu's study was published in the July 17, 2006 issue of *Annals of Internal Medicine*. Interestingly, there was another childhood obesity study that released about this same time that concluded the best way to treat childhood obesity is with prescription drugs and behavior therapy. Are these people out of their minds? Kids don't need medications and psychobabble to help them lose weight! What they need is leadership from their parents about the right way to eat and exercise. We need to stop relying on the pharmaceutical companies to come up with a pill to solve all of our problems and start taking better care of ourselves with the blessings God has given us to watch over. Weight loss is needed at any age and parents can make this happen for their families.

Childhood obesity is dead serious lethal, but you have the power to change that destiny for your child. You might even consider livin' la vida low-carb for that precious little child you love and care about so much. It's a way of eating that they will thank you for teaching them for many years to come. And it is something they will pass on to your grandchildren someday. What a low-carb legacy that would be!

Three of the world's largest health advocacy groups — the World Health Organization, the Centers for Disease Control and Prevention and the American Academy of Pediatrics — put out a warning call in September 2006 regarding rising obesity rates among babies and it reminded me of an e-mail I received from one of my blog readers that may help shed some light on why this is happening.

The e-mailer told me she hadn't heard anyone deal with this topic and it seemed all too obvious to her as someone who has been livin' la vida low-carb for a while now. It has to do with what we are feeding our babies. That's right, there's something about baby food that may in fact be contributing to the rise in childhood obesity rates. My reader wrote the following regarding baby food and formula:

"One of the first ingredients in almost every baby formula is corn syrup in some shape or form. It seems like everyone has been baffled about why bottle-fed babies are more likely to be overweight later in life and have diabetes, and the connection is so obvious to me now. It just screams for the world to know. Well, duh! We are addicting our bottle-fed babies to corn syrup long before they can make any choices. How rotten is that! I did it without even knowing it, as 99% of the population probably does as well."

Have you ever thought about this before? I don't have any kids yet, so this didn't immediately pop into my head. But it really does make sense when you stop to think about it. Have you ever really read those nutritional labels on the baby food and formula you are giving to your child? Or do you just trust baby food companies are giving your baby exactly what is needed to be healthy and strong?

The unfortunate thing is people who buy baby food in those distinctive jars may be depriving their little ones of the essential nutrients he or she needs to grow up to be a strong kid and healthy adult. I'm no expert on this subject, but it seems the children who are breast-fed by their mothers tend to be less likely to become obese because they are not exposed to the carb-heavy baby food that is on our shelves today. You don't believe me that today's baby food is unhealthy for your child? Just take a look at the macronutrient ratio on that jar the next time you go to the grocery store. What you will find is a TON of carbohydrates with very little protein and fat. It is not uncommon for the fat/protein/carbohydrate ratio to be around 5/10/85 or even worse. EEEK! Go see for yourself! It really will open your eyes.

Even more egregious are the ingredients in these baby foods which contain so much corn syrup as my reader wisely noted in her e-mail to me. All of that sugar and the obvious lack of protein and fat which is sorely needed to help growing babies develop properly is one of the reasons why I think we have seen obesity among children and even babies become increasingly worse. Food companies have been steadily sneaking in sugar and its evil twin high fructose corn syrup (HFCS) into the vast majority of foods we eat for a long time now and it's starting to catch up to us with rising obesity and health problems. Even worse is the facade that feeding babies foods such as rice, sugary fruits, and starchy veggies is healthy. It is not! Most of these foods are jam-packed with so many carbohydrates it makes those poor little babies start becoming addicted to carbohydrates long before they can even talk.

Additionally, the lack of protein and fat in these baby foods don't allow the baby to develop as well as he or she should because they aren't getting the essential building blocks that come from these macronutrients responsible for healthy brain function, strong bones, and muscle growth, too! And whatever you do, don't neglect the role of saturated fat in a baby's development because it plays a vital role in their brain health as well. And where are the omega-3 essential fatty acids?

Essentially what you are doing if you are feeding your baby out of a jar is putting him or her on a low-fat, low-calorie diet that is sugar and carbohydrate-heavy — a far cry from the excellent nutrition provided by the mother's breast milk full of healthy fats. That's some food for thought to chew on, especially if you have the thrill of bringing a baby into your home or will soon be hearing the sweet sound of pitter-patter and the cackle of a happy little one grateful for loving parents. Enjoy that precious gift that God has given to you, but be aware that the food companies don't care if they are addicting your kids to sugar or not. As long as they are making a buck, they don't care what happens to your baby. Sadly, it's the same philosophy they take with adult food, too! You have been fairly warned.

In a September 2006 report by the Institute of Medicine's Committee on Progress in Preventing Childhood Obesity entitled "Progress in Preventing Childhood Obesity: How Do We Measure Up?," the panel looked at childhood obesity to see if any progress had been made over the previous two years regarding turning the tide of weight increases in children as the trend had been. What they found is that the problem is getting worse despite attempts on the federal government level to implement pro-active ways to combat it.

One of the key findings of the IOM panel was that one out of every five children in the United States will likely become obese by the year 2010. Because of this, the experts at IOM who participated in this report lament the seeming lack of financial backing for programs that have been implemented to help combat childhood obesity.

Lead panelist Dr. Jeffrey P. Koplan, former U.S. Centers for Disease Control (CDC) director, chairman of the IOM Committee on Progress in Preventing Childhood Obesity and the current vice president of Academic Health Affairs at Woodruff Health Sciences Center at the Atlanta-based Emory University, said he was encouraged by the number of initiatives that have been sprouting up in pockets across the country to help reduce childhood obesity, but admits they still don't know which programs are working the best to help kids lose weight and get healthy.

Dr. Koplan added that a task force was needed to determine the best methods for bringing about the necessary changes that need to happen and that national health leaders need to step up to the plate to help with this "major health problem."

"Is this as important as stockpiling antibiotics or buying vaccines? I think it is," Dr. Koplan exclaimed. *"It's of a different nature than acute infectious threats, but it needs to be taken just as seriously."*

Absolutely, Dr. Koplan! But why do we expect childhood obesity rates to change when the same old dietary recommendations that have been used for the past three decades have remained unchanged? There are many reasons why childhood obesity has not gotten any better, not the least of which is our government's lack of acknowledging that we have a problem in the first place. However, even if they do fess up to the fact that our kids are getting fatter and fatter, all we get from our government are gimmicks like the Kid's Food Pyramid that doesn't translate into sound nutritional advice for children to adhere to. Kids these days are bombarded with junk food ads but it is the parents who need to take ownership of this problem by becoming responsible for their children's eating and fitness routine.

Dr. Koplan is right to be concerned about the issue of childhood obesity because he knows the problems that lie ahead for those children who cannot manage their weight heading into adulthood. This is extremely serious business and real changes need to be implemented as soon as possible. But throwing more money at the problem isn't gonna help. I disagree with Dr. Koplan on this point because pumping more tax dollars into programs that are dubious at best will do nothing but waste the funds that are supposed to be helping educate kids about proper nutrition and fitness. Pointing fingers at budget cuts certainly does not address the root cause of the problem either.

This issue reminds me of the subject of education spending. People get in such a tizzy when you talk about cutting funding for schools and education. But you can't do that, it's for our children, they say. Yes, it is for the children which is important, but there are ways to better maximize the use of those funds in a manner that will produce better results with less burden on the taxpayers. And the same goes for childhood obesity. Increasing the budget for programs like VERB, a $59 million government marketing campaign created in 2005 to make exercise look "cool" to tweens, is unrealistic to sustain over the long-term without a measureable difference seen in childhood obesity rates. Nevertheless, the IOM panel said the withdrawal of funding for VERB shows the lack of "commitment to obesity prevention within government."

Oh please, no it doesn't. It simply means the government wants to get more bang for their buck with the tax dollars spent on such programs and they didn't see that happening with this particular one. If childhood obesity was cut in half because of VERB, then you had better believe they'd be lined up with the funding quicker than you could say "rockin' results!" But Dr. Koplan contends that the VERB program was working well enough and that the funding was pulled from it prematurely. Now, the CDC is urging state and local governments to take the lessons learned from VERB to apply in every area of the country to see if childhood obesity rates can come down any at all. There is also a school snack program where they were pushing more fruits and vegetables that was implemented in 14 states, but again there was whining from the bureaucrats that there just isn't enough money to get the word out.

If the people who truly cared about childhood obesity would simply stop their bellyaching just long enough to realize how ignorant they sound asking for more money to address a problem they themselves admit they don't know the answer to, then perhaps they would start to see there are viable and effective solutions to help curb childhood obesity that exist right under their noses. Here are just a few of my proposed suggestions:

1. Parents need to stop turning a blind eye to their child's obesity problem. This is an issue that needs to be addressed by the mother and father of that obese child, even if it means they need to do something about their own weight problem as well.

2. We need to stop fooling kids into thinking they have to eat a low-fat diet to be healthy. With all the negative effects that sugar and refined carbohydrates have on our bodies, it's certainly not a bad idea to get children used to eating a controlled-carb diet with nutritious meals loaded with essential nutrients their growing bodies need without the excessive amounts of sugar, high fructose corn syrup and just plain junk food that they are stuffing in their mouths these days.

3. While many believe a 100 percent obesity rate is inevitable In America, it doesn't have to be if each individual family unit does what it has to do to bring about lifestyle changes that need to happen within themselves. Why wait on a government education program to tell your kid how to eat and exercise right when you can do it right now?!

This most certainly isn't the end of this discussion about childhood obesity, but rather a good starting point that government and health leaders in the United States should be focusing their attention on rather than the next great "cool" ad campaign. Please stop bemoaning about how things aren't changing quickly enough and start looking at why the advice we've been spoon-fed for generations has been such a miserable bust! This is the coveted answer to the childhood obesity crisis that could be reversed in very short order if we would enact meaningful changes like the ones I have suggested in this chapter. I remain hopeful, but realize the chances of this happening anytime soon are slim to none.

Recently McDonald's Corp. agreed to make the $2 million donation to fund childhood obesity and diabetes research in 2006. No, I'm not kidding, they really did donate money to look into why kids are getting chubby. Obviously feeling the public pressure regarding their high-carb, junk food offerings, McDonald's decided it was time to partner up with biomedical scientists at the California-based Scripps Institute for the first time in their company's history to look into ways to curb childhood obesity rates.

McDonald's President and Chief Operating Officer Ralph Alvarez said it is the goal of McDonald's to "make a difference in the lives of children."

"The collaboration with Scripps Research is an extension of McDonald's long-standing commitment to the well-being of children around the world," he said. "Everything that we keep on seeing is the whole issue of childhood obesity and the early onset of Type 2 diabetes has grown exponentially. We felt we needed to get greater education in this area."

Am I the only one who sees the incredible irony in this? Here we have the head of the #1 fast food company in the entire world talking about how much his company cares about the health of kids while at the same time they are aggressively marketing products directly to children that are arguably one of the root causes of the childhood obesity epidemic. The fact that they threw a few pennies of their hundreds of billions of dollars in sales at obesity research does not get them off the hook from their culpability in the debate over rising childhood obesity. They hope it does, but it very clearly does not.

Fried junk food consumption has doubled among kids and another study showed that eating fast food makes you one-third fatter. Anyone who denies the contributing role of fast food in the current childhood obesity epidemic is either ignorant to the facts staring them in the face or they are simply protecting the financial interests of an industry that has a lot of explaining to do. Meanwhile, McDonald's is working overtime trying to come across as a caring company when it comes to healthy living by doing such meaningless gestures as removing the "Super Size" from the menu and showing an "active" Ronald McDonald playing sports in their television ads.

You will have to do better than that if you're going to convince people like me that you are really serious about improving the health and weight of the children you claim to care so much about. Ever since documentary filmmaker Morgan Spurlock released his *Super Size Me* movie about McDonald's in

2004, the company with the golden arches has been on a mission to convince the public that their food can be a part of a healthy diet. We've seen people go on a McDiet to show how you can lose weight eating at Mickey D's, too, including comedian Tom Naughton in his 2009 documentary film entitled *FAT HEAD* (FatHead-Movie.com) demonstrating how you can eat healthy even at fast food restaurants. While I don't think fast food is solely to blame for rising obesity, their unique role in marketing this garbage food cannot be overlooked. If that's being too hard on McDonald's, then that's their problem because it's the truth!

So what does Alvarez think about the irony of McDonald's supporting scientific research into childhood obesity when most people universally agree that they are part of the problem?

"Ironic or not we're going to make a difference," he said in a Reuters story. "You won't see those benefits short-term, in one to three years, because habits change over time. But as a major restaurant company, we need to be on the cutting-edge of what's happening."

Okay, so McDonald's gives a little bit of money to childhood obesity research — now what? What is going to change at the restaurant level, Mr. Alvarez? Anything? Sure, you come up with high-sugar Apple Dippers that are about as unhealthy as everything else on your menu. But don't you market them as one of your healthy new products? Where's the integrity in that? Is that really all McDonald's can do is push some high-carb, low-fat products and think they're helping improve the health of children?

McDonald's certainly has the right to sell whatever they deem necessary to turn a profit, but what are the logical consequences of continually feeding that market with more and more junk year after year? Obesity rates will just keep going through the roof with no end in sight. But McDonald's can proudly say they donated $2 million to childhood obesity and diabetes research, can't they? What good does that do when people are still getting obese and unhealthy eating their foods?

We need better education for children about what is causing them and their parents to get so fat. Wake up America! We don't need to be eating fast food as part of our healthy lifestyle changes. We are partially to blame, too, because we keep subsidizing this garbage that companies like McDonald's are serving daily. It's not the fat in the foods we are eating, but the excessive amounts of refined carbohydrates, starchy vegetables, white flour, and most of all SUGAR! Ironically, all of these things are very prevalent in the foods at McDonald's. How does someone like Alvarez keep a clear conscious about what his company is doing to children and adults while spouting off the company line that McDonald's cares about the kids? That's just a big load of corporate crap and he knows it!

The ultimate responsibility about what children are eating still falls on the parents and they need to practice restraint even when their children beg and plead to go to McDonald's. Trust me, when they get older and have a healthy body because of your wise decision to avoid McDonald's as much as possible, they will thank you for it. Maybe if my mom had skipped taking us kids to McDonald's so much, then maybe we wouldn't have all ballooned into the morbidly obese adults that we all became. These are the unintended consequences of the existence of companies like McDonald's. Whether they give $2 million, $20 million, or $200 million to childhood obesity research, nothing is going to change the fact that they are one of the primary reasons obesity is as bad as it is today. Call me whatever you want for saying that, but I challenge anyone to tell me it isn't true.

Oh, but we should herald that bastion of nutritional and fitness goodness known as McDonald's for offering kids and parents the very best food money can buy for a healthy lifestyle such as Big Macs, French fries, Coca-Cola, chocolate milkshakes, Chicken McNuggets, and so much more. I can't believe we have such an out-of-control obesity epidemic in this country with such a strong example coming from the Golden Arches!

You know I'm kidding, right?

But that's the EXACTLY the kind of image I believe the corporate executives in the upper echelons of the McDonald's empire want people to have in their minds when they think about the world's #1 fast food restaurant chain. They seem to have been have been working very diligently to shape and mold themselves as a company that t truly cares about the overall health and well-being of its customer base. That's like a drug dealer putting a filter on that marijuana cigarette he sells you to make it "better" for you. It's superficial change at best that still results in damage to your health. Nevertheless, McDonald's has certainly been trying to convince the public that they have seen the error in their ways and are ready to make things right.

Now we can add another element to the rebuilding of the McDonald's image with the introduction of their new "R Gym" concept in December 2006. The days of kids playing around in a public pool of balls and crawling around in tubes like lab rats are numbered as a new generation of children will have a full workout activity room to climb a rock wall, ride on a stationary bike hooked up to a video game, and shoot some hoops — all while dining at McDonald's! The popular restaurant chain is dead serious about this and has already added an "R Gym" to selected units in California, Oklahoma, Colorado and Illinois. They hope to open many more in other states in the coming years based on the positive feedback they have been receiving from customers about the improved exercise facilities for kids.

Bill Whitman, a McDonald's spokesman said the company has every intention of expanding the "R Gym" concept as long as there is a "benefit in it."

"We have for many years supported programs that promote physical activity, and we will continue to do that," he said.

While it is admirable that a company like McDonald's supports exercise as part of their business model, Mr. Whitman, there's only one problem with your company's position. You assume that weight gain is only prevented through the implementation of physical activity and has nothing at all to do with a child's diet. Am I the only one who notices this glaring factual omission?

Perhaps McDonald's should rethink some of those menu items they believe are good for kids and adults to eat. Having a fun and exciting place like the "R Gym" for kids to look forward to when they visit McDonald's is a great way to market your food. With this knowledge, how about offering some menu items that children and adults can not only enjoy eating, but are also good for them as well, McDonald's? Company spokeswoman Jennifer Smith believes they are already doing that with such menu items as low-fat milk and yogurt, for example.

"The R-Gym is just another example of McDonald's dedication to helping customers live balanced, active lifestyles," she said.

These people just don't get it, do they? We don't need to remove the fat out of everything McDonald's sells to make the food healthy. How about offering some low-carb and/or sugar-free options as well to reach a broader base of health-conscious consumers who have children with insulin resistance, celiac disease or diabetes? Why does McDonald's refuse to cater to this segment of their customer base?

Here are just a very few low-carb suggestions I have off the top of my head:

1. Grilled chicken strips with green beans and a side salad
2. Hamburger steak and onions with cauliflower and a side salad
3. Breakfast bowl with eggs, bacon, sausage, and cheese
4. Sugar-free ice cream or cheesecake with berries
5. Ham or turkey w/cheese in low-carb wraps

These are very simple and deliciously healthy additions to the menu at McDonald's that would attract people like me and others who support livin' la vida low-carb. Why must we be subjected to the Dr. Dean Ornish-approved low-fat specialty salads that contain gobs of sugar or apple dippers that feature high-fructose corn syrup in the caramel dipping sauce as the "healthy" options at McDonald's? Fixing these major menu problems would go a lot further in showing the public that you mean business when it comes to tackling childhood obesity.

Upon hearing about this new concept at McDonald's, the "R Gym" may sound like a good idea because it encourages kids of all ages — with sections for toddlers, elementary school aged, and pre-teens — to move their bodies and shake off those calories they just consumed. But how many parents are actually going to just sit around inside of McDonald's for hours on end while their kids use the "R Gym?" Not many, which doesn't give kids much time to use these facilities in a meaningful way to burn very many calories. I can see the following scenario playing out now:

Johnny finishes his meal and goes to play in the "R Gym."
(Five minutes later)
MOM: *"Johnny, drop the basketball it's time to go."*
JOHNNY: *"Aw, mom, can't I keep playing, this is so much fun."*
MOM: *"Did you eat all of your 9-piece Chicken McNuggets and fries?"*
JOHNNY: *"Yes, ma'am, and I even drank every drop of my large Coke, too!"*
MOM: *"That's good, but we need to go now. We'll be back again soon."*
JOHNNY: *"Oh, alright. Can I get the Big Mac meal next time?"*
MOM: *"Of course, honey, because you'll play it off in the 'R Gym!'"*

JOHNNY: *"Yeeaaaah! I just LOVE McDonald's!"*

You may be laughing at my fictitious interaction between a mother and her child, but somebody tell me that's not exactly what is going to play out in the real world concerning these "R Gym" facilities. Even worse is the fact that kids will start whining and complaining to their parents about going to McDonald's to "play," so moms and dads will rationalize to themselves that eating there is healthy so their kids can get some exercise. Can you see how twisted this marketing ploy by McDonald's has become?

And riddle me this, Batman: McDonald's is not in the business of offering a place for kids to just come hang out and play, are they? No, they're not. Instead, their goal is to make lots of money while addicting their customers to fast food and counting on this addiction to keep them as customers when they reach adulthood. Fast food addiction is very hard to break (I know because I used to visit McDonald's and other fast food restaurants more than five times a week!). But it is possible to lose your desire for those disgusting carb-loaded foods if you simply refuse to settle for putting junk like this into your body ever again. Believe me when I say it is so much more pleasurable to eat healthy than it is to eat fast food. Give it up for 30 days and start eating real food for once and you'll see exactly what I mean.

As healthy as McDonald's is trying to make their restaurants appear to the consumer, the fact is they still peddle garbage food. Nobody will ever argue this point because it is a universal truth that everyone already agrees with. In other words, just because McDonald's has come up with the "R Gym," that is no reason to start bowing down to them as a great example of how to combat the growing obesity problem. They still have a long way to go. Case in point comes from an *Orange County Register* column that shared about the opening of one of these "R Gym" facilities at a local McDonald's there. In the middle of the story, you will see the following shocking announcement about the opening of the "R Gym" facility:

"The McDonald's at 1526 W. Edinger Ave. in Santa Ana is celebrating the debut of the R Gym, as well as the restaurant's remodel, at 11 a.m. today. Ronald McDonald will be giving out free cookies and balloons."

Yep, you read that right: Ronald McDonald is giving out sugary cookies — oh joy! Gee, that's really healthy, isn't it? It's the irony of all ironies — opening a kid's mini-gym and celebrating that by giving out free cookies. Ugh! And we wonder why childhood obesity lingers!

My wife Christine and I are really big fans of DreamWorks' *Shrek* movies. We think Mike Myers and Eddie Murphy are a hilarious comedy duo and the computer animation in these movies is simply spectacular. DreamWorks has been able to bankroll the rest of their entire lineup of films just with the profits they've made from the *Shrek* machine. Because of the very high marketability of the lovable characters from the movie, particularly Shrek and Donkey, all sorts of companies have lined up to use them in a cross-promotional effort to push their products. I was watching television last year and noticed they put some well known candy cartoon characters together with Shrek and Donkey in a 30-second spot. It was a cute commercial despite the high-sugar product that was being peddled.

When *Shrek The Third* was released in May 2007, promotions for foods like candy, soda, sugary cereal, toaster pastries, cheese crackers, cookies and even a fast food meal. With all this high-carb garbage being recommended by Shrek and his pals, it was more than a bit unusual to read about another surprising "product" Shrek was asked to represent — EXERCISE! This was not a joke!

Sponsored by the U.S. Department of Health and Human Services, the Small Step Kids campaign had Shrek with his big chubby face and body jumping up and down. There was also Donkey's Jumping Jacks, Fiona's Sit Ups, Puss In Boots Push Ups, Hopping With Gingy (the Gingerbread Man!), and The Running Of The Pigs. All of this is supposed to encourage kids to get in one hour of exercise daily. Hmmm.

Let me just say that I can appreciate the good intentions of this government-endorsed *Shrek* promotion of exercise. But you can't help but think about how confusing this must be to little Johnny or Jane who sees their favorite movie characters eating foods like junky kids meals from fast food places, sugary cereals and candy and then those same character encouraging exercise.

So which is it, Shrek? Healthy or unhealthy habits?

Well, I'm not alone in my concerns. A group called The Campaign for a Commercial-Free Childhood (CommercialExploitation.org) said these close ties between Shrek and the unhealthy foods makes the popular animated character a poor choice to represent exercise. They even organized a petition drive to then-Health and Human Services Secretary Mike Leavitt for him to "Fire Shrek" and to "start getting serious about combating childhood obesity." Commercial-Free Childhood campaign director Susan Linn, a psychiatry professor at Harvard, wrote a letter to Secretary Leavitt in May 2007 stating the use of Shrek in their exercise promotion to kids demonstrates "an inherent conflict of interest between marketing junk food and promoting public health."

"Surely Health and Human Services can find a better spokesperson for healthy living than a character who is a walking advertisement for McDonald's, sugary cereals, cookies and candy," she exclaimed.

But Health and Human Services spokesperson Bill Hall said at the time that the Shrek promotion had been underway for several months and that nothing was going to change. The public service announcement television ads were also a part of the efforts by the Ad Council's Coalition for Healthy Children. In fact, Hall said there was nothing at all wrong with using Shrek in these ads.

"Shrek is a very well known character in the target population of this campaign," he remarked. "We have always promoted a balanced, healthy diet, which does not necessarily exclude the occasional treat."

Occasional treat, Mr. Hall? Of ALL of those foods promoted by Shrek, guess how many of them are NOT loaded with sugar, sugar, and more sugar? Just one — the Cheez-Its — but even that product has so much flour in it that the carbs turn into sugar in your body which then leads to such an insulin release that obesity and disease are soon to follow. To purport that a "balanced, healthy diet" includes these products is naive.

You and I both know that kids eat these foods as their primary source of energy, not as the "occasional treat." When they see Shrek on the television or on the packaging of these food products, children immediately start screaming "Mommy, Mommy, I've got to have the Shrek cereal and toaster pastries! Please, please, please?!!" Of course, that's what marketing is supposed to do and the parents give in. Welcome to modern day capitalism!

If the Shrek endorsement of these products only brought about a nominal increase in sales, then they wouldn't use that character again in future ads. But the fact is Shrek is very influential on young impressionable minds, which is why Linn says the conflicting messages about healthy living is confusing to little kids who idolize and trust whatever their favorite movie star tells them.

"Why would young children follow Shrek's advice about healthy living and ignore his entreaties to eat Happy Meals and Pop-Tarts?" she wrote in her letter. "If government agencies are serious about combating childhood obesity, they should stop cozying up to industry and start taking real steps to end the barrage of junk food marketing aimed at children."

I don't personally have an issue with using Shrek to promote healthy choices such as exercising for an hour a day. That's excellent advice in this generation of video games, computers, and other non-physical activities that our children are engaging in. But it should not be used in conjunction with these other ads promoting junk foods. That is where the conflict of interest arises. But don't tell that to the then-Health and Human Services deputy assistant secretary.

"Shrek is a good model, especially for children who can benefit from more exercise," then-Deputy Assistant Secretary Penelope Royall responded. "He doesn't have a perfect physique, he's not a great athlete. We hope children will understand that being physically fit doesn't require being a great athlete."

Yep, you read that right. Royall said Shrek is a "good model" for healthy activity and living. The character stuffs his mouth nonstop with all kinds of nasty stuff while his big ole belly and butt hang out like some kind of tumor. It's what makes Shrek the character funny, but most definitely not a role model for children when it comes to health. Royall said the purpose of the ads was to get children to exercise, not eat right.

But how can you promote health by pushing activity and not diet, Ms. Royall? That's a strange way to combat childhood obesity if that is indeed your goal with this ad campaign. The best approach would be two-pronged — promote healthy nutrient-dense foods along with moderate and fun activities that will get their heart rates up and burn calories.

DreamWorks said they just want to be "responsible marketers" in all of this with their *Shrek* brand. Well, you've failed miserably at that and the almighty dollar seems to supersede all your good intentions. If you had Shrek promoting sugar-free chocolates or eggs, then perhaps you could be seen as more "responsible" — but not now. And McDonald's once again is put right smack dab in the middle of this debate, too.

When is the craziness gonna end with these cross-promotions between block-buster films aimed at children and fast food restaurants? We wonder why childhood obesity isn't getting any better and yet we continue to see such blatant abuse of the love and trust kids have in these characters they see on the silver screen. Prior to the movie release in May 2007, McDonald's teamed up with DreamWorks to use the Shrek character to try to promote "healthy" kids meals to encourage children to eat better. So an ogre who eats anything and everything in sight wants kids to do as he says not as he does. I see.

The Shrek Happy Meal gave the following "healthy" food choices for children — Chicken McNuggets (breaded and packed with carbohydrates), Apple Dippers with Caramel Dipping Sauce (as if the sugar from the apples wasn't bad enough, you have to give them a high-fructose corn syrup dip, too — oh yeah, it's LOW-FAT!), low-fat milk (um, that's not exactly healthy for you, I hate to break it to the head honchos at Mickey D's!) and a Shrek toy (well, at least SOMETHING is carb-free). The worst part of all is McDonald's thumped its chest at how responsible they were to offer such "healthy" options for their young customers when they did no such thing. Of course, they played it up by claiming their Shrek marketing strategy was the "single biggest global promotion" of fruits, vegetables, and low-fat milk in the company's history.

You've GOT to be kidding me!

McDonalds has yet to cater to the low-carber on their menu while they've followed the nutritional advice of people like Dr. Dean Ornish. Even HE told me in a podcast interview with him that they should be doing more. Why is that, McDonald's? What's wrong with putting even a few token "low-carb" items on your menu so that we can find something healthy to eat when we are on the road? Grilled chicken nuggets, blueberries and cream, sugar-free low-carb cookies, anything! Do you even care about having people who eat low-carb as customers?

Nevertheless, marketing promotions like the one with Shrek remain to give kids "choices." Sigh. While Shrek may be telling kids to "Go for Green," I have a feeling they'll keep on going for carbs instead. A 2007 American Diabetes Association dietary trends report for children ages 2-19 years found the following vegetable consumption among kids (don't pass out when you see this!):

Fried potatoes — 46%
Others — 22%

Other potatoes — 10%
Tomatoes — 9%
Dark green/orange — 7%
Legumes/beans — 6%

Almost two-thirds of the "healthy" vegetable consumption by the future of our society is made up of potatoes. SAY WHAT?! These extremely starchy, carb-loaded foods are as harmful to your child's weight and health as eating table sugar by the spoonful! Carbs, carbs, and more carbs. Can you see how the McDonald's culture has so gripped our nation's youth that nearly half of their vegetable intake is from French fries? Yikeseroo! And this is what I'm talking about when I say it's a copout to generically say "eat your fruits and vegetables." Without a qualifying statement to explain what you mean, then it is not necessarily a good thing and the resulting action is kids eat more of the poor choices instead.

In fact, I think it should be criminal to make the claim that a potato is even a vegetable. Here's the truth about potatoes — it's poison for your blood sugar! You don't need it, you'll never need it, and you won't miss having it. Trust me on this, you won't. And this isn't just an American problem either as McDonald's took their Shrek campaign to over 100 nations worldwide. So, by all means go watch Shrek, Donkey, The Gingerbread Man, Puss in Boots, and Fiona in their magical tales on the silver screen. But tell your kids about what healthy eating is really about by celebrating with a meal fit for a low-carb king. But it's not gonna be found at McDonald's, I can assure you of that.

I don't really like talking about politics within the context of my health and weight loss writings, but sometimes these two worlds inevitably collide. In 2006, five of the top junk food vending machine companies — PepsiCo, Mars Inc., Kraft Foods Inc., Campbell Soup Co. and Dannon Co. — vowed to take their high-carb, high-fat products out of the schools in favor of "healthier products" (we'll get into what that means in a moment). The voluntary agreement was made possible by the ever-present elder statesman himself, former President Bill Clinton, along with the American Heart Association (AHA). They wanted to help make the nutritional choices for kids better while they are in school because many blame these foods on the rise in childhood obesity rates.

But if any politician is sincerely interested in helping protect kids from the junk food that entices them, why not get Congress to pass a law to make it mandatory to ban these from schools? If they really want these junk foods out of schools, then make it a requirement with a law. That would certainly add more teeth to the argument that you care about improving the health of children if you think the presence of junk food is the culprit.

Gary Ruskin from the non-profit childhood obesity education group Commercial Alert (CommercialAlert.org) had a rather terse response for Clinton questioning the "healthy alternatives" that will be allegedly offered as well as what's in this deal for the former president.

"Who is Bill Clinton kidding? Baked potato chips and sweetened bars are not substitutes for apples and carrots, beans and greens," Ruskin exclaimed. "Has the Clinton Foundation received any contributions from any of the companies that are a party to this agreement? How about the American Heart Association?"

This isn't the first time Clinton and the AHA have come together in a similar arrangement regarding junk food in schools. In early 2006, they got the Coca-Cola Co., PepsiCo and Cadbury Schweppes PLC to stop selling non-diet soft drinks in schools since so many kids were chug-a-lugging on sugary sodas during the daytime. Now they will be guzzling sugary pseudo-fruit juices and energy drinks instead. Like I said where are the meaningful changes?

I remember those snack food machines and the vendors during lunch when I was in high school in the mid-to-late 1980s and never gave a second thought about the nutritional value of what I was eating. If it tasted good and I wanted it, then I bought it. Of course, that may explain how I eventually got to be 400+ pounds as an adult, too. While I like the idea of giving kids a choice of better food options while at school, this agreement does not stop kids from going by their local corner convenience store on the way to or on the way home from school. It's like banning the sale of drugs on school grounds. That's all well and good until the students step off of school property and is on the streets. At that point, all bets are off and the net result is the same as it was before.

An agreement like this one from Clinton and the AHA is like having a non-smoking section in a restaurant that allows smokers to puff away without the use of a ventilation system. You can ban smoking all you want in the nonsmoking section, but you and I both know that doesn't keep the smoke from traveling into that section, thus rendering the distinction between the two sections completely irrelevant.

Okay, let's just pretend for a moment that these changes WILL make a difference. What are they asking these companies to alter about their products to make them "healthier?" Here are the new criteria for allowable foods sold at schools under the agreement:

1. Calories from fat limited to 35 percent
2. Calories from saturated fat limited to 10 percent
3. Sugar by weight is limited to 10 percent
4. Sodium is limited to 480mg, except for soup

Again we see the continuing ramifications of how scared people are of fat and even saturated fat. While it is noble they are limiting sugar to 10 percent by weight, that's still not doing anything about the excessive carbohydrates that many of these products contain which then turn into sugar when it is absorbed by the body. As for salt, it is mostly a non-issue except for those who are salt-sensitive.

Even low-fat diet advocate Dr. Dean Ornish said in my interview with him that he doesn't like the influx of low-fat and fat-free snack food products because they are still not healthy choices for people to consume.

"People are going out and eating the Snackwell cookies and the fat-free desserts and cakes that may be very low in fat, but very high in sugar — I've never recommended that which is why I've been more explicit in clarifying that," Ornish said during the podcast interview.

Despite all of this, data has been collected by the AHA and the Clinton Foundation to measure the impact of these changes through 2010. Again, any changes will be minimal at best until we get a better handle on what is causing obesity — namely the excessive consumption of carbohydrates, including those found in low-fat products like baked potato chips, pretzels, 10% fruit juices, and so much more. Selling these as "healthy" foods is wrong. Now the junk food companies involved in this agreement are going to begin "taking steps to make snacks more nutritious."

What do we have to look forward to? How about low-fat, whole wheat Twinkies sweetened with aspartame in them? Or perhaps we'll see, as one of my readers shared with me, vendor sandwiches made with Wonder Bread, anti-bacterial-sprayed bologna slices, and eggless Miracle Whip? Who are we kidding? Kids won't go for this stuff unless they are educated better about why they shouldn't eat the junk food.

We're stuck in a nutritional abyss nowadays and there doesn't seem to be an easy way out of it. Childhood obesity can be prevented, but that won't happen until some major barriers are torn down for good — namely that eating fat is bad for you, eating excessive carbohydrates is good for you, and that there are no consequences to eating junk food. All of these so-called axioms in our society are as WRONG as wrong can be. We must continue to share with others the truth.

We've always heard that kids need to get ample exercise to ward off obesity, but what if that bit of conventional wisdom was dead wrong? In a study published in the October 2006 issue of the *British Medical Journal*, lead researcher Dr. John J. Reilly from the Division of Developmental Medicine at the University of Glasgow along with his fellow researchers wanted to look at the effectiveness of physical activity on the prevention of childhood obesity in a randomized controlled trial. Specifically, they were looking at the reduction in the body mass index (BMI) of preschool-age children over a one-year period.

The research included 545 children from 36 preschools in Glasgow, Scotland with a mean age of 4.2 years old when the study began. They were required to participate in three 30-minute exercise sessions each week in the first six months of the study as well as health education courses in the home to foster increased physical activity among the young study participants outside of school rather than doing such slothful activities such as watching television, playing video games, or any other non-exercise activities. While the primary focus of the study was on BMI, Dr. Reilly also wanted to see how much exercise the children got versus their sedentary behavior and whether that made any measurable difference.

The results? No significant effect was made on BMI after six months and twelve months! The control group and study group were virtually the same with a standard deviation score for BMI at 0.46 after six month and 0.41 after twelve months. The control group BMI was exactly the same at 0.43 after six and twelve months. However, one difference seen was the kids who had increased exercise did have significantly better motor skills than their control counterparts when adjusted for sex and baseline performance. As a result, Dr. Reilly and his researchers concluded that physical activity is not a factor in weight loss among children. They stated that perhaps other changes are necessary to turn the tide of obesity among young children.

"Successful interventions to prevent obesity in early childhood may require changes not just at nursery, school, and home but in the wider environment," the researchers found. *"Changes in other behaviors, including diet, may also be necessary."*

So all the talk about kids needing to sneak in more exercise has been just a smokescreen to avoid dealing with the real culprit in childhood obesity — a poor diet! This study by Dr. Reilly clearly shows exercise alone is not the answer and that it must be in correlation with other changes, including what we are feeding kids. Whether people realize it or not, this is a very serious issue that has potentially lethal consequences for overweight and obese children when they mature into adulthood. Fat babies make fat adults and there's no getting around that fact. If we can stop the obesity epidemic while children are still young, then a lot of the health problems that are plaguing the adult population today can be avoided.

But the changes in diet have to make good nutritional sense for our children as well. Kids these days are eating way too much sugar and other refined carbohydrates for their bodies to use for energy. Considering the state of childhood obesity is where it is today, it may not be a bad idea for parents to start looking at the low-carb lifestyle for their children and themselves for that matter. It's certainly something worth a closer look in light of the failure of what we are doing right now. Clearly, something is not working, so making measureable and meaningful changes in the diet we are feeding our kids is sorely needed. Your children can exercise to their heart's content and that's a good thing — a very good thing! But if you keep feeding your family garbage foods that are doing nothing to add value to their health, then all that exercise is negated.

Of course, critics of Dr. Reilly's study will claim the children did not get the 30-minutes-a-day minimum amount of moderate-to-vigorous physical activity recommended recently by the American Heart Association. But it may not make a difference if they're still eating all those high-carb, high-sugar foods that tend to plague our diet in modern times. Incidentally, the study was paid for by the British Heart Foundation, the Glasgow City Council, and the Caledonian Research Foundation.

Although the late, great Dr. Robert C. Atkins is no longer with us, his work is still making a huge impact on the most important health issues of the day — including childhood obesity. In an official presentation at the 2007 California Childhood Obesity Conference in Anaheim, CA, The Dr. Robert C. and Veronica Atkins Foundation (AtkinsFoundation.org) agreed to pledge $10 million to the Center for Weight and Health at the University of California-Berkeley for research into eradicating childhood obesity. The center's co-founder Pat Crawford, who is also co-director of the center, Cooperative Extension Nutrition Specialist in the Department of Nutritional Sciences, and Adjunct Professor in the School of Public Health and Department of Nutritional Sciences and Toxicology, was thrilled by the donation from the widow of Dr. Atkins and agreed to rename the center the Dr. Robert C. and Veronica Atkins Center for Weight and Health (cnr.berkeley.edu/cwh) as a small gesture of her appreciation for the much-needed funds.

"What distinguishes our center is our focus on the prevention of pediatric obesity, and we are so grateful that the Atkins Foundation is supportive of that," she said. *"With this pledge, we'll be able to continue the important work we've been doing to help reverse the troubling epidemic of childhood obesity in this country."*

Stephen M. Shortell, who serves as dean of the School of Public Health, said the timing of this pledge could not have been better to continue on the legacy of Dr. Atkins and the center for the "generations" to come.

"The Atkins Foundation support will significantly strengthen our ability to solve one of the nation's most intractable problems — the growing percentage of Americans who are overweight and obese," he said. *"The foundation's commitment means that we will be able to touch thousands more lives with our interdisciplinary research and teaching that ranges from basic science research to community-wide interventions."*

Veronica Atkins has been quite the philanthropist since her husband's passing providing funding to solid nutritional research that furthers the cause that Dr. Atkins was pursuing — namely eliminating obesity, diabetes, cancer, heart disease and more through the use of sound scientific methodology. Other benefactors of these dollars include The University of Connecticut, The University of Texas-Southwestern, and Dr. Atkins' alma mater at The University of Michigan. While funding alone is not the answer to the childhood obesity problem that plagues our nation, I like the way Mrs. Atkins is being discerning about who gets the money and who doesn't. If the potential recipients are unwilling to even consider the positive benefits of livin' la vida low-carb as the starting point for their research, then it's a sure bet the funding will go elsewhere.

While the Dr. Robert C. and Veronica Atkins Center for Weight and Health does not actually promote or advocate the Atkins low-carb nutritional approach in its research, they are most certainly open to a wide variety of ways for handling the obesity problem from different perspectives customized to the individual. The researchers there are adamant that obesity be examined at every point in the proverbial food chain, including where the food is produced and distributed, how it is handled in the process of bringing it to the market, and the unique role played by the health industry, public education and even the pesky media who has a knack for conveniently leaving out pertinent facts regarding the treatment of obesity.

Right now, there are 30 different ongoing research projects, including a program aimed at poor black children with Type 2 diabetes, the removal of sugary soft drinks from public schools, and the impact of the frequency of meals on the weight of teenage girls. These are the kind of studies that will be funded thanks to the generous donation from Mrs. Atkins.

"The center at UC Berkeley is a tribute to my husband's belief in the power of influencing public health outcomes, particularly in the battle against obesity," Veronica Atkins stated at the obesity conference on Wednesday evening. "On behalf of the Atkins Foundation, I am proud to partner with a center as active and accomplished as Berkeley's, and excited to support the ongoing advances of its outstanding researchers."

Mrs. Atkins was especially drawn to the preventative nature of the research being done at UC Berkeley and how those measures could be clearly explained to the public for easy implementation. In other words, Atkins Foundation executive director Abby Bloch said, it's more than just coming up with a few theories for dealing with obesity, but actually identifying solutions that will have a greater impact over the long-term.

"The researchers at the center are out in the trenches, in the community, working hands-on to help people have healthier lifestyles," she noted. "The commitment of these researchers to this area of research and the translational

application into the community are very much on target with the mission and goal of the foundation."

The center will continue to be funded by $500,000 grants from the College of Natural Resources and the School of Public Health until Veronica Atkins passes away. At that time, the center will inherit her $10 million gift. Lost in the debate over the long-term health benefits of livin' la vida low-carb is the fact that the science is indeed coming proving the veracity of this way of eating. All those people who thumb their nose up at low-carb smugly proclaim that there are no real studies showing low-carb is a healthy diet over the long-term. But because of the generosity of the lovely and gracious Veronica Atkins and the money her husband made from the sales of his books and products, the next 5, 10, and even 20 years should be very exciting to watch as we continue to learn more about how safe and effective the Atkins diet is not just for weight loss, but improving overall health in both children and adults. Ready or not, here it comes!

But a sugar-free grassroots movement has already begun to happen within schools as a result of studies like one that came out of Sweden in 2007. Lead researcher Claude Marcus, professor of Pediatrics at the Stockholm, Sweden-based Karolinska Institute, wanted to see if an across-the-board ban on all sweets, junk food, and sodas in ten area schools would make a difference in the number of overweight children at those schools. These high-carb sugary garbage foods were replaced by high-fiber, lower-fat, low-carb foods. Over a four-year period, the number of overweight or obese 6-10 year old children in the project called STOPP (Stockholm Obesity Prevention Project) dropped markedly from 22 percent down to 16 percent. WOW! That's a full six percentage points simply by removing the sugar option from the foods available at school.

So what happened to the control group that changed nothing? These sugar-eating, high-carb junk food-ingesting children saw the number of overweight or obese children RISE from 18 percent to 21 percent. This is not at all surprising to those of us who are livin' la vida low-carb. The results of Marcus' study were presented at the 15th European Congress on Obesity in Budapest, Hungary in April 2007. STOPP was financed by the Stockholm County Council with contributions from the Swedish Research Council and the Masonic Home for Children in Stockholm. Interestingly, Marcus said his study showed it is indeed possible to tackle childhood obesity without adding any extra expenditure to the existing school budgets.

"Our results show that programs to reduce the increasing rate of obesity can be carried out within the schools' existing budgets," he said.

Sweet! So much for the excuse that serving kids healthy alternatives to junk food is too expensive and unappealing. As long as those "healthy" alternatives have enough fat and protein to make them good for the kids, it shouldn't be a problem economically or nutritionally. That seems to be what this study indicates and the proof is in the astounding results. There was one positive impact that the example from the sugar-free schools had when the children got home.

"We also interpret the results to mean that clear regulations in schools can help parents to set standards for their children and improve dietary habits at home," the study indicated.

What an excellent point! When parents who want to feed their kids the right kind of foods get reinforcement when their children go to school, then they are better able to effectively bring about improvements in their child's health without the fear of being undercut by the peer influences at school. We need something like this to be implemented in the United States — ASAP! And the good news is it is happening in one Georgia school thanks to a brave forward-thinking principal named Dr. Yvonne Sanders-Butler.

Whenever most people hear about the subject of childhood obesity, they tend to get pessimistic about it because they feel the next generation is too far gone to do anything about it. If we simply give up on trying to educate kids about making healthier choices in their diet, then what do you think they'll eat all day? Hamburgers, pizza, candy bars, sugary soda, candy, potato chips, and anything else they can get their hands on. Why? Because they think that's real food and how they are supposed to eat based on what they've been allowed to do for so long.

But what would happen if adults actually took back control of the schools where the parents, administrators, principals, teachers, and educational staff decided to lay down the law and set rules that the kids would have to abide by in terms of their diet? For example, what if one of the mandates was to ban all sugary, processed, junk food from being served on campus? Well, we don't have to wonder about that because it's been happening at an elementary school in Lithonia, Georgia since 1998.

Browns Mill Elementary School is currently leading the way as one of the only schools in America where the children do not participate in any school fundraiser bake sales, do not celebrate birthdays of their classmates with cup-cakes, and never get served cookies or ice cream in the cafeteria or anything like that. Why? Because sugar is not allowed at the school! That's right — Browns Mill Elementary School is what they call "a Sugar Free Zone." All soda and junk food vending machines have been long removed from school grounds and the cafeteria only serves real food like broccoli (the most popular veg-gie) and peaches for dessert. This cutting-edge concept was the brainchild of Dr. Sanders-Butler. She has the only sugar-free school in America and has been lauded for her visionary tactic for dealing with the problem of childhood obesity for more than a decade.

"We have received many positive phone calls, letters, and emails from across the country applauding the children, parents and Browns Mill Staff for do-ing such an outstanding job of keeping our school environment free of foods laden with sugar," Dr. Sanders-Butler writes on the school web site at www. dekalb.k12.ga.us/brownsmill.

It's a simple measure to take, but only Browns Mill has been willing to enact it school-wide...and with AMAZING results! Describing childhood obesity as "our [Hurricane] Katrina," Dr. Sanders-Butler says she dismisses any criticism people may have for her about this decision to make Browns Mill Elementary School sugar-free because the children are worth teaching something invalu-able that will benefit them long after they reach adulthood.

"If we're really thinking about the best interests about the young people today, then we will take a stand," she noted.

In addition to the sugar-free food policy, the kids at the school also engage in one hour of cardiovascular exercise disguised as play. From jumping jacks to just dancing around to some hip-hop music, the school gets the blood pump-ing early.

"When students are healthy, they do their best work," Dr. Sanders-Butler ex-plained. "We want to make sure we're providing foods that will not only nourish the body, but also brain foods."

They follow the nutritional guidelines provided by the United States Depart-ment of Agriculture (USDA) as found in the U.S. Food Pyramid. Although you know how I feel about the low-fat, high-carb Food Pyramid for kids, I think it's better to have children eating closer to optimum than allowing their diet to be

dominated by junk foods that are full of sugar. And the kids seem to love it —
especially the non-starchy vegetables.

"One of the most requested vegetables now is broccoli," the principal revealed.
"Can you believe that? The kids love broccoli."

The tangible benefits started pouring in quickly after the sugar-free zone was
introduced over a decade ago — disciplinary incidents fell by nearly one-
fourth, counseling referrals dipped 30 percent in just six months, standardized
test scores by which all public schools are measured for their performance
rose 15 percent in the reading category, and Browns Mill Elementary School
was named a national blue ribbon school and a Georgia school of excellence in 2005. Data has not been gathered from the school records by any
researcher yet to determine if obesity rates have fallen, but you would have to
assume they have.

Even if the children resumed consuming sugar when they got home from
school and on weekends, the positive impact of cutting it out for those few
hours during the day had to make some sort of an impact on their weight and
health that could not be ignored by caring parents. Nevertheless, the success
at Browns Mill has encouraged at least 17 other public schools in the state of
Georgia to try to follow their lead. GREAT NEWS!!!

And the long-term effects of the school going sugar-free is still being felt over
ten years later from a junior in college who was in the fifth grade when Dr.
Sanders-Butler implemented this sudden change.

*"I was one of the heavier students in elementary school, so I really lost a lot
of weight and just became healthier overall with the changes,"* confessed former student Simone Davis. *"Kids were hyper, bouncing off the wall and those
things changed."*

This brave decision to go sugar-free was not without controversy for Dr. Sanders-Butler, but she knew it was the right thing to do after battling obesity and
a stroke at the age of 39 years old. And it seems she was way ahead of her
time now that schools all across the country are removing vending and soda
machines and replacing them with better alternatives. The most effective part
of the sugar-free program at Browns Mill Elementary School today is probably
peer pressure. Think about all the kids who have gone before in this environment where sugar is not allowed. The new children don't know any different

and just believe that's the way things are supposed to be. So they willingly choose to eat fruit instead of chocolate cake. See how quickly the paradigm can shift if the environment is changed to create healthier choices?

One kid said it best: *"Junk food makes my stomach hurt."* This is awesome! I publicly applaud Dr. Yvonne Sanders-Butler and her staff at Browns Mill Elementary School in Lithonia, Georgia. Bravo on a job well done! Keep up the GREAT work and I look forward to seeing more incredible results from this idea of cutting sugar out of your school. Who knows, you might just start a national trend that will catch on! We can only hope.

Seeing examples like this encourages me that we can do something constructive to battle childhood obesity in the United States, but then I see studies like one that was published in the March 2009 issue of the *Journal of Happiness Studies*. Have you heard about this one? The researchers attempted to examine the childhood obesity epidemic and wanted to look at the relationship between unhealthy eating and how children feel about themselves. For their study, they looked at how fast food and soda impacted body weight and their happiness level. Not surprisingly, the more fast food and sugary soda the kids ate, the fatter they got. At the same time, though, the kids also got happier.

I guess this begs the question: is it better for kids to be fat and happy than thin and unhappy? And what's to say that these kids couldn't find happiness in eating something healthier than junk foods? One more question — what kind of happiness will those fast food eating kids have about themselves when they grow into morbidly obese adults? Just something to think about and yet more evidence that we still have a long ways to go before we can make a real dent in childhood obesity rates. If we don't do it now, then it may be too late once these kids grow to become adults someday.

And that's exactly what happened to my beloved older brother Kevin who is the subject of the final and I would argue most important lesson of all I have to share with you in this book.

LESSON #21
The early death of a brother or loved one may not be prevented

"The death of a brother or any other close family member can certainly derail or alter one's life journey that one might not even understand. Having just lost my brother, role model, and inspiration for my weight loss, I feel I have lost one of the anchors in my own life. Whether or not it is expected or unexpected, the loss has an impact; however, realize this loss is only temporary. If you believe in a higher power and life after death as I do, then you realize you can indeed see your loved one again. The challenge is therefore for the living to use any regrets or remorse over past actions or actions never taken as fuel to improve one's relations with those still around you. You can't change the past or bring back the loved one, but you can definitely change the future and ensure others see your love for them in word and in deed."

— **Kent Altena**, 200-pound Atkins weight loss success story, popular low-carb blogger (Network-Admin.net) and YouTube videographer (YouTube. com/Bowulf)

As I have prepared to write this final "lesson" in my book, I do so with a very heavy heart because of someone who was, is, and always will be very near and dear to me in my life — my only full-blooded brother, Kevin Lee Moore. Those of you who read Chapter 5 of my first book and have regularly visited my blog over the past few years know that Kevin, like me for most of my life, had struggled with his weight and allowed it get up to a very dangerous level of morbid obesity. In fact, he experienced a series of heart attacks in the span of one week in 1999 that nearly took his life at the age of 32. But by the grace of God he survived that ordeal, lost weight and was doing so well. Unfortunately,

Kevin quickly started neglecting his health by scarfing down junk food, sweets and snacks and his weight went back up again — way up! — all the while his health condition just kept getting worse and worse.

When my wife and I visited my family in Florida during Christmas 2004, I could not believe eyes when I saw my brother had gotten as big as he had. He had to weigh at least 400-450 pounds when we saw him. Of course, he saw how much weight I had lost that year on my low-carb lifestyle and I was hopeful that my example might spur him on to do something about his weight. Unfortunately, he had already decided that attempting to lose weight was probably a lost cause, a pointless endeavor and started gaining some more. That's the ruthless cycle far too many people needlessly go through in their life attempting to follow the "recommended" diet.

One year later on a Sunday night in November 2005, my brother went to dinner with my sister Beverly and he told her he wasn't feeling very well. That night he checked himself into the hospital and they discovered that every single one of the arteries that had been cleared just six years prior following his heart attacks were fully blocked again and there were several new ones. When they asked Kevin how much he weighed since none of their scales could weigh him, he responded, "I'm 365." I understand denial about your weight because that is how I got up to 410 pounds. But Kevin was probably much heavier than he thought. His doctor told my mother at the time that if Kevin didn't make any changes in his lifestyle with either his diet or exercise routine that he would be dead within a year. That hit my mom like a baseball bat to the forehead and she was both angry and concerned.

When I heard the news via telephone (I live 500 miles from Florida), I sat dumbfounded for several minutes. Why is my brother having such a hard time with this? Doesn't he even care that he is killing himself? I love the big goof, but he really needed to stop playing with his life and get going with this — fast! As I wrote about in my first book, Kevin's situation was one of the reasons I started livin' la vida low-carb in the first place. I didn't want to be subjected to a life of taking a big handful of medications everyday and relying on a machine in my chest to keep me alive. That's not what Kevin needed or deserved either.

Ironically, Kevin was a gentle giant with a big loving heart. But his decision to ignore his weight problem was catching up to him fast and he had a clear choice — continue on the same path and die or make some attempt to lose weight and lots of it. Most people would say Kevin was given plenty of opportunities to get his weight and health under control. If the heart attacks he had in 1999 didn't wake him up, then what would? You just have to shake your head at people (even family members) who don't allow circumstances to jar them back into reality.

For much of his life, Kevin shunned doing anything about his weight. He was discharged from the Army in his early 20's because of his weight and it was all downhill from there. He was in a very bad marriage with an ex-wife who literally abused him both mentally and physically that drove him to eat, eat, and eat some more just to comfort himself. It really was a very sad situation that led him down the path to morbid obesity. Others may see Kevin's story as an extreme circumstance, but I believe he is more typical than people want to admit. While many overweight and obese people can be happy in life and everything seems fine, there are ways that life could be so much better if they could bring their weight under control.

Before I started livin' la vida low-carb and lost all of my weight in 2004, most people would have described me as a pretty happy-go-lucky kinda guy. Not much bothered me and I always tried to bring a smile to the faces of the people I encountered. Life itself couldn't have been better. But that nagging feeling within me to do something about my weight never seemed to go away even when I feigned like I didn't care. Of course I cared, but what could I do? It seemed so very hopeless from my vantage point. To the glory of God, I was able to find solace in the low-carb lifestyle and the rest is history. But I could have very well been in the same boat as Kevin and the millions more who have the "I don't care about my weight" mentality had I not found my low-carb answer.

It's almost impossible to talk about Kevin without discussing the somewhat tumultuous childhood we grew up experiencing. Our mom and dad got divorced at the age of 21 when I was nearly two years old and Kevin was six years old. Both of my parents then remarried and we went to live with my mother in Florida with her new husband while my father remarried and stayed in Tennessee. Two years later, my mom had my half-sister Beverly while my dad birthed his third and final son Nathan (my half-brother) four years after that. Not long after these new children came into the world, both mom and dad divorced their spouses — again! They then ended up remarrying their third spouses and my mom even briefly divorced and then remarried her third husband. UGH!

Today I use all of this as a joke at parties. Have you played that game where you write on a sheet of paper something about yourself that people don't know about and then exchange the papers reading them aloud trying to figure out who wrote it? Well, nobody has ever figured out that Jimmy Moore is the one who has been through six marriages! HA! People are so shocked and then I tell them my parents divorced a lot when I was a kid. You can say that again!

As for describing my siblings, I tell people I have one full-blooded brother named Kevin, a half-sister who is my mother's second husband's daughter named Beverly, and a half-brother who is my father's second wife's son named Nathan. Is your head spinning yet? Yeah, I've had some fun with my genealogy over the years.

Needless to say, this is not exactly what people would describe as the "ideal" way to raise children in the United States although my experience is unfortunately not a unique one with divorce so normal these days. That's why I told my wife Christine when I married her in 1995 that we're cutting the word divorce out of the dictionary because it's not even an option to me. She might have to kill me first, but we're not getting a divorce no matter what. So far, so good because I'm still here.

Kevin and I both bounced between Florida and Tennessee every year growing up as kids traveling back and forth between Pensacola, Florida and Bolivar, Tennessee for six weeks in the summer, two weeks at Christmas, and one week during Spring break. However, it wasn't until I turned 14 when my mom and her third husband (the one she divorced and then remarried) decided they didn't want me in their house anymore that I moved to live with my father in Tennessee. They devised a plan to have me go visit my father for the Christmas holidays and then he dropped the bombshell on the day I was supposed to go home to Florida that I'd be living there with him in Tennessee permanently. I was devastated and cried for hours after this transpired for several reasons.

First, I was enjoying my classes in high school and making lasting friendships with people I shared common interests with and now that was all gone. Second, life had somewhat normalized and enabled me to begin thinking clearly about what I wanted to do with the rest of my life but now that was being taken away from me, too. Finally, my father had shown himself to be a very dominating and angry figure that I was terrified to be in the house with because you never knew what was going to set him off. My distress about living there was quickly confirmed and I realized I was walking into a living nightmare at a very impressionable age.

Over the next three years of my life until I turned 17, graduated from high school, and began attending college, I endured physical, mental, and emotional abuse that took me many years of reflection, prayer and forgiveness to overcome. There are times even now when I still have flashbacks of the horror I went through with my father that can literally make my body tremble. I remember this man I called my dad once got so mad at me that he threw me up against the wall inside his brand new house that my head literally left a big dent the size of a basketball in the sheet rock. Another time, when he was teaching me how to drive with a stick shift, I was driving down the road with him in the passenger seat and he started hitting me on the side of my head repeatedly because he didn't like something I said to him. I feared for my life and just knew I was going to crash into an oncoming car or a building. Sadly, this was the norm week in and week out for most of my high school days.

Sure I got a lot of spankings that left red "handprint" welts from where my dad made me pull down my pants to beat my butt, but sometimes he'd even resort to punching me in the face so hard with his closed fist that I'd have a black eye (when my friends would ask me who beat me up, I'd tell 'em I tripped and fell). As if the physical abuse wasn't bad enough, the mental and emotional abuse scarred me even more.

He'd say such things to me like the following:

"You're not good enough."
"You'll never amount to anything."
"What are you, a faggot?"
*"I'm gonna beat that a**."*
*"You're nothing, you worthless piece of sh**."*
*"Why the He** were you even born."*

Was this painful? Do you even have to ask? It was by far the worst period of my entire life having to live with my dad through that traumatic experience during high school. This paralyzed me from ever having the courage to ask a girl out on a date, make friends, or do anything social. Although I brought home excellent grades in school and worked hard to please my father as much as I possibly could, none of it ever seemed to be good enough.

Looking back on it now, I realize this very difficult experience I endured has made me a stronger person than I would have ever been without going through it so that maybe I can help others who are also dealing with their own horrific past. But for many years after leaving home to start my own life with my wife Christine, the memories of my childhood years kept me from dealing with some issues that needed to be handled — namely my weight problem (ah, you knew I'd get around to weight loss at some point, didn't you?!).

While you are probably thinking what an awful dad I had for doing this to me over two decades ago, I can't and don't blame him for it because that's exactly how his dad treated him and his siblings growing up. My grandfather Richard, who I never knew because he died before I was born, was an alcoholic drunk who would come home at night after work and start flying into fits of rage randomly beating the living daylights out of whoever was in his way, his wife (my Memaw Luerene who died in 2007) included.

Abuse was what my dad saw from his dad on a daily basis. So my dad was merely mimicking what he had learned from his dad. This is a ruthless cycle that so many generations of families go through until one person in that chain is able to climb out of the deep, dark pit of despair that was dug so long ago and finally say enough is enough. I am hoping to be that person in my family to buck the trend and overcome the pain of the past. There's just no excuse for continuing the abuse.

So far, the plan is working quite well in recent years and I have not shown the same abusive character traits of my dad and granddad to my darling wife Christine. That's not to say I didn't struggle with this early on in our marriage when I would get angry at times and grab her by the wrists when she'd get upset at me. But by the grace of God I have never once hit her during our marriage and would never think of doing something like that. In fact, perhaps it has been the Lord's perfect timing to hold off on granting us children for a time to help me mature even more into the man He would have me to be before giving me the privilege of becoming a father. It'll happen someday when it is finally meant to be within His perfect will. I really want to be a daddy.

Looking back on all those years after high school that I wasted looking over my shoulder wondering if my dad was watching my every move with disappointed disdain, I can only shake my head now wondering how much sooner I could have truly beaten my obesity. While I'm not saying I reached over 400 pounds all because of my father, it would be foolish to say my experience with him in those few years I lived with him didn't serve as a residual causal factor in the fact that I got that big. Plus, look at Kevin. Could his morbid obesity have been caused in part by some of the pain of his past with abusive relationships with his dad and wife?

How about you? Do you feel like you've been plagued by your past because of abuse you endured from your father or another family member? Believe me, I know that constant fear can grip you like nothing else and paralyze you from moving forward with your life. It took me over ten years to finally stop living in the past and to start living for me and my family in the here and now. Once I did, I was able to regain proper control over my weight and health for good thanks to livin' la vida low-carb. And now I'll never be the same again.

I suppose you must be wondering what my relationship with my dad is like today. I'm pleased to report that we are on good speaking terms and talk regularly by telephone. About a year and a half ago after my 180-pound weight loss in 2004, I noticed my dad said something to me that I'll never forget during one of our conversations that I had never heard him utter before. Here's what he said: *"Son, I'm proud of you for what you have accomplished. I love you."*

He may never even realize just how powerful those simple words were that he spoke to me that day. I literally choked up and couldn't respond back except to somehow say, "Thank you." But you know what? Every time we have talked since then, my dad has made it a point to tell me "Son, I love you" at the end of the call. In fact, Kevin told me around the same time that dad did the same thing with him and it made him ball his eyes out. I now proudly and sincerely tell my dad back that I love him, too. Now that he is older, dad may even realize and feel guilty about what he did to me and Kevin when we were growing up and is perhaps just now getting over the pain that his dad inflicted on him when he was young. This was all a part of the healing process that had to take place after going through such hard times.

Despite what happened all those years ago, the weighty influence that my big bad dad had on me is one that I have no doubt made me into the man I am today. I have learned to appreciate what life brings me now and am passionate about the things that I believe are most important (like helping people deal with their weight issues, too!). Would I have those traits had I not gone through what I did? I don't know. But life's circumstances mold and shape us into the people we become as adults. Dad was, is, and always will be one of the most generous people you will ever meet in your life and he regularly did things (and still does) for other people without charging them a single penny for his services. That's just the kind of stand-up guy he is.

Now that you know a little bit of our family background, let's turn back to the subject of my brother Kevin again. He continued to have health problems over the past few years because of his morbid obesity, heart disease, and diabetes. Just as he had done on every previous time he attempted weight loss or anything in his life, Kevin was gung ho about it...for a while. But then it happened to him — he would start feeling a little bit better thinking he was gonna be okay, stop doing those things that were essential for improving his weight and health, and then go into complete denial about his morbid obesity. Sure, he'd had some difficult life experiences, including a horrific marriage to a woman who basically made his life a living Hell when he had his heart attacks in 1999 and was no longer able to work. Thankfully he got out of that relationship a few years ago, but the lingering effects of that toxic marriage had been done.

Like many people who are hurting and their life seems to be in such turmoil, Kevin undoubtedly turned to food to comfort himself. And not just a little food. I mean an out-of-proportion gargantuan amount of grub that would make most people's eyes bug out. For example, he used to tell me how he would go to McDonald's and get 5 Big Macs with 3 large orders of French fries and 10 cookies. EEEEEK! What would be unreasonable to most, this was the reality for my brother.

Here was my own flesh and blood killing himself with his diet — a man that I grew up with as my Big Bro and I always looked up to. Yeah, he was my stupid, ugly butt hole older brother and he thoroughly enjoyed taunting me as every older brother does, but it was only because he was my brother. We shared a lot of happy memories wrestling (he used to say, "let's me and you rassel!") on the ground or playing pool at the local game room (I always beat him and he hated that!). We endured divorces galore that both of our parents went through and lived as normal a life as we possibly could with the hand life dealt us as kids. What we went through was "normal" for us.

Fast forward a few years to 2004, I decided to take control of my weight and health for real and stopped wallowing in the past with all the genuine hurt and pain that I had endured for my entire life. It was at that point there were no more excuses for the way I was living my life NOW and I did something about it. My old eating habits would have to be radically changed and exercise would need to become my friend rather than my foe.

As you know, I did it — I lost 180 pounds that year and avoided the obesity-related health decline that hit my brother like a 2X4 upside the back of his head. My brother was a contributing motivating factor for me to do it for real this time for a couple of reasons. First, I wanted desperately to avoid experiencing what he had since his heart attacks. Second, and even more importantly, I thought my example to my only full-blooded brother would get him going again. More than anything, I wanted to motivate my own brother to get his life back too.

Unfortunately, I learned the hard lesson that you can't make anyone lose weight that is unwilling to do it for themselves. You just can't and Kevin is the prime example. He read my first book, he saw me in person after my weight loss, I gave him practical advice about the changes he could make in his life if he truly wanted to lose weight and restore his health — but he ignored it all.

In October 2006, Kevin was again hospitalized as he had been hundreds of times the previous seven years, but this time was quite different. The stent they put in his heart valve before was completely blocked again. He had two other arteries that were 90 percent blocked as well. He was very weak and fatigued when I spoke with him on the telephone at the time, but he was hopeful the doctors could do something for him as they had so many times before.

The doctors he saw said they were too afraid to do open heart surgery on him because they feared he may not be strong enough to come back if they put him under. Do I even need to tell you how upsetting this was to me and my family? It's something no parent or sibling should ever have to go through because it was all so preventable. But we all have choices to make in our lives and Kevin made his. He simply accepted that he was fat and would always be fat for the rest of his life. That's what I used to think, too, but I instinctively knew better. Why do people fall into this self-imposed trap about their weight? There is always a way.

Now you realize why I remain so vigilant and passionate about sharing what has happened to me through my weight loss experience because this subject just hits too close to home. My mom has dealt with her obesity with gastric bypass surgery and my half-brother Nathan was able to take off the pounds with a low-carb-styled diet and exercise program which was also a motivating factor in my decision to start on Atkins in 2004. But this is something that had completely eluded Kevin and the price for that decision, conscious or otherwise, was going to have to be paid someday.

One of my low-carb blogging friends and triple-digit low-carb weight loss success Richard Morris (BreadAndMoney.com) sent me the following e-mail of encouragement about Kevin after I wrote about his declining health on my blog in 2006:

Hi Jimmy,

I just read your article about your brother. Wow. First of all, I didn't know you had a brother and I just assumed that everyone within range of your infectious enthusiasm would be just as gung-ho on healthy living as you are.

After a short bit of reflection though, I realized that the situation with your brother makes perfect sense. You see, I have an older sister who is morbidly obese as well. Like you, I've done everything to try to help her. She spent two months with my family a while back and had really started to change physically and mentally, but then she returned home out West and went back to her old lifestyle.

Like you, I've received numerous emails from people who have attended my workshops, read my book or visited the web site and have had their lives transformed, and yet when it comes to family, it seems that those closest to us are the hardest to reach. I've heard variations of this same story from other people who can't seem to get a brother, sister or parent to see the nutritional light and walk therein.

I just thought I'd share this perspective. I think sometimes people think there's something about them or the relationship they have with a loved one that prevents that person from taking charge and making change, but the fact is that your situation with your brother is fairly common.

I'm so sorry to hear that his condition has worsened. I'll keep him in my thoughts and prayers.

Peace,
Richard

THANKS Richard and to everyone else who has offered thoughts and prayers for Kevin over the years — from the bottom of my heart, I am grateful to know that so many of you have shown me and my family genuine and loving concern at this time. God bless you!

In 2006, Kevin needed open-heart surgery according to the doctors, but they didn't want the liability of his death in case he didn't survive it. He was only 39 years old at the time and we knew Kevin would need a miracle at that point. The doctors tried two things — a harness to wrap around his thigh that was supposed to help pump the blood through the heart when the flow became weak and an experimental new oral medication designed to break up blockages in the arteries. I had never heard of either one of those treatments, but these seemed to be some of the latest advances in medical technology they were using on him.

The subject of my brother Kevin came up quite often at my blog over the past few years and one of the people who read about him was a heart specialist who works with Olympic-level athletes to get them into tip-top shape. He personally offered to help "save" Kevin free of charge if he would be willing to share his typical daily routine, including the medications he was taking at the time. When I presented this offer to Kevin, he seemed very excited about it initially and I was delighted that perhaps the dark cloud of despair that had hovered over him the previous few years would finally begin to clear up.

Unfortunately, though, in typical fashion Kevin squandered this golden opportunity by being less than forthright about his condition. When I requested some basic information about his health, here are the mendacious answers he gave to me along with the cold hard facts:

Height — 6'0" (TRUE)
Weight — 373 pounds (FALSE, he had to weigh well over 400 pounds)
Waist — 62 inches (Perhaps, but he had a really big belly)
Calories Consumed Daily — 1800 (Maybe for breakfast)
Exercise — 2 miles daily (Not likely with only 15% of his heart functioning)

After Kevin had a series of heart attacks in 1999, he had 4 stints put in. In 2005, an ICD implant was put in to prevent heart failure and he was declared a Type 2 diabetic. Here is a list of the prescription medications he was taking as of October 2006:

GLUCATROL 2.5 MG
PRINAVIL 10 MG
POTASSIUM CHLORIDE 10 MG
PLAVIX 75 MG
COUMADIN 10 MG

ASPIRIN 81 MG
IMDUR 60 MG
COREG 37.5 MG
LASIX 80 MG
ALLOPURINOL 100 MG
TOPROL 50 MG

As you can see, Kevin was still in pretty bad shape and I feared he would stay that way as long as he kept lying to himself about his weight and health. Some people criticized me for claiming people with obesity are in deep denial about their weight problem, but Kevin is the prime example of this. He hadn't even turned 40 yet and was convinced that he was eating and exercising the healthy way. He earnestly believed that there was no way he could possibly do anything more for himself. If that's NOT denial in light of what he had learned from my low-carb example, then I don't know what is!

While the circumstances about how he got to be morbidly obese are one thing, the truth for him and anyone else in the same circumstance is that they need to make weight loss a priority and JUST DO IT! Stop saying it's too hard, and for goodness sake stop pointing the finger of blame waiting for somebody else to do it for you. There's no arguing that genetics or a propensity to being fat in some people is a reality. But far too many people are using those lame excuses as a crutch to wiggle out of making the right choices for themselves.

When I spoke with Kevin's roommate about what he had eaten one day, she told me Kevin had a bowl of oatmeal with a banana, a glass of fat-free skim milk and orange juice for breakfast, she didn't see him at lunch so she didn't know, and for supper he had a big bowl of grits with eggs and sausage. Then he went out with friends and she was unaware of what he ate, but suspected he ate something. He was obviously eating way too many carbohydrates and calories even though he was supposed to be trying to eat lower-carb and allegedly sticking to 1800 calories. This was so incredibly frustrating for me to watch happening right before my very eyes!

The longer Kevin ignored the grave reality of his condition, the longer he remained morbidly obese and slowly kept chipping away at his life. Seeing the devastation of Kevin's condition has kept me focused these past few years on what I am doing to help educate, encourage and inspire others to get this part of their life headed in the right direction. It's not my fault if people like Kevin don't listen, but it won't stop me from trying. I'll never quit if for no other reason than to help spare others the pain of having to go through the drama of seeing a loved one eating his way to an early grave. If we can save just one person from doing that, then all the thousands of hours I have invested in my blog will have been worth it!

When I went to visit my family for Thanksgiving in 2006, I was shocked when we sat down to watch a movie together as a family and mom had made a big batch of brownies. The aroma in the air was just too much for Kevin to bear, so he went and loaded up his plate with 4 large blocks of brownies with ice cream on top. Keep in mind he was a Type 2 diabetic and morbidly obese! Oh, you don't know how much I wanted to scream out, "No! You don't need that Kevin!" But I bit my tongue and remained silent. I learned a long time ago that you can't force someone to change who isn't ready to change. They have to be ready and it's our job to serve as an example until they are. That's all I had left to hope for at that point. Kevin was a 39-year old man at the time that didn't need someone like his little brother holding his hand about what to do about his weight and health. He alone made the decisions about his life and he would have to face the consequences of his actions at some point.

In the spring of 2008, mom called me again and said hospice had been called in for Kevin who was given only a few more months to live. While on the outside he looked fine, the inevitable impact of years of morbid obesity was catching up with my brother. The hospice nurse would administer oxygen and morphine for Kevin so he would be comfortable in the final few months he was expected to live.

Needless to say, Christine and I visited him one last time in Pensacola, Florida in July 2008. We had an awesome time seeing him and my family in a week I will never forget for the rest of my life. Kevin only had one artery functioning at the time and it was 95% blocked with stents no longer doing any good. He was too high-risk for any surgery and he had pretty much given up on changing his diet and lifestyle anyway.

The thing that struck me about seeing Kevin was how "normal" he looked. Yes, he was a very large man weighing in at about 350-400 pounds or so. But he was out and about doing the things he loved the most — playing Texas Hold 'Em, bingo, flirting with the ladies, and singing at the local karaoke bar. We did a little bit of everything he enjoyed during that week (sans the flirting for me since I already have my woman!). And yet he was on morphine and oxygen for comfort because he was easily out of breath and sweating profusely even in a well air-conditioned room. This was Kevin's life in the final days. We made some great memories together that I'll not soon forget.

We stayed with my beautiful sister Beverly for the week who was a very gracious host making us homemade meals, driving us around everywhere we wanted to go with Kevin, and just being a good little sister. In fact, Kevin came and stayed with Beverly during the week we were there. Since we all grew up together as kids, it was pretty neat all being under the same roof again as a family for what would be the final time. That had been a rarity since we all became adults. When we went over to mom's house for dinner to watch some of ventriloquist Jeff Dunham DVDs together, Kevin was laughing so hard I was worried about him. But it was great seeing him enjoying himself so much considering what would happen just three months later.

Although it was not unexpected, my brother Kevin started rapidly declining in health in October 2008. I received a telephone call from my dad in Tennessee who was passing on the message to me from my mom who was so shaken up by the news that she couldn't bear to call me directly about it. It turned out Kevin went to the hospital on a Friday evening because his defibrillator went off twice. The doctors were keeping him overnight for observation and early on that Saturday morning he had a heart incident that did not trigger the defibrillator to go off. They had to shock his heart 10 times to revive him and he severely bloodied his lip and tongue from biting them as they were doing this. Major damage was done to his already weakened heart and now he was in a "coma" state in intensive care for a variety of reasons. Things looked very bleak and we knew it was only a matter of days for Kevin to live.

He was hooked up to a ventilator and was heavily sedated with seven medicines being pumped into his body so he couldn't be awake. His body would start gagging if he were conscious with all the tubes running down his throat. Plus, they had to go in and do a heart cath after administering plasma to thicken up his blood and doctors found that there was really not much else they could do for him with virtually every single artery completely blocked. Additionally, the pressure on his heart was supposed to be 15, but his registered at 40. It was as if his heart was about to explode and the doctors were helpless to do anything about it. They were trying to wait it out for a few days to see if his condition would improve on its own.

As you can imagine, this was a very difficult time for my family and I did get to speak with my mom about it. She was obviously very shaken up by this sudden turn for the worse with Kevin's health. Yes, we knew this day would come for a while, but now that it was here it seemed so much more real to all of us. I could not imagine what both my mom and dad were thinking about this seeing their 41-year old son on the verge of taking his final breath on Earth. Never in a million years did either one of them expect to outlive any of their children, but their worst-case scenario nightmare was unfolding right before their eyes with their first child.

Although Mom told me to stay home in South Carolina until something "worse" happened to Kevin, I just felt like I needed to be with my family through this difficult time. No, there was nothing I could do for Kevin to make his situation better and he wasn't even aware that people were in the room with him when he was unconscious from the medications. But Mom told me she sat with Kevin holding his hand and telling him "I love you" during visiting hours. I ached for her because I knew she was taking this very hard. That was one reason I wanted to be there to let her know that her other son was there to share in the grief of this situation. I'm very grateful to have had the chance to spend some quality time with Kevin in July 2008 and those are memories I'll cherish forever — it was the most fun we had experienced together in years.

Kevin was only looking at a few more hours of life before the good Lord decided it was time to take him home. And thankfully Kevin was a Christian and had Jesus in his heart. We can rest assured that the perfect healing happened for him and that he went to a place where there's no more suffering, no more pain, and no more crying. Knowing this gave me a peace in my heart about what happened on those few grueling days in mid-October 2008.

The pulmonary doctor gave us the grim truth of the situation — Kevin's kidneys were shutting down from the efforts to keep his blood pressure and heart rate reduced since he suffered cardiac arrest on that previous Saturday. They were hoping keeping him in a drug-induced coma would help his heart heal, but his other organs were beginning to fail. They turned off his defibrillator and on that Wednesday morning they took him off of the ventilator since they expected more organ failure and increased pressure in his heart.

The doctors said he would live as little as a few minutes or up to a few days when they did this. At this news, I saw something I'd never seen before in my entire life — my dad walked off to the side towards the wall turning his head away from everyone and started sobbing uncontrollably. I mean I'd never even seen the man cry before and there he was with tears rolling down his cheeks.

I wrapped my arms around his neck and held him close to console him. It was something I never want to see again because I knew this was breaking dad's heart to watch happening to his son just a few months after he had quintuple heart bypass surgery himself.

For the first few hours Kevin was off the ventilator, he was in and out of consciousness but breathing on his own and somewhat alert. The nurse told us that when they shocked his heart back on Saturday that he may have sustained some brain damage. It was probably only minor, she added, but it could impact his ability to talk. But as the day progressed, Kevin's ability to communicate improved quite dramatically right before our eyes. Despite having no nourishment for his body since that previous Friday, taking him off of all blood pressure and heart rate machines, and keeping him on a morphine drip and oxygen alone, Kevin did something that was a pleasant surprise to all of us — he smiled.

It happened kind of by accident when I got locked inside of the bathroom adjacent to the hospital room they put him in. When I finally got out, my sister Beverly said, "Hey Kevin, Jimmy got locked in the bathroom!" Hearing this, the biggest, most beautiful smile bloomed on Kevin's face teeth and all and it was a joyful time for the family to know he was still with us for however much longer God would allow. We got Kevin to laugh a few more times in the next few hours, especially when my mom accidentally introduced me as Kevin's "sister" to a visitor — Kevin couldn't stop grinning because I know he was laughing his butt off on the inside with that one.

At 4:30am on Thursday, October 16th, 2008, our loving son, brother, and friend went home to be with the Lord. He passed away peacefully in his sleep in the early morning hours. I'll never forget that big grin on his face as we shared memories and funny moments throughout the day. My dad was with Kevin when he took his final breath and we were all there at the hospital bed within a few minutes of learning he was gone. It was very difficult on all of us as my mom, sister Beverly, dad, and others were openly sobbing in the hours after we all let what happened sink in all the while telling our favorite stories about Kevin. By the grace of God, I was able to keep it together fairly well and it took some time to hit me fully. Eventually we had to say goodbye to Kevin's body and we had the assurance that we would see him again someday in heaven.

Watch my Kevin tribute video on YouTube: http://www.youtube.com/watch?v=mbVGhnmx_y4

It wasn't until we were on The 2nd Annual Low-Carb Cruise to Mexico in January 2009 when I was speaking to the group of low-carbers on board the Carnival Ecstasy cruise ship about my low-carb story and winding down my talk when my wife Christine chimed in, "Hey Jimmy, why don't you tell them about your brother Kevin?" Within seconds, my voice quivered and the floodgate of tears opened up for the first time since he had died just a few months before and it made me realize at that moment he was gone forever. Kevin was really gone. That infectious, goofy laugh of his would no longer be heard and my Big Bro would no longer be there for us to visit when we go to Florida. It all makes me very sad to think about, but I'm also encouraged to know that there is still hope for other Kevins out in the world today.

You see the early death of a brother or loved one may not be prevented no matter how much of an example you are. But that shouldn't stop you from trying to make a difference in the lives of everyone you come into contact with. The health of these people we call our own is just too important to simply give up on them — even if they seem to give up on themselves. If you have friends or family members who are overweight or obese that you love and care about very much, then you owe it to them to do everything you can to help them overcome this obstacle in their life by confronting them about it.

Let me get one thing out of the way about what I mean by "confronting" them. No, I don't mean walking up to that person and bluntly telling them, "You know you're pretty fat and should go on a diet or something!" Besides lacking any tact or taste, that's just plain rude. And you're basically making a bad situation even worse by degrading that person to the point that they feel even worse than they already do about themselves while angering them to the point that they give up even trying to lose weight. Not good and I never would have done that to Kevin.

As tempting as it is to just tell it to them straight up like that, there are much better ways to get the message across. And, no, nagging or whining is not one of them. My dear wife Christine used to shed tears over my weight problem. She would cry and cry until her eyes got all puffy telling me with a voice of genuine concern, "But honey, I don't want you to die of a heart attack! Please lose some weight!" While I could see how hurt she was and I believed she was sincere in her reasons for wanting me to lose weight, I just felt like I was being emotionally guilt-tripped into losing weight just to make her stop crying. Again, not good.

It wasn't until Christine stopped the "nagging" about my weight and just kept on loving me for who I was — all 410 pounds of me! — that I eventually determined on my own that weight loss was what I needed to do. It wasn't an overnight decision, but there were the small events that made me decide that it was time to lose the weight.

The snide comment from the kid in my class.
The inability to climb the rock wall.
The ripped pants getting in my car.
The difficulty breathing comfortably.
The three prescription drugs I was taking.

All of these things brought me to my breaking point and led me to begin the low-carb journey via the Atkins diet and the rest, they say, is history! However, I would have never made it to where I am today without the gentle show of love and support that I received when I was an obese man. That right there is the key!

Don't try to be too overbearing about your "concern" over their "problem." Trust me, obese people are not stupid! An overweight or obese person knows when you are trying to lecture them about their weight and their brain will shut you down before you even get started talking. They don't need someone to tell them they are fat. Tell me something I don't know.

There are ways to get your message to these people without offending them or ticking them off. For example, I remember talking to this very nice lady who I see almost every single day and most people would say she has a fairly serious weight problem. I guesstimate that she weighs at least 150 pounds over her ideal weight and that's probably on the low side. Every single time I see her, my heart aches for what she is going through because I am reminded of what I felt like not that long ago. You don't know how tempting it has been to blurt something out to her about her weight, but I have said nothing to her out of the blue.

We were talking about this and that one day and I brought up something about a trip I was taking to an obesity conference or something. When this woman asked what the trip was about, that opened the door for me to talk about my weight loss success and how I've been involved in staying on top of the latest research behind low-carb diets for producing weight and health improvements. I didn't push anything on her about livin' la vida low-carb, never mentioned that

I write books about my weight loss, nary a discussion further about it. I just left it at that for her to ponder more if she so desired and when the right moment comes she'll know where to turn.

But, but, but...shouldn't you have pursued that further when you had the opportunity? Nope! Incrementally, we'll make a mention here and there on my weight loss and health improvements and just allow her to approach me about the subject if she desires to talk about it in greater detail. Being fat is embarrassing enough and the last thing you want to do is open yourself up for more ridicule and scorn. Perhaps knowing that there is someone who has not only been where you are and has been able to overcome it gives me a little bit of an advantage over most people when it comes to confronting the obese about their weight.

Being available with a listening ear is an invaluable asset to helping the obese when they are ready to do something about their weight and health. Having a shoulder to cry on and someone they can trust and look to for support when they make the effort is your job as the loved one of these precious individuals. It all starts with building those relationships with people and, more than anything, acknowledging that they are human by befriending them and showing them that you consider them your equal. Unfortunately, whether we will admit it or not, the overweight and obese are looked down upon by our society as a whole. There must be something wrong with you if you allow yourself to get so fat, people reason in their minds. Don't you even care enough about yourself to control your weight?! The blatant discrimination that fat people must endure sickens me to no end!

If only it were as easy as snapping your fingers and making the weight disappear. Ha! Don't we wish! In reality, it takes a whole lot of blood, sweat, and tears on the part of the person who needs to lose weight to make it happen. Although it isn't easy, it can and will happen if you commit to it 100%, find the support of people who will be there for you, implement a sound strategy that includes a healthy diet and exercise plan, and then keep doing that lifestyle change forever. Weight loss is not that complex, but it does take time and dedication.

They didn't build Rome in a day and I didn't lose 180 pounds in a week. Slow, methodical, day-by-day living and you'll get there. If you lose one pound per week for the next two years, that's over 100 pounds lost forever it doesn't seem so hard when you think of it those terms now, does it? Can you just lose one measly pound per week, which amounts to a teeny tiny 4 pounds per month? Of course you can! Now, go do it.

So how do you approach the obese about their weight? In a nutshell, you be-friend them, you love them, you prove you can be trusted, you share openly and honestly without casting judgment, and then you wait for them to come back to you. When that happens, will you be ready to help? You had better be because their life may literally depend on it! It won't work with everyone as the sad story about my brother Kevin demonstrates, but it's certainly worth a shot with your friend or loved one.

And that, my friends, is the single biggest life lesson I have learned from this low-carb journey and I hope it encourages you as you continue your own low-carb path to better health. There are so many more "lessons" I've learned in the few short years since I've been low-carbing that I'd like to share with you in future books, so never stop growing and transforming yourself into that person deep down inside who has been just screaming to come out and shine for all the world to see. And remember; never ever, ever, ever give up! You really can do this if you do what you can to make it happen! Whatever you do, just keep on livin' la vida low-carb, baby!

Recommended Low-Carb Reading and Resources

Dr. Atkins' New Diet Revolution and *Atkins for Life* by Dr. Robert C. Atkins

Atkins Diabetes Revolution by Dr. Mary C. Vernon and Jacqueline Eberstein, RN

Protein Power and *6-Week Cure for the Middle-Aged Middle* by Drs. Mike & Mary Dan Eades

Good Calories, Bad Calories by Gary Taubes

Living Low Carb and *The 150 Healthiest Foods On Earth* by Dr. Jonny Bowden

The Stubborn Fat Fix by Dr. Keith Berkowitz and Valerie Berkowitz, RD

The Primal Blueprint by Mark Sisson

The Omnivore's Dilemma and *In Defense of Food* by Michael Pollan

Strong Kids, Healthy Kids and *The Slow Burn Fitness Revolution* by Fred Hahn

The Brain Trust Program by Dr. Larry McCleary

The Silver Cloud Diet by Dr. John Salerno

The Great Cholesterol Con by Dr. Malcolm Kendrick

SUGAR SHOCK! by Connie Bennett

Genocide! by Dr. James E. Carlson

Carbohydrates Can Kill by Dr. Robert Su

Track Your Plaque by Dr. William Davis

The Metabolism Miracle by Diane Kress, RD

Real Food and *Real Food for Mother And Baby* by Nina Plank

The Diet Cure by Julia Ross

Eat Fat, Lose Fat and *Nourishing Traditions* by Dr. Mary Enig and Sally Fallon

A Life Unburdened by Richard Morris

Body by Science by Dr. Doug McGuff
Men's Health TNT Diet by Dr. Jeff Volek and Adam Campbell
Lights Out! by T.S. Wiley
Malignant Medical Myths by Dr. Joel Kauffman
Sweet Poison by Dr. David Gillespie
Sugarettes by Dr. Scott Olson
The Metabolic Code Diet by Dr. James LaValle
The Zone Diet and *Toxic Fat* by Dr. Barry Sears
Natural Health & Weight Loss and *Trick and Treat* by Dr. Barry Groves
The True You Diet by Dr. John Briffa
Refuse To Regain by Dr. Barbara Berkeley
The Truth about Beauty by Kat James
CARB WARS by Judy Barnes Baker
How I Gave Up My Low-Fat Diet and *500 Low-Carb Recipes* by Dana Carpender
The Diabetes Diet: Dr. Bernstein's Low-Carbohydrate Solution by Dr. Richard Bernstein
Eating Stella Style and *George Stella's Livin' Low-Carb* by George Stella
Life Without Bread by Dr. Christian B. Allan and Dr. Wolfgang Lutz
The Schwarzbein Principle by Dr. Diana Schwarzbein
Fat: An Appreciation of a Misunderstood Ingredient by Jennifer McLagan
The Sugar Fix by Dr. Richard Johnson
FAT HEAD documentary DVD by Tom Naughton
My Big Fat Diet documentary DVD by Dr. Jay Wortman and Mary Bissell
In Search of the Perfect Human Diet documentary DVD by C.J. Hunt

Jimmy Moore's Favorite Low-Carb Diet and Health Web sites

ABOUT.COM LOW-CARB DIETS — lowcarbdiets.about.com
DR. MIKE EADES' HEALTH AND NUTRITION — proteinpower.com/drmike
TOM NAUGHTON'S FAT HEAD — fathead-movie.com
MARK SISSON'S DAILY APPLE — marksdailyapple.com
DANA CARPENDER'S HOLD THE TOAST — holdthetoast.com
DR. JONNY BOWDEN'S BLOG — jonnybowden.com/blogger.htm
DR. WILLIAM DAVIS' HEART SCAN BLOG — heartscanblog.blogspot.com
FRED HAHN'S SERIOUS STRENGTH BLOG — slowburn.typepad.com
AMY DUNGAN'S HEALTHY LOW-CARB LIVING — lovinglowcarblife.blog-spot.com
FEMALE FITNESS AND NUTRITION — cassandraforsythe.blogspot.com
REGINA WILSHIRE'S WEIGHT OF THE EVIDENCE — weightoftheevidence.wordpress.com
JUDY BARNES BAKER'S CARB WARS — carbwars.blogspot.com
DR. JOHN BRIFFA'S BLOG — drbriffa.com/blog
DR. DUANE GRAVELINE'S WEB SITE — spacedoc.net
JACKIE EBERSTEIN'S CONTROLLED CARBOHYDRATE NUTRITION — controlcarb.com
KENT ALTENA'S ATKINS DIET BLOG — network-admin.net
DR. BARRY GROVES' SECOND OPINIONS — second-opinions.co.uk
DR. RICHARD FEINMAN'S METABOLISM SOCIETY — nmsociety.org
SALLY FALLON'S WESTON A. PRICE FOUNDATION — westonaprice.org
DR. RICHARD BERNSTEIN'S DIABETES SOLUTION — diabetes-book.com
KAREN RYSAVY'S TRULY LOW-CARB — trulylowcarb.com

KUDOS FOR BALANCED FITNESS & LIFESTYLE — kudosforlowcarb.blog-spot.com

BRIAN CORMIER'S LOW-CARB DUDE — lowcarbdudecom.blogspot.com

ADAM CAMPBELL'S MEN'S HEALTH FITNESS INSIDER — thefitnessinsider.menshealth.com

DAVE DIXON'S SPARK OF REASON — sparkofreason.blogspot.com

PETER'S HYPERLIPID — high-fat-nutrition.blogspot.com

RICHARD NIKOLEY'S FREE THE ANIMAL — freetheanimal.com

METHUSELAH'S PAY NOW LIVE LATER — paynowlivelater.blogspot.com

SUGAR-FREE SHEILA — sugarfreesheila.com

KALYN DENNY'S KITCHEN — kalynskitchen.blogspot.com

LINDA'S LOW-CARB MENUS & RECIPES — genaw.com/lowcarb

VALERIE'S VOICE: FOR THE HEALTH OF IT — valerieberkowitz.wordpress.com

THE VERONICA ATKINS FOUNDATION — veronicaatkinsfoundation.org

DOKTOR DAHLQVISTS BLOGG (Swedish) — blogg.passagen.se/dahlqvistannika

BIG DADDY D'S LOW-CARB BLOG — lowcarbohydrate.blogspot.com

J.P. FANTON'S HEALTHY FELLOW — healthyfellow.com

SHERRIE'S PINCH OF... — pinchof.blogspot.com

LOW-CARB FOR YOU — lowcarb4u.blogspot.com

NATHAN ELLISON'S THE PEOPLE'S CHEMIST — thepeopleschemist.com/blog

LOW-CARBING AND GENERAL HEALTH NEWS — low-carb-news.blogspot.com

HEALTHY INDULGENCES — healthyindulgences.blogspot.com

THE LOW-CARB LOSER — thelowcarbloser.blogspot.com

PJ'S THE DIVINE LOW-CARB — thedivinelowcarb.blogspot.com

CLEOCHATRA'S THE LIGHTER SIDE OF LOW-CARB — cleochatra.blogspot.com